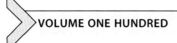

VOLUME ONE HUNDRED

ADVANCES IN
VIRUS RESEARCH

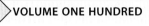

VOLUME ONE HUNDRED

Advances in
VIRUS RESEARCH

Edited by

MARGARET KIELIAN
Albert Einstein College of Medicine,
Bronx, New York, United States

THOMAS C. METTENLEITER
Friedrich-Loeffler-Institut,
Federal Research Institute for Animal Health,
Greifswald – Insel Riems, Germany

MARILYN J. ROOSSINCK
Center for Infectious Disease Dynamics,
Pennsylvania State University, University Park,
Pennsylvania, United States

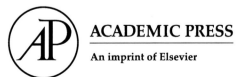

ACADEMIC PRESS

An imprint of Elsevier

Academic Press is an imprint of Elsevier
50 Hampshire Street, 5th Floor, Cambridge, MA 02139, United States
525 B Street, Suite 1800, San Diego, CA 92101-4495, United States
The Boulevard, Langford Lane, Kidlington, Oxford OX5 1GB, United Kingdom
125 London Wall, London, EC2Y 5AS, United Kingdom

First edition 2018

Notices
Knowledge and best practice in this field are constantly changing. As new research and
experience broaden our understanding, changes in research methods, professional practices,
or medical treatment may become necessary.

Practitioners and researchers must always rely on their own experience and knowledge in
evaluating and using any information, methods, compounds, or experiments described
herein. In using such information or methods they should be mindful of their own safety and
the safety of others, including parties for whom they have a professional responsibility.

To the fullest extent of the law, neither the Publisher nor the authors, contributors, or editors,
assume any liability for any injury and/or damage to persons or property as a matter of
products liability, negligence or otherwise, or from any use or operation of any methods,
products, instructions, or ideas contained in the material herein.

ISBN: 978-0-12-815201-0
ISSN: 0065-3527

For information on all Academic Press publications
visit our website at https://www.elsevier.com/books-and-journals

  **Working together
to grow libraries in
developing countries**

www.elsevier.com • www.bookaid.org

Publisher: Zoe Kruze
Acquisition Editor: Ashlie
Senior Editorial Project Manager: Jo Collett
Production Project Manager: James Selvam
Senior Cover Designer: Matthew Limbert

Typeset by SPi Global, India

CONTENTS

7. So What Have Plant Viruses Ever Done for Virology and Molecular Biology? 145

George P. Lomonossoff

8. Hosts and Sources of Endemic Human Coronaviruses 163

Victor M. Corman, Doreen Muth, Daniela Niemeyer, and Christian Drosten

CONTRIBUTORS

Aulia Annisa
Institute of Plant Science and Resources (IPSR), Okayama University, Kurashiki, Japan

Pavithra Aravamudhan
University of Pittsburgh School of Medicine, Pittsburgh, PA, United States

Rogier Bodewes
Utrecht University, Utrecht, The Netherlands

Maria Bottermann
MRC Laboratory of Molecular Biology, Cambridge, United Kingdom

Victor M. Corman
Charité–Universitätsmedizin Berlin, corporate member of Freie Universität Berlin, Humboldt-Universität zu Berlin, and Berlin Institute of Health, Institute of Virology; German Center for Infection Research (DZIF), Berlin, Germany

Terence S. Dermody
University of Pittsburgh School of Medicine, Pittsburgh, PA, United States

Mareike Dörr
Paul-Ehrlich-Institut, Langen, Germany

Christian Drosten
Charité–Universitätsmedizin Berlin, corporate member of Freie Universität Berlin, Humboldt-Universität zu Berlin, and Berlin Institute of Health, Institute of Virology; German Center for Infection Research (DZIF), Berlin, Germany

Jackson Emanuel
Laboratory of Virology, National Institute of Allergy and Infectious Diseases, National Institutes of Health, Hamilton, MT, United States

Heinz Feldmann
Laboratory of Virology, National Institute of Allergy and Infectious Diseases, National Institutes of Health, Hamilton, MT, United States

Michael M. Goodin
University of Kentucky, Lexington, KY, United States

Bradley I. Hillman
Plant Biology and Pathology, Rutgers University, New Brunswick, NJ, United States

Leo C. James
MRC Laboratory of Molecular Biology, Cambridge, United Kingdom

Thijs Kuiken
ErasmusMC, Rotterdam, The Netherlands

George P. Lomonossoff
John Innes Centre, Norwich, United Kingdom

Yongxu Lu
University of Cambridge, Cambridge, United Kingdom

Andrea Marzi
Laboratory of Virology, National Institute of Allergy and Infectious Diseases, National
Institutes of Health, Hamilton, MT, United States

Caitlin Milligan
Division of Human Biology, Fred Hutchinson Cancer Research Center; Medical Scientist
Training Program, University of Washington School of Medicine, Seattle, WA, United
States

Juan A. Mondotte
Institut Pasteur, Viruses and RNA Interference Unit, CNRS Unité Mixte de Recherche
3569, Paris, France

Doreen Muth
Charité–Universitätsmedizin Berlin, corporate member of Freie Universität Berlin,
Humboldt-Universität zu Berlin, and Berlin Institute of Health, Institute of Virology;
German Center for Infection Research (DZIF), Berlin, Germany

Daniela Niemeyer
Charité–Universitätsmedizin Berlin, corporate member of Freie Universität Berlin,
Humboldt-Universität zu Berlin, and Berlin Institute of Health, Institute of Virology, Berlin,
Germany

Julie Overbaugh
Division of Human Biology, Fred Hutchinson Cancer Research Center; Medical Scientist
Training Program, University of Washington School of Medicine, Seattle, WA, United
States

Daniel Pérez-Núñez
Centro Biología Molecular Severo Ochoa, CSIC-UAM, Madrid, Spain

Kristin Pfeffermann
Paul-Ehrlich-Institut, Langen, Germany

Yolanda Revilla
Centro Biología Molecular Severo Ochoa, CSIC-UAM, Madrid, Spain

Juergen A. Richt
Diagnostic Medicine/Pathobiology, Center of Excellence for Emerging and Zoonotic
Animal Diseases (CEEZAD), College of Veterinary Medicine, Kansas State University,
Manhattan, KS, United States

Maria-Carla Saleh
Institut Pasteur, Viruses and RNA Interference Unit, CNRS Unité Mixte de Recherche
3569, Paris, France

Jennifer A. Slyker
University of Washington, Seattle, WA, United States

Geoffrey L. Smith
University of Cambridge, Cambridge, United Kingdom

Danica M. Sutherland
Vanderbilt University School of Medicine, Nashville, TN, United States

Nobuhiro Suzuki
Institute of Plant Science and Resources (IPSR), Okayama University, Kurashiki, Japan

Callum Talbot-Cooper
University of Cambridge, Cambridge, United Kingdom

Marc H.V. Van Regenmortel
School of Biotechnology, CNRS, University of Strasbourg, Strasbourg, France

Veronika von Messling
Paul-Ehrlich-Institut, Langen, Germany

Florian Zirkel
Paul-Ehrlich-Institut, Langen, Germany

PREFACE TO VOLUME 100: HISTORY AND LOOKING FORWARD

1. DISCOVERY OF VIRUSES: THE FIRST "GOLDEN AGE" OF VIROLOGY

Viruses were discovered in the 1890s by the work of Dimitri Iwanowsky (1864–1920), Martinus W. Beijerinck (1851–1931), Friedrich Loeffler (1852–1915), and Paul Frosch (1860–1928). While the former two analyzed tobacco mosaic disease in plants, Loeffler and Frosch worked on foot-and-mouth disease of cloven-hoofed animals. Viruses were first identified as novel infectious agents since they were able to pass through kieselgur (diatomaceous earth) and porcelain filters of pore sizes considered to withhold all then-known bacteria. Thus, the initial differentiating characteristic of the novel class of infectious agents was "filterability" and "filterable viruses" became a defining name (reviewed in Mettenleiter, 2017; Murphy, 2014). Virology is now widely considered to have started in 1898, since in this year Loeffler and Frosch as well as Beijerinck published their seminal works (Calisher and Horzinek, 1999). By the start of the First World War (WWI) the infectious agents of ca. 30 diseases had been characterized as "filterable viruses." The first extensive reviews on "filterable viruses" were published in 1908 in English by M'Fadyean, who in 1900 had discovered filterability of the African Horse Sickness agent (M'Fadyean, 1908), in 1911 in German by Loeffler (Loeffler, 1911), Doerr (Doerr, 1911), and Giovanni Valillo (Valillo, 1911), and in English in 1912 by S. B. Wolbach from Harvard Medical School (Wolbach, 1912). Valillo specifically mentioned that "This new area of research encompasses the science of the filterable viruses." Loeffler's expanded review, written before WWI, finally appeared in the textbook "Lehrbuch der Mikrobiologie" edited by Ernst Friedberger and Richard Pfeiffer, in 1919 (Friedberger and Pfeiffer, 1919). The reviews of Wolbach and Loeffler listed 30 and 39 diseases caused by "filterable viruses," although in hindsight not all of them turned out to be caused by viruses. Most of them were diseases of animals or zoonotic infections, since proof of infectivity required the repeated infection of the natural host of the agents. It is worth noting that the first human virus discovered, yellow fever virus, was indeed isolated from and tested in humans with sometimes fatal consequences (Reed, 1902). Thus, by the beginning of the WWI, the new class of infectious agents had been firmly established.

Although a chapter on "filterable viruses" had been included in the microbiology textbook edited by Friedberger and Pfeiffer (1919), the first textbook solely dedicated to "filterable viruses" appeared in 1928; it was edited by Thomas M. Rivers (Rivers, 1928a,b) based on a review he wrote the preceding year (Rivers, 1927). In 10 chapters it covered areas from "general aspects of filterable viruses" to "virus diseases of bacteria— bacteriophagy." It summarized the extensive knowledge that was amassed on animal, human, plant, and bacterial viruses in the preceding 30 years. It also contained an impressive bibliography with 539 publications referenced in its first, general chapter written by Rivers himself. This textbook marked a milestone in the emancipation of virology as a separate discipline and is regarded as the predecessor of many similar oeuvres to follow.

In the subsequent years, virology went through a series of technological breakthroughs including size determination of viral particles (Schlesinger, 1932) using ultracentrifugation developed by Theodore Svedberg (Svedberg, 1927), the crystallization of tobacco mosaic virus (TMV) by Wendell Stanley (1935), sparking debates on whether viruses are "alive," and the first visualization of viruses after the development of "hypermicroscopy," i.e., electron microscopy by Ernst and Helmut Ruska and colleagues (Krüger et al., 2000). In 1938 the first electron micrograph of a virus, ectromelia virus, was published (von Borries et al., 1938), whereas in 1939 TMV was imaged for the first time (Kausche et al., 1939). Virus isolation and propagation was accomplished in embryonated chicken eggs (Woodruff and Goodpasture, 1931) or in ex vivo organ cultures to allow the confirmation of etiology required by the Henle–Koch–Loeffler postulates (Loeffler, 1884). Bacteriophages were identified by d'Herelle and Twort during WWI (d'Herelle, 1917; Twort, 1915). Studies on these bacterial viruses resulted in the identification of nucleic acid as the genetic material (Hershey and Chase, 1952) and laid the groundwork for understanding genetics not only of viruses (Luria, 1945). X-ray diffraction led to much improved structural models of viruses, and in 1958 Rosalind Franklin designed a molecular model of TMV for the World's Fair in Brussels (see chapter 11, Fig. 2). These studies marked the beginning of what we today designate as molecular virology (Enquist and Racaniello, 2013). Thus, by the 1950s, virology had come of age and had found a distinct place in science. Actually, some authors consider this later period as the "real" start of virology as a scientific discipline (van Helvoort, 1996). Therefore, the time was ripe for giving virus research greater visibility and impact.

2. THE WORLD'S OLDEST REVIEW SERIES IN VIROLOGY: *ADVANCES IN VIRUS RESEARCH*

In August 1953 Volume 1 of a new review series, *Advances in Virus Research (AVR)*, was published under the editorship of Kenneth M. Smith and Max A. Lauffer. This represented the first series exclusively devoted to comprehensive reviews on all aspects of virus research.

It is worthwhile to have a look at the preface to Volume 1, which gives insight into the motivation to start this first review series in Virology:

> *Virus research is carried out by individuals representing widely diversified specialties in the physical and in the biological sciences. Man, higher animals, insects, plants and bacteria are susceptible to virus infection. Therefore, it is natural that physicians, veterinarians, entomologists, plant pathologists and bacteriologists should all be interested in the study of viruses and of virus diseases. Furthermore, viruses lend themselves to fundamental investigations by the methods of biochemists, biophysicists, serologists, geneticists and others. The natural result is that the findings in this area are published in a great number of journals reflecting the backgrounds of the individual investigators. Even review articles are widely scattered. ADVANCES IN VIRUS RESEARCH is planned to help surmount this obstacle encountered by those who attempt to follow virus literature. The focus of interest in this series is to be the virus, not the disease. The editors intend to bring together critical review articles which include discussions incorporating the authors' own views and which cover all types of viruses as studied from many different aspects. Occasionally articles on special techniques will appear. Articles merely descriptive of new virus diseases will not be included.*
>
> *The first volume serves to indicate the intended scope of this series. Included are essays on various viruses which affect man, animals, insects, plants and bacteria. Some of the reviews have been written by animal biologists, some by plant biologists, some by biochemists and some by biophysicists. It is hoped that this and subsequent issues will afford virus researchers a comprehensive up-to-date view of virology as a whole.*

In the preface to Volume 2, this was supplemented by the following:

> *In Volume 2 of Advances in Virus Research, the editors are attempting to carry out their policy, announced in the Preface to Volume 1, of bringing together critical review articles, written from various points of view, on representative viruses causing diseases of man, of animals (including insects), of plants, and of bacteria. The present volume contains two chapters on plant viruses, two on viruses causing diseases of animals and of man, one on the chemical constitution of viruses, and three on biophysical aspects of virus research. Already published in Volume 1 are a chapter on bacteriophages, two chapters on plant viruses, one on insect*

viruses, two on viruses affecting man, one on viruses affecting animals and one on virus nucleic acids.

The combined contributions of Volumes 1 and 2 come closer to fulfilling the editors' goal than do the specific chapters included in either volume. The editors have attempted and will continue to attempt to achieve balance in each volume, but they are obviously limited by the inability of authorities on some of the subjects which ought to be included to find the time to prepare chapters. Nevertheless, the editors feel confident that over the course of several years, they will be able to present a comprehensive survey of the field of virology.

Advances in Virus Research is planned as an annual review series. The contributions are written by experts, some with backgrounds as biologists, and some with backgrounds as physical scientists, each of whom presents his subject matter in his own style. It is the editors' view that it would be impossible, and undesirable even if possible, to mold the contributions in a particular volume into a homogeneous unit resembling a monograph. It is their aim, however, that, as the volumes accumulate, the reviews appearing in Advances will provide the individual scholar with the material he needs to synthesize his own view of virology as a whole.

This "mission" of *AVR* was stated 65 years ago but is still valid today. Transdisciplinarity was its goal as it was considered the basis of successful virus research exemplified by the variety of professions contributing to virus research from human and veterinary physicians to physicists, chemists, and biologists. Of course, in the meantime an ever-increasing number of journals of widely differing impact publish reviews on virology and related sciences. Also, the concept of focusing on reviews in virus research as initiated by *AVR* was taken up and carried forward by a number of other periodicals. While today there is a plethora of journals and reviews to choose from, *AVR* continues to serve an important purpose by its broad focus on viruses of bacteria, plants, and animals including insects, and its distinctive international bent.

Over the years a number of virologists with different backgrounds and expertise have served as editors (Fig. 1). The inaugural editors were Smith and Lauffer. Kenneth Manley Smith (1892–1981; Fig. 1A) was a plant virus researcher at Cambridge, United Kingdom, working at the Potato Virus Station. He identified the potatovirus X and Y complex and several other potato viruses. He teamed with Max A. Lauffer (1914–2012; Fig. 1B), from 1949 the first chair of the biophysics department of the University of Pittsburgh and Dean of the Division of Natural Sciences from 1956. In 1963 Smith (then aged 70) joined Lauffer at Pittsburgh before returning to Cambridge in 1969.

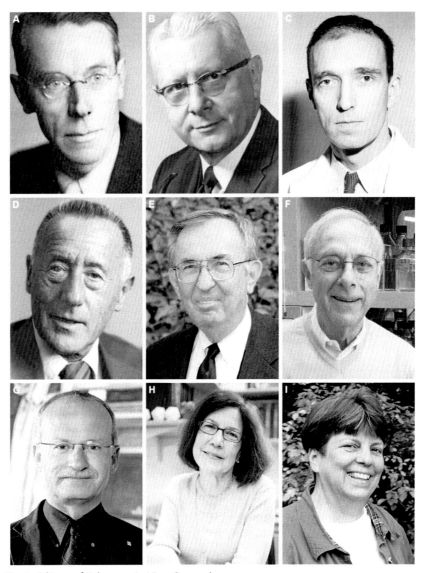

Fig. 1 Editors of *Advances in Virus Research*.

Starting with Volume 15, Smith and Lauffer were joined by Frederik B. Bang (1916–1981; Fig. 1C), a pioneer in applying marine biology to medical research. He worked on viral as well as parasitic infectious diseases. Bang was for 35 years a member of the faculty of Johns Hopkins and chairman of the pathobiology department of the Hopkins School of Hygiene and

Public Health. He was one of the pioneers in using electron microscopy to analyze viruses.

Karl Maramorosch (1915–2016; Fig. 1D), an eminent entomologist, plant pathologist, and virologist, joined the group from Volume 18 onward. He served the longest as serial editor until the age of 100! Karl Maramorosch was born in Vienna, Austria, and educated in Poland. He fled with his wife to Romania during the Second World War, and in 1947 emigrated to the United States. Transiting through Rockefeller University in New York City and the Boyce Thompson Institute in Yonkers, NY, he joined Rutgers University in New Jersey in 1974. Maramorosch pioneered work on insect-transmitted plant viruses.

After the departure of Smith, Lauffer, and Bang, in 1983 Frederick A. Murphy (Fig. 1E) and Aaron J. Shatkin (1934–2012; Fig. 1F) joined Karl Maramarosch. Frederick A. Murphy, a veterinarian, worked at the CDC since 1964 as chief of the viral pathology branch, then director of the division of viral and rickettsial diseases before moving in 1991 to the University of California–Davis School of Veterinary Medicine. Since 2005 he is professor at the department of pathology, University of Texas Medical Branch, Galveston, TX. Frederick A. Murphy is probably best known for his first electron micrographic demonstration of Ebola virus, a picture which hit the news then and still does. Aaron J. Shatkin, a chemist–virologist, specialized in reoviruses, working first at the National Institutes of Health before moving to the Roche Institute of Molecular Biology in Nutley, NJ. In 1985 he became founding director of the Center for Advanced Biotechnology and Medicine at Rutgers University, NJ. Studying reovirus transcription, Aaron J. Shatkin discovered many basic principles of mRNA transcription, processing, and translation.

After Shatkin's death and Murphy's retirement, Thomas C. Mettenleiter (Fig. 1G) was recruited in 2014 as serial editor. A biologist by training he has been active in studying molecular biology of viruses of veterinary importance since the early 1980s. He is currently president of the Friedrich-Loeffler-Institut, the oldest virus research facility worldwide having been founded by Friedrich Loffler in 1910. He was joined in 2015 by Margaret Kielian (Fig. 1H), professor of cell biology at the Albert Einstein College of Medicine and Samuel H. Golding Chair in Microbiology (New York). Kielian works on the entry and exit of enveloped animal viruses, with a focus on alphaviruses and flaviviruses. In 2016 the current team was completed by Marilyn J. Roossinck (Fig. 1I), professor of plant pathology and environmental microbiology at Pennsylvania State University. Roossinck studies virus ecology and evolution, using plant and fungal viruses as models, and has focused recent work on beneficial viruses.

3. VIROLOGY TODAY: ANOTHER GOLDEN AGE IN VIRUS RESEARCH

Our understanding of viruses has escalated amazingly from Volume 1 to 100 of this series. It is interesting to consider how current scientific advances will impact virology as they enable new questions to be addressed.

From their outset, electron microscopy and structural biology have greatly contributed to our understanding of viruses. The 2017 Nobel Prize in Chemistry was awarded to Dubochet, Frank, and Henderson for their contributions to the field of cryo-electron microscopy (Nobel Prize Announcement, 2017), and it is worth noting that many of the early cryo-EM studies were based on imaging of viruses (e.g., Adrian et al., 1984). Recently there has been an amazing "quantum leap" in the field of cryo-electron microscopy, based on improved microscopes, detectors, and computational methods (reviewed in Kühlbrandt, 2014). Within the past few years, symmetrical viruses whose structures were once determined to a "state-of-the-art resolution" in the range of $25\,\text{Å}$ have been solved to $3\text{--}4\,\text{Å}$. The new advances in cryo-EM mean that the structures of many proteins including viral proteins can be addressed without crystallization and that asymmetric structures can more readily be determined. The resolution of cryo-EM tomography also continues to advance rapidly, and has already contributed to our understanding of more pleomorphic virus structures (e.g., Grunewald et al., 2003), and to the study of viruses during host cell entry, replication, and exit (Welsch et al., 2009).

Virology has been strongly impacted by the advances in the genomics of viruses and hosts. From the virus side, this has enabled studies of the functions of novel viral gene products and advanced our understanding of the genetic relationships among viruses. From the host side, we can now readily characterize changes in host gene expression during virus infection. Methods such as siRNA, CRISPR–Cas9, or haploid genetic screens allow querying the requirements for virus infection, leading to the identification of host factors involved in the promotion or inhibition of the virus lifecycle (Perreira et al., 2016). Advances in our understanding of cell biology then permit detailed studies of the functions of such host factors. In addition, the development of fluorescent protein-labeled viruses has enabled virus tracking in live cells in culture or in the host organism. Application and development of these methods will be central to advancing our understanding of virus–host cell interactions.

Lastly, it has become apparent that sophisticated methods of "virus hunting" will be of continued importance in the future. These are a far cry from early studies that relied on recovery of viruses from field samples by infection of model organisms or cell cultures followed by virus identification using serology and other methods. State-of-the-art sequence analysis enables the identification of virus sequences in nature, helping to define virus reservoirs, changes in virus distribution, and emergence and evolution as pathogens. Deep-sequencing technologies allow the identification of viruses from environments never explored before, and we are becoming aware of the vast numbers of viruses in the oceans (estimated at 10^{31} virus particles (Suttle, 2013)), terrestrial environments, plants, and animals. The International Committee for the Taxonomy of Viruses has recently concluded that in some cases viruses can be declared new species by sequence determination alone (Simmonds et al., 2017). Advanced sequence determination has also led to a plethora of whole genome sequences of hosts, and these all contain integrated virus sequences. The identification of these molecular fossils of past virus infections has led to the new discipline of paleovirology.

While it is difficult to predict the future, it is safe to say that the study of viruses will continue to be fascinating, surprising, and important. We can surmise that sequencing, structural, and visualization methods will continue to advance. Nanotechnology, while tangentially related to virology, will also help to drive many of these new technologies. *Advances in Virus Research* will continue to aim to provide broad background, authoritative commentary, and interdisciplinary views for established virologists, and to excite and engage new researchers to contribute to the future of virology.

ACKNOWLEDGMENTS

The immense help on discussing historical aspects of virus research provided by former series editor Frederick A. Murphy as well as providing his compilation of photographs of previous *AVR* editors (part of Fig. 1) is greatly appreciated.

Editors of AVR
Kenneth M. Smith (1892–1981): Volumes 1–27
Max A. Lauffer (1914–2012): Volumes 1–29
Frederik B. Bang (1916–1981): Volumes 15–27
Karl Maramorosch (1915–2016): Volumes 18–95
Frederick A. Murphy: Volumes 30–91
Aaron J. Shatkin (1934–2012): Volumes 30–84
Thomas C. Mettenleiter: Volumes 92–present
Margaret Kielian: Volumes 93–present
Marilyn J. Roossinck: Volumes 97–present

REFERENCES

Adrian, M., Dubochet, J., Lepault, J., McDowall, A.W., 1984. Cryo-electron microscopy of viruses. Nature 308, 32–36.

Calisher, C., Horzinek, M., 1999. 100 Years of virology—the birth and growth of a discipline. Arch. Virol. Suppl. 15.

d'Herelle, F.H., 1917. Sur une microbe invisible antagoniste des bacilles dysentériques. C. R. Acad. Sci. 165, 373–375.

Doerr, R., 1911. Über filtrierbares Virus. Centralbl. Bakteriol. 1, 13–23, 1. Abt. Beiheft.

Enquist, L.W., Racaniello, V.R., 2013. Virology: from contagium fluidum to virome. In: Knipe, D., Howley, P.M. (Eds.), Fields Virology, sixth ed. Wolters Kluwer, Lippincott Williams & Wilkins, Philadelphia, pp. 1–20.

Friedberger, E., Pfeiffer, R., 1919. Lehrbuch der Mikrobiologie. Fischer Verl., Jena.

Grunewald, K., Desai, P., Winkler, D.C., Heymann, J.B., Belnap, D.M., Baumeister, W., Steven, A.C., 2003. Three-dimensional structure of herpes simplexvirus from cryo-electron tomography. Science 302, 1396–1398.

Hershey, A.D., Chase, M., 1952. Independent functions of viral protein and nucleic acid in growth of bacteriophage. J. Gen. Physiol. 36, 39–56.

Kausche, G.A., Pfannkuch, P.F., Ruska, H., 1939. Die Sichtbarmachung von pflanzlichem Virus im Übermikroskop. Naturwissenschaften 27, 292–299.

Krüger, D.H., Schneck, P., Gelderblom, H.R., 2000. Helmut Ruska and the visualization of viruses. Lancet 355, 1713–1717.

Kühlbrandt, W., 2014. The resolution revolution. Science 343, 1443–1444.

Loeffler, F., 1884. Untersuchungen über die Bedeutung der Mikroorganismen für die Entstehung der Diphtherie beim Menschen, bei der Taube und beim Kalbe. Mittheilungen aus dem kaiserlichen Gesundheitsamte 2, 421–499.

Loeffler, F., 1911. Über filtrierbares Virus. Centralbl. Bakteriol. 1, 1–12, 1. Abt. Beiheft.

Luria, S.E., 1945. Mutations of bacterial viruses affecting their host range. Genetics 30, 84–99.

Mettenleiter, T.C., 2017. The first 'virus hunters'. Adv. Virus Res. 99, 1–16.

M'Fadyean, J., 1908. The ultra-visible viruses. J. Comp. Pathol. Therap. 21, 58–68, 168–175, 232–242.

Murphy, F.A., 2014. The Foundations of Medical and Veterinary Virology: Discoverers and Discoveries, Inventors and Inventions, Developers and Technologies. http://www.utmb.edu/virusimages/.

Perreira, J.M., Meraner, P., Brass, A.L., 2016. Functional genomic strategies for elucidating human-virus interactions: will CRISPR knockout RNAi and haploid cells? Adv. Virus Res. 94, 1–51.

Reed, W., 1902. Recent researches concerning the etiology, propagation, and prevention of yellow fever, by the United States Army Commission. J. Hyg. 11, 101–119.

Rivers, T.M., 1927. Filterable viruses—a critical review. J. Bacteriol. 14, 217–258.

Rivers, T.M., 1928a. Some general aspects of filterable viruses. In: Rivers, T.M. (Ed.), Filterable Viruses. The Williams & Wilkins Co., Baltimore, pp. 3–54.

Rivers, T.M., 1928b. Filterable viruses. The Williams & Wilkins Co., Baltimore.

Schlesinger, M., 1932. Die Bestimmung von Teilchengröße und spezifischem Gewicht des Bakteriophagen durch Zentrifugierversuche. Z. Hyg. Infektionskr. 114, 161–176.

Simmonds, P., Adams, M.J., Breitbart, M., Benkö, M., Briste, J.R., Carstens, E.B., Davison, A.J., Delwart, E., Gorbalenya, A.E., Harrach, B.Z., Hull, R., King, A.M.Q., Koonin, E.V., Krupovic, M., Kuhn, J.H., Lefkowitz, E.J., Nibert, M.L., Orton, R., Roossinck, M.J., Sabanadzovic, S., Sullivan, M.B., Suttle, R., Tesh, B., van der Vlugt, R.A., Varsani, A., Zerbini, F.M., 2017. Virus taxonomy in the age of metagenomics. Nat. Rev. Microbiol. 15, 161–168. https://doi.org/10.1038/nrmicro.2016.177.

Stanley, W.M., 1935. Isolation of a crystalline protein possessing the properties of tobacco mosaic virus. Science 81, 644–645.

Suttle, C.A., 2013. Viruses: unlocking the greatest biodiversity on Earth. Genome 56, 542–544.

Svedberg, T., 1927. The Ultracentrifuge. Nobel Lecture, May 19, 1927.

The Nobel Prize in Chemistry, 2017. Scientific Background: The Development of Cryo-electron Microscopy. http://www.nobelprize.org/nobel_prizes/chemistry/laureates/2017/advanced.html.

Twort, F., 1915. An investigation on the nature of ultra-microscopic viruses. Lancet 186, 1241–1243.

Valillo, G., 1911. Filtrierbare virus. Z. Infekt. Krankh. Haustiere IX, 433–479.

van Helvoort, T., 1996. When did virology start? ASM News 62, 142–145.

von Borries, B., Ruska, E., Ruska, H., 1938. Bakterien und Virus in übermikroskopischer Aufnahme. Klin. Wochenschr. 17, 921–925.

Welsch, S., Miller, S., Romero-Brey, I., Merz, A., Bleck, C.K., Walther, P., Fuller, S.D., Antony, C., Krijnse-Locker, J., Bartenschlager, R., 2009. Composition and three-dimensional architecture of the dengue virus replication and assembly sites. Cell Host Microbe 5, 365–375.

Wolbach, S.B., 1912. The filterable viruses—a summary. J. Med. Res. 27, 1–25.

Woodruff, E.M., Goodpasture, E.W., 1931. The susceptibility of the chorio-allantoic membrane of chick embryos to infection with the fowl-pox virus. Am. J. Pathol. 7, 209–222.

FURTHER READING

Beijerinck, M.W., 1898. Über ein Contagium vivum fluidum als Ursache der Fleckenkrankheit der Tabaksblätter. Verhandelingen Koninklijke Akademie van Wetenschappen te Amsterdam (Tweede Sectie) 6, 3–21.

Loeffler, F., 1898. IV. Bericht der Kommission zur Erforschung der Maul- und Klauenseuche bei dem Institut für Infektionskrankheiten in Berlin. Centrabl. Bakteriol. 24, 569–574, 1. Abt.

Loeffler, F., 1919. Filtrierbare Virusarten. In: Friedberger, E., Pfeiffer, R. (Eds.), Lehrbuch der Mikrobiologie, II. Band, Spez. Teil, pp. 1091–1155.

Loeffler, F., Frosch, P., 1898. Berichte der Kommission zur Erforschung der Maul- und Klauenseuche bei dem Institut für Infektionskrankheiten in Berlin. Centrabl. Bakteriol. 23, 371–391, 1. Abt.

THOMAS C. METTENLEITER
Friedrich-Loeffler-Institut, Greifswald – Insel Riems, Germany
MARGARET KIELIAN
Albert Einstein College of Medicine, Bronx, NY, United States
MARILYN J. ROOSSINCK
Pennsylvania State University, Philadelphia, PA, United States

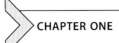

CHAPTER ONE

The Species Problem in Virology

Marc H.V. Van Regenmortel[1]

School of Biotechnology, CNRS, University of Strasbourg, Strasbourg, France
[1]Corresponding author: e-mail address: vanregen@unistra.fr

Contents

Abstract

Virus classification deals with conceptual species classes that have viruses as their members. A virus species cannot be *described* but can only be *defined* by listing certain species-defining properties of its member. However, it is not possible to define a virus species by using a single species-defining property. The new 2013 official definition of virus species is not appropriate because it applies equally to virus genera. A nucleotide motif is a chemical part of a viral genome and is not a species-defining property that could be used for establishing new virus species. A virus classification based solely on nucleotide sequences is a classification of viral genomes and not of viruses. The variable distribution of species-defining properties of a polythetic species class is not itself a single common property of all the members of the class, since this would lead to the paradox that every polythetic class is also a monothetic one.

1. INTRODUCTION

The species problem is not unique to virology since 150 years after the publication of Darwin's *On the Origin of Species*, biologists still did not agree about what constitutes a microbial, plant, or animal species. Although the term species is used as the lowest category in all hierarchical biological classifications, what a species actually is, namely its ontology, remains an unresolved issue in the philosophy of biology (Claridge et al., 1997; Ghiselin, 1997; Stamos, 2003). Mayr (1982) declared: "There is probably no other concept in biology that has remained as consistently controversial as the species concept," and in 1997 during an international conference on species, no less than 22 different species concepts were discussed (Mayden, 1997).

Although viruses are usually not considered to be alive (Van Regenmortel, 2016a), they are recognized as biological entities and are classified using the categories species, genus, family, and order universally used in biology. The question of what a virus species actually is, is a problem of logical and lexical semantics. In the case of genera and families, virologists readily admit that these categories are conceptual, abstract constructions of the mind, and they do not confuse them with the real objects they encounter in their daily handling of viruses. They are fully aware that a virus family, for instance, cannot be purified by centrifugation, sequenced, or visualized by electron microscopy since it is an imaginary, conceptual creation of the mind, and not a physical entity.

The situation is different with virus species since virologists often view them as more "real" than genera and families because they tend to think of a virus species as an individual kind or type of virus that is able to infect a particular host. This confusion between a species as a concrete kind of object and as an abstract category in a classification is actually prevalent in the whole of biology and is exacerbated because the vast majority of individual organisms in botany, zoology, and microbiology do not have common names different from the Latin name of the species to which these organisms belong. As a result, biologists will write that a person has been infected with *Escherichia coli* (in italics because it is a species name) which suggests that a conceptual category is able to infect a physical organism. There are about 800,000 species of insects on earth but as very few members of these species have a common name, virologists will write that dengue virus is transmitted by the species *Aedes aegypti* and not by a living but nameless member of that species. Such a formulation unfortunately blurs the logical distinction between concrete objects and abstract concepts. Although a tongue-in-cheek solution to this problem has been proposed (Calisher and Van Regenmortel, 2009), it is unlikely that such a solution will ever be implemented.

It is noteworthy that virologists are the only biologists who could easily avoid this type of logical confusion since every infecting virus has a common name that differs from the species name to which the virus belongs. It would thus be easy for virologists to say that it is a particular virus that causes a disease and not an abstract species category, but this of course assumes that they can readily distinguish concepts from objects which is a task that turns out to be much more difficult than could have been anticipated (Van Regenmortel, 2003). Since all humans share with all viruses the property of having an individual name, this led Calisher (2010) to quip: "What is the difference between a virus species and a virus? The same as the difference between *Homo sapiens* and you."

The root of the term classification is "class" and virus classification deals with several abstract classes of viruses, one of them being virus species. The most important characteristic of a species class is that it has members which are the concrete viral objects studied by virologists, and the species is actually defined by listing certain properties of the viruses that are its members. Since whatever is said about a thing ascribes a property to it, properties and classes are related entities (Quine, 1990, p. 22). Viruses, however, should not be confused with species that are conceptual constructions of human minds and not real objects.

Class membership is the logical relation that allows a bridge to be established between the two logical categories of physical objects and conceptual constructs. This membership relation is different from the part–whole relationship that exists between two concrete objects, one being a part of the other, in the way a limb is part of a body. A viral object cannot to be a physical part of a mental species construct nor can a concept be a part of a material object. The question whether virus species exist as real biological entities independent of any human conceptualization is still the subject of intense debate (Claridge, 2010; Mishler, 2010). If one accepts that real, phenomenal, and conceptual modes of existence actually exist (Bunge, 2016), it is possible to say that virus species have at least a conceptual existence.

2. THE LOGIC OF HIERARCHICAL VIRUS CLASSIFICATION

Virus classification follows the logic of the Linnaean system (Buck and Hull, 1966) which consists of a hierarchy of taxa from species to the higher taxa of genera, families, and orders. The viruses that are members of a species are also members of taxa above it, and the relation between a lower taxon and a higher taxon immediately above it is called class inclusion. Class inclusion obviates the need to repeat the properties used for defining higher taxa in the definition of the lower taxa that are included in them. The "defining" properties of a genus are thus always present in all the members of the species that are included in the genus, although they are not species-defining properties that allow species to be differentiated.

Since higher taxa such as families and orders are defined by a small number of stable properties of their members (such as virion structure and virus replication strategy) that are both necessary and sufficient for establishing membership, these classes, which are usually considered to be universal classes, are much easier to define than species classes. Higher taxa have more virus members than species taxa, and they require fewer defining properties than species taxa for establishing membership. This follows the logical principle that increasing the number of required qualifications decreases membership (Buck and Hull, 1966). This principle also invalidates the currently fashionable claim that a single property could be sufficient for defining a virus species.

3. DEFINITIONS OF VIRUS SPECIES

Biological species have been traditionally considered to be populations whose members can only breed among themselves and are reproductively isolated from those of other populations (Mayr, 1970). Since this biological species definition applies only to organisms that reproduce sexually, it was later modified to make it applicable to asexual organisms as follows: *A species is a reproductive community of populations, reproductively isolated from others, that occupies a specific niche in nature* (Mayr, 1982).

In the 1980s, plant virologists rejected the view that there could be virus species because they thought that the biological species concept could not be applied to viruses that replicate as clones (Milne, 1984). These virologists also opposed the introduction of virus species because they believed that such a move would bring about the use of Latin species names which they refused to accept (Matthews, 1983, 1985). The use of a Latinized viral nomenclature had initially been advocated by the International Committee on Taxonomy of Viruses (ICTV) (Fenner, 1976; Wildy, 1971), but Latin names were never introduced, and the rules regarding the use of Latin in virus taxonomy were later removed (Francki et al., 1991).

Another reason for rejecting the use of species in virus classification was that the ICTV had never been able to agree on a definition of virus species. Many definitions had been proposed over the years (Van Regenmortel, 2016b), but only in 1991 did the ICTV endorse the following definition of virus species: *A virus species is a polythetic class of viruses that constitute a replicating lineage and occupy a particular ecological niche* (Pringle, 1991). This definition indicated that the members of a virus species are not simply similar objects devoid of a common origin but are collections of objects related by common descent. It also incorporated the notion of a shared ecological niche (Colwell, 1992) used by Mayr in his species definition, which is a relational, functional property of an organism or a virus rather than a vacant space waiting to be occupied (Mahner and Bunge, 1997, pp. 181–185). However, the main novelty of the species definition endorsed in 1991 was that it included the notion of polythetic class which by then had become generally adopted by taxonomists (Beckner, 1959; Hull, 1976; Van Regenmortel, 2010). Whereas monothetic classes are universal classes defined by one or a few properties that are both necessary and sufficient for membership in the class, polythetic classes are defined by a variable combination of properties, none of which is a defining property necessarily present in every member of the class. This means that (1) each member of a polythetic species shares a certain number of properties, (2) each property is present in a large but unspecified number of members, and (3) no property is necessarily present in all the members of the class and absent in the members of other classes (Fig. 1). It should be stressed that the term polythetic only describes a particular distribution of properties present in a class and that the members of a class do not themselves possess polythetic or monothetic properties.

	A	B	C	D	E	F	G	H
1	+	+	+					
2	+	+			+			
3	+		+	+				
4		+	+	+				
5					+	+	+	
6					+	+	+	
7					+	+		+
8					+	+		+

Fig. 1 Distinction between polythetic and monothetic classes in the case of eight individuals (1–8) and eight properties (A–H). The possession of a property is indicated by a *plus sign*. Individuals 1–4 constitute a polythetic class, each member possessing 3 out of 4 properties with no common property being present in all the members. Individuals 5–6, 7–8, and 5–6–7–8 form three monothetic classes with, respectively, 3, 3, and 2 properties present in all the members (Van Rijsbergen, 1979; see also: http://www.iva.dk/bh/lifeboat_ko/CONCEPTS/monothetic.htm).

The term species is used to refer to the thousands of virus species taxa that have been established by taxonomists (Adams et al., 2016), but it also refers to the species category which is the class of all the species taxa. This category is the lowest one in a classification, below the genus, family, and order categories.

The concept of polythetic class, also known as a cluster class (Pigliucci, 2003), has been used successfully by ICTV Study Groups for establishing many new virus species (Ball, 2005). In recent years, a few virologists (Gibbs and Gibbs, 2006) objected to virus species being called polythetic classes because they claimed that the term polythetic was obscure and poorly understood by virologists and they proposed instead that virus species should be defined monothetically using certain features present in the genome sequences of individual viruses. In 2004, it had been reported that the RNA genome sequence of all the viruses that were members of the species *Tobacco mosaic virus* possessed a unique, combination nucleotide motif (NC) of 47 nucleotides present in the viral polymerase. It was suggested that this NC motif could be used for identifying all the members of that species and for distinguishing them from members of other species in the *Tobamovirus* genus. Unfortunately, this proposal of using a nucleotide motif as a diagnostic marker for identifying the members of a previously established species was actually confounded with the activity of taxonomists when they establish a new polythetic virus species using species-defining properties (see Section 4). This confusion gave rise to the illusion that virus species could be "created" by taxonomists on the basis of a single characteristic feature of a viral nucleotide sequence.

In 2012, four members of the ICTV Executive Committee (A. King, M. Adams, E. Lefkowitz, and E. Carstens) posted on the ICTV website the following new definition of virus species: *A virus species is a monophyletic group of viruses whose properties can be distinguished from those of other species by multiple criteria* (King et al., 2012). Although it was acknowledged that these criteria could be genome properties or any other phenotypic properties of viruses, the earlier requirement that a virus species had to form a polythetic class defined by the absence of a single defining property present in all the members of the species was abandoned. As a result, it became possible to establish a species as a monophyletic group of viruses that shared only one common defining property. For instance, if two anelloviruses possessed only 65% nucleotide identity in their genomes, this sole criterion was sufficient to allocate them to two different species even in the absence of any known difference in biological or other phenotypic properties. Furthermore, since every species and genus can be considered to be a monophyletic group, the new definition was in fact a definition of both virus species and virus genus. Another reason why monophyly is not an adequate criterion for species demarcation is the common occurrence of recombination and reassortment among parts of many viral genomes which produces chimeric viruses with polyphyletic genomes (Calisher et al., 1995) and makes it impossible to accurately represent such multidimensional phylogeny in a monophyletic scheme (Ball, 2005).

Many other shortcomings of the proposed new species definition have been posted on the ICTV website (King, 2012) and were described in detail by a group of six ICTV Life Members and eight other senior virologists (Van Regenmortel et al., 2013). For instance, the proposers of the new definition had claimed that the term "class" could only be used to denote a category in the classification hierarchy, namely the one situated above the category order and below the category phylum, although such a category is not used in virus classification. This preposterous claim (King, 2012) ignored the fact that "class" is the root of the term classification and is universally used in all biological classifications because it allows a logical link to be established between an abstract class and the concrete organisms or the viruses that are members of a class. The proposers of the new definition also objected to virus species being called polythetic classes, and they defined a species as a "group" of viruses that make up a collection of viral objects linked to each other by part–whole relations instead of by the membership relation. These criticisms were ignored by the authors of the new species definition who claimed that the species definition endorsed by the ICTV in 1991 was based on specious reasoning and on meaningless terms such as polythetic class, replicating lineage and ecological niche! An acrimonious debate involving many virologists ensued which has been recorded in full on the ICTV website (King, 2012), but the ICTV Executive Committee was undeterred and had their new species definition ratified by a fast-track approval process which reduced the time available for posting further objections on the ICTV website. The result of the ballot was 45 in favor, 21 against, and 2 abstentions (Adams et al., 2013). A glaring example of the pernicious consequence of allowing new virus species to be established only on the basis of a single percentage of genome divergence (in this case a threshold of 91%) is the 307 species of begomoviruses (out of a total of 3704 species taxa in the current ICTV Master Species List; Adams et al., 2016) that have recently been recognized (Brown et al., 2015). This included 42 different species of *Tomato leaf curl virus* that were all very similar biologically and were differentiated only by including in the species name the geographical location of the first isolate of each species. No evidence was presented that these 42 species all differed in their biological properties and since the location where one isolate is found is not a relevant property of a virus, a new nomenclature was allowed to take precedence over a new taxonomy. In contrast, the two species *Bean golden mosaic virus* and *Bean golden yellow mosaic virus*, for instance, differed in the tissue tropism of their members. Obviously, it would have been preferable to consider the 42 species of *Tomato leaf curl virus* as strains of a single species.

This new classification (Brown et al., 2015) was based on pairwise sequence comparisons of all available begomovirus genome sequences which produce plots of the frequency distribution of pairwise identity percentages showing multimodal distributions of several peaks (Van Regenmortel, 2007). Some of these peaks could have been attributed to genera, species, subspecies, strains, or serotypes (Van Regenmortel, 2011), if phenotypic traits of the viruses were taken into account for producing biologically meaningful categories. Instead of opting for a species demarcation criterion of 91% it would, for example, have been possible to use the small valley observed at 71% pairwise identity in the twin peaks in the region of 62%–82% pairwise sequence identity (Brown et al., 2015) as a cutoff point for differentiating between strains and species. It should be noted that in the genus *Mastrevirus* in the same *Geminiviridae* family, a more appropriate cutoff point of 75% sequence similarity in DNA-A sequences was used which led to the creation of only 12 separate species (Fauquet and Stanley, 2005).

4. DIAGNOSTIC MARKERS USEFUL FOR VIRUS IDENTIFICATION ARE NOT SPECIES-DEFINING PROPERTIES

It should be stressed that concepts and abstract species classes, like any abstraction, can only be "defined," whereas the individual members of a species or any other concrete object can only be "described" (Ghiselin, 1984). A species class itself cannot possess any intrinsic property such as a chemical composition, and the class can only be defined by listing properties of its concrete members. The definition or meaning of a species taxon is known in logic as its intension, whereas the viruses that the species class refers to are known as its extension or referents that are the concrete instances that satisfy the membership conditions of the class. Since the extension of a class can only be determined if one can distinguish members from nonmembers, the definition or intension of a species taxon must first be established by taxonomists before it becomes possible for virologists to determine its actual extension. In other words, the intension must precede the extension (Mahner and Bunge, 1997, p. 227) since it is otherwise not possible to ascertain if a sufficient number of species-defining properties are present in an individual virus to make it a member of the species. The proposal that a monothetic species class can be established by relying on a single defining property such as a nucleotide motif found in viral genomes (Gibbs et al., 2004) overlooks the fact that it would be necessary to know beforehand that this motif is present in all the members of the species and absent in other species which implies that the extension would have to precede the intension which is impossible (Van Regenmortel, 2011, 2016b).

Properties useful for distinguishing individual species within a genus obviously cannot be invariant, genus-defining properties but must be species-defining properties such as natural host range, cell and tissue tropism, pathogenicity, mode of transmission, and small differences in genome sequence. These properties which can be altered by a few mutations also vary considerably in different members of a species which is the reason why species are defined polythetically by a variable combination of properties rather than by a single conserved property present in all the species members. It is unfortunate that some virologists confound the identification of a virus isolate as a member of a species using a single diagnostic maker such as a particular nucleotide motif (Van Regenmortel, 2011) with the unfeasible task of establishing a new species using a single character since the intensional definition of a species cannot be derived from its extension.

The technique known as barcoding (Hebert and Gregory, 2005) is sometimes presented as a useful method for establishing new species, although it is only a tool for identifying members of existing species. Nucleotide motifs cannot be used for distinguishing or establishing new species from millions of genomes of potential species that have not yet been recognized on the basis of phenotypic criteria (Ebach and Holdrege, 2005; Van Regenmortel, 2016c).

It is sometimes assumed that when virus species are demarcated only on the basis of genome sequences and a derived plausible phylogeny, this will produce a classification that is more correct, relevant, or useful than a classification based on all the phenotypic properties of viruses (Calisher et al., 1995). However, genome characteristics do not by themselves justify taxonomic allocations and the aim to record phylogeny should not overshadow the relevance of biological and phenotypic characteristics that are the main reason why virologists engage in species demarcation.

Some proponents of a monothetic definition of virus species also make the bizarre claim that since a species corresponds to a replication lineage, it cannot possibly be a polythetic class since all its members must have inherited one or more properties from a common ancestor which must therefore make the class a monothetic one. However, a polythetic class is defined by a variable distribution of properties in the members of the class together with the absence of a single common species-defining property in all its members, and such a combination of properties does not itself constitute a single common property of all the virus members of the class. If it did, it would lead to the paradox that every polythetic class is also a monothetic one. This paradox is similar to the well-known Russell paradox of the improbable barber who only shaves all those men in the village who do not shave themselves, since this implies that the barber would have to shave himself only if he does not do so (Quine, 1990, p. 227). Concrete membership conditions determine a class but since a class is not a concrete object, it cannot itself figure as a candidate for membership of the class. Classes of viruses can only admit viruses as members but cannot admit themselves as members which means that nonself membership is not an acceptable membership condition (Quine and Ullian, 1978; Van Regenmortel, 2016b).

5. ONLY VIRUSES BUT NOT THEIR GENOME SEQUENCES CAN BE CLASSIFIED INTO SPECIES AND GENUS CLASSES

Although viruses are currently classified using a combination of structural, chemical, biological, and genetic properties, it has recently been suggested that nucleotide sequences obtained from viral metagenomic data could be used for establishing new virus species and for incorporating them in the existing virus classification system (Simmonds et al., 2017). This suggestion arose because tens of thousands of previously unrecorded viral sequences representing a metagenomic consensus sequence instead of a single viral haplotype have been found in various marine and biological environments.

Viruses have been described as living or nonliving processes corresponding to a replication cycle (Dupré and Guttinger, 2016), and it could be argued that the genome sequence constitutes the stable, continuing property of an individual viral process. However, the genome is only a part of the virion and it is difficult to attribute a constant property to a process. Furthermore, the persistence of a viral nucleotide sequence during the replication cycle arises from many interactions between individual viral genes and various gene products of hosts and vectors and the alleged persistence may thus not be the cause but rather the consequence of numerous dynamic processes involving the virus and its environment (Van Regenmortel, 2016c).

It should also be recognized that the most conspicuous and overwhelming purpose of a phylogenetic virus classification is mainly to satisfy an intellectual curiosity about the evolutionary history of viruses on our planet, and such knowledge may not necessarily be the major concern of laboratory virologists involved in the study of present day viruses. It is also ironic that RNA viruses are said to form so-called quasispecies, since the term species in this context is borrowed from chemistry where chemical species always consist of identical molecules. It should be evident that no virus species can ever correspond to a chemical species and referring to virus species as imperfect, quasispecies simply reflects a confusion between chemical and biological categories (Van Regenmortel, 2011).

The notion of what is a trait, a character, an attribute or a property of a concrete object that could be used for classifying it, has been called the central problem of taxonomy (Inglis, 1991). Although a part of an object is often confused with a property, a part of a thing is a thing and not a property. The possession of a certain part may perhaps be interpreted as a property of an object but certainly not the part itself. It is not clear if a complete genome sequence, a particular NC motif or the presence of a certain nucleotide in the genome, should count as a single character (Van Regenmortel, 2007).

It is often overlooked that the genomic DNA or RNA sequence present in a virion is part of the virus phenotype since it is part of the virion chemical composition and structure. A virus classification based on nucleotide sequences found in virions can thus be viewed as a phenotypic classification that relies on the properties of molecular sequences instead of on the biological and functional properties of viruses. The nucleotide sequence of a virus is clearly an essential constituent part of a virus in the same way that an engine is an essential constituent part of a motor car. If one classifies car engines, the result will be a classification of engines and not of motor cars. Similarly, it is possible to classify the nucleotide sequences found in viruses on the basis of characteristics such overall genome organization, genome compositional features, gene content and order, particular nucleotide motifs, and inferred replication strategies, but this would produce a classification of nucleotide sequences or of viral genomes and not a classification of viruses (Van Regenmortel, 2016c).

5.1 The Phenotypic Properties of a Virus Cannot Be Inferred From Its Genome Sequence

Although it is usually claimed that the properties of a virus are largely or entirely encoded by its genome, it is actually not possible to infer all the phenotypic and biological characteristics of a virus simply from its nucleotide sequence. One reason for this is that genome sequences are not causally linked to particular phenotypic traits since alternative splicing and the discarding of introns produces unpredictable RNA transcripts as well as proteins that interact with vector and host gene products through numerous mechanisms that have not been elucidated. Causal connections between viral genes and the development of complex phenotypic traits are always indirect and are contingent upon many other unknown causal factors that eventually result in the development of a viral phenotype. Treating viral genes as representatives of phenotypic traits or as instructions for producing them reduces the role of these other causal factors to a simple nonspecific support for reading genomic information imbedded in undefined regions of the viral nucleotide sequence (Griffiths and Tabery, 2013). It is well known that small DNA and RNA viruses are composites of replication and structural gene modules that are reorganized during their evolutionary histories and can lead to changes in host range and other properties (Simmonds, 2015). The presence of structurally homologous capsid proteins in many DNA and RNA viruses suggests that the evolutionary history of structural genes is distinct from that of nonstructural genes (Koonin and Dolja, 2013). In reality, we have no information on the multiple causal mechanisms that arise from complex interactions between parts of the viral genome and the biological environment of viral vectors and hosts, although phenotypic traits arise from these interactions (Van Regenmortel, 2016c).

The argument that certain viral phenotypic properties are not deducible from the viral genome may seem to be contradicted by the considerable success of metagenomic approaches in reliably predicting protein structures from nucleotide sequences using for instance the Rosetta server (Ovchinnikov et al., 2017). Such methods that rely on the accurate prediction of individual residue–residue contacts using millions of metagenomic protein sequences together with coevolutionary analyses have indeed made it possible to identify many novel protein families. Successful predictions of protein structures from a viral genome sequence will no doubt allow us in future to allocate a newly discovered viral genome to a viral order or family since membership in such categories can be decided on the basis of very few conserved structural features. However, this is not the case when one allocates a virus to a species using a combination of genetically variable properties instead of by the presence of a single and stable structural property that may indeed be predictable from the genome sequence.

Links between genotypes and phenotypes are also obscured because many epigenetic factors, such as DNA methylation, histone modifications, and DNA silencing mediated by noncoding microRNAs, are known to regulate the interactions between the virus and its host and vectors, thereby influencing viral phenotypes (Galvan et al., 2015; Gómez-Díaz et al., 2012; Kettler et al., 2007; Milavetz and Balakrishnan, 2015; Ovchinnikov et al., 2017). It is also known that all the members of a virus species do not necessarily share the same genes with the result that it may be difficult to ascertain which nucleotide stretches of the so-called pangenome cause a phenotypic trait. Although it is possible, by analyzing the nucleotide composition of a virus, to show that it is an insect virus (Kapoor et al., 2010), this does not mean that it possible to identify the actual insect host that a virus is able to infect.

Although certain nucleotide motifs in the genome of a virus may be correlated with the virus being a member of a particular species or genus, correlation is not causation and such motifs are not causally linked to the phenotype of the virus. Although the seasonal appearance of storks in Strasbourg is sometimes correlated with increased numbers of human births, this does not justify a belief in fairy tales. In the absence of phenotypic information on the viruses themselves, there is little justification for trying to incorporate new species taxa proposed on the basis of metagenomic data in the current official system of virus classification (Van Regenmortel, 2016c).

6. THE CURRENT DEBATE ON NON-LATINIZED BINOMIAL NAMES OF VIRUS SPECIES

Assigning names to virus taxa is the responsibility of the ICTV, and the names of virus genera, subfamilies, families, and orders have for many years been written in italics with a capital letter which is a different typography from that used by the *Biological Code of Nomenclature* (Greuter et al.,

2011). The ICTV has always followed its own rules and Code and did not follow the traditions that exist in the rest of biology such as the use of Latin species names (Matthews, 1983) or the formation of binomial species names using the order genus name first/species identifier second, instead of the reversed order (species-first/genus-second) introduced in virology 50 years ago (Fenner, 1976).

Non-Latinized binomial names (NLBNs) have been used since the 1970s in plant virology papers and books (Bos, 1999; Brunt et al., 1990; Matthews, 1971) as well as in ICTV Reports (Fenner, 1976; Matthews, 1979, 1982). Italicized species names are formed by replacing the terminal word "virus" occurring in all common English virus names with the genus name to which the virus belongs, which also ends in virus. Measles virus, for instance, becomes a member of the species *Measles morbillivirus*. Such a system which does not require the creation of new species names since it combines known virus names with known genus names would also avoid the introduction of thousands of newly created Latin species names which certain taxonomists, for some obscure reason, consider to be preferable. English has replaced Latin as the international language of science (Van Regenmortel, 2003), and it seems unlikely that virologists would welcome having to start using thousands of unpronounceable Latin species names instead of using names that are already familiar to them (Van Regenmortel and Fauquet, 2002).

In 1998, the ICTV Executive Committee unfortunately decided to ratify English names of viruses as species names after italicizing them to indicate that they were taxonomic classes like italicized genera and families (Mayo and Horzinek, 1998).

As a result virus names and species names now differed only by typography and virologists were constantly forced to decide whether they wanted to refer to a real virus or to a taxonomic class, a distinction that many of them found difficult to make (Calisher and Mahy, 2003; Drebot et al., 2002; Kuhn and Jahrling, 2010; Van Regenmortel, 2007). Virologists would often write that *Measles virus* or *Cucumber mosaic virus* (instead of the viruses) had been isolated, transmitted to a host or sequenced, disregarding the fact that taxonomic creations of the mind obviously cannot have hosts, vectors, or sequences.

Virologists have come to realize that NLBNs for species would be preferable since binomial names in biology are always associated with taxonomic entities, and this makes it easier not to confuse the names of viruses with the names of species. It is also evident that NLBNs which include the genus name provide useful additional information on the species members, which of course was the reason why Fenner started to use NLBNs already in 1976. In 2002, two ballots held in the United States and in France showed that a significant majority of the 250 virologists who expressed an opinion voted in favor of NLBNs for species (Mayo, 2002; Van Regenmortel, 2016b; Van Regenmortel and Fauquet, 2002). In recent years, large numbers of NLBNs were introduced in several virus families such as the *Arenaviridae, Bornaviridae, Filoviridae, Nyamiviridae, Rabdoviridae, Paramyxoviridae*, as well as in the order *Mononegavirales* (Amarasinghe et al., 2017; Bukreyev et al., 2014; Kuhn et al., 2015) and it is to be hoped that the ICTV will eventually introduce NLBNs for all virus species.

ACKNOWLEDGMENTS

The author owns the copyright of the paper "Classes, taxa and categories in hierarchical virus classification: a review of current debates on definitions and names of virus species" published in 2016 in Bionomina 10: 1–21 (Magnolia Press, Auckland, NZ). Several paragraphs of this paper have been reproduced in the present review and are referenced under Van Regenmortel, 2016c, copyright M. Van Regenmortel.

A few paragraphs from the paper "Only viruses, but not their genome sequences, can be classified into species and genus classes" published in Current Topics in Virology 13: 59–68 have been reproduced in this review and are referenced under Van Regenmortel, 2016b, with the permission of the copyright owners Research Trends (P) Ltd., Kerala, India.

The author is grateful to Florence Diemer (CNRS, Strasbourg) for her secretarial assistance.

REFERENCES

Adams, M.J., Lefkowitz, E.J., King, A.M.Q., Carstens, E.B., 2013. Recently agreed changes to the international code of virus classification and nomenclature. Arch. Virol. 158, 2633–2639.

Adams, M.J., Lefkowitz, E.J., King, A.M., et al., 2016. Ratification vote on taxonomic proposals to the International Committee on Taxonomy of Viruses. Arch. Virol. 161, 2921–2949.

Amarasinghe, G.K., Bào, Y., Basler, C.F., et al., 2017. Taxonomy of the order Mononegavirales: update 2017. Arch. Virol. 162, 2493–2504. https://doi.org/10.1007/s00705-017-3311-7.

Ball, L.A., 2005. The universal taxonomy of viruses in theory and practice. In: Fauquet, C.M., Mayo, M.A., Maniloff, J., Desselberger, U., Ball, L.A. (Eds.), Virus Taxonomy: Eight Report of the International Committee on Taxonomy of Viruses. Elsevier Academic Press, Amsterdam, pp. 3–8.

Beckner, M., 1959. The Biological Way of Thought. Columbia University Press, New York.

Bos, L., 1999. Plant Viruses, Unique and Intriguing Pathogens—A Textbook of Plant Virology. Backhuys Publishers, Leiden.

Brown, J.K., Zerbini, F.M., Navas-Castillo, J., et al., 2015. Revision of begomovirus taxonomy based on pairwise sequence comparisons. Arch. Virol. 160, 1593–1619.

Brunt, A., Crabtree, K., Gibbs, A., 1990. Viruses of Tropical Plants. CAB International, Wallingford.

Buck, R.C., Hull, D.L., 1966. The logical structure of the Linnaean hierarchy. Syst. Zool. 15, 97–111.

Bukreyev, A.A., Chandran, K., Dolnik, O., 2014. Discussions and decisions of the 2012–2014 International Committee on Taxonomy of Viruses (ICTV) Filoviridae Study Group, January 2012–June 2013. Arch. Virol. 159, 821–830.

Bunge, M., 2016. Modes of existence. Rev. Metaphys. 70, 225.

Calisher, C.H., 2010. What is the difference between a virus species and a virus? The same as the difference between *Homo sapiens* and you. Rev. Pan-Amaz Saude 1, 137–139.

Calisher, C.H., Mahy, B.M.J., 2003. Taxonomy: get it right or leave it alone. Am. Soc. Trop. Med. Hyg. 68, 505–506.

Calisher, C.H., Van Regenmortel, M.H.V., 2009. Should all other biologists follow the lead of virologists and stop italicizing the names of living organisms? A proposal. Zootaxa 2113, 63–68.

Calisher, C.H., Horzinek, M., Mayo, M.A., et al., 1995. Sequence analyses and a unifying system of virus taxonomy: consensus via consent. Arch. Virol. 140, 2093–2099.

Claridge, M.F., 2010. Species are real biological entities. In: Ayala, F.J., Arp, R. (Eds.), Contemporary Debates in Philosophy of Biology. Wiley-Blackwell, Chichester, UK, pp. 91–109.

Claridge, M.F., Dawah, H.A., Wilson, M.R. (Eds.), 1997. Species. The Units of Diversity. Chapman & Hall, London.

Colwell, R.K., 1992. Niche: a bifurcation in the conceptual lineage of the term. In: Keller, E.F., Lloyd, E.A. (Eds.), Keywords in Evolutionary Biology. Harvard University Press, Cambridge, MA, pp. 241–248.

Drebot, M.A., Henchal, E., Hjelle, B., et al., 2002. Improved clarity of meaning from the use of both formal species names and common (vernacular) virus names in virological literature. Arch. Virol. 147, 2465–2471.

Dupré, J., Guttinger, S., 2016. Viruses as living processes. Stud. Hist. Philos. Biol. Biomed. Sci. 59, 109–116.

Ebach, M.C., Holdrege, C., 2005. More taxonomy, not DNA barcoding. Bioscience 55, 822–823.

Fauquet, C.M., Stanley, J., 2005. Revising the way we conceive and name viruses below the species level: a review of geminivirus taxonomy calls for new standardized isolate descriptors. Arch. Virol. 150, 2151–2179.

Fenner, F., 1976. The classification and nomenclature of viruses. Second report of the International Committee on Taxonomy of Viruses. Intervirology 7, 1–115.

Francki, R.I.B., Fauquet, C.M., Knudson, D.L., Brown, F., 1991. Fifth report of the International Committee on Taxonomy of Viruses. Arch. Virol. Suppl. 2, 450.

Galvan, S.C., García Carrancá, A., Song, J., Recillas-Targa, F., 2015. Epigenetics and animal virus infections. Front. Genet. 6, 48.

Ghiselin, M.T., 1984. Definition, character, and other equivocal terms. Syst. Zool. 33, 104–110.

Ghiselin, M.T., 1997. Metaphysics and the Origin of Species. State University of New York Press, Albany.

Gibbs, A.J., Gibbs, M.J., 2006. A broader definition of the 'virus species'. Arch. Virol. 151, 1419–1422.

Gibbs, A.J., Armstrong, J.S., Gibbs, M.J., 2004. A type of nucleotide motif that distinguishes tobamovirus species more efficiently than nucleotide signatures. Arch. Virol. 149, 1941–1954.

Gómez-Díaz, E., Jordà, M., Peinado, M.A., Rivero, A., 2012. Epigenetics of host-pathogen interactions: the road ahead and the road behind. PLoS Pathog. 8. e1003007.

Greuter, W., Garrity, G., Hawksworth, D.L., 2011. Draft BioCode (2011). Principles and rules regulating the naming of organisms. New draft, revised in November 2010. Bionomina 3, 26–44.

Griffiths, P.E., Tabery, J., 2013. Developmental systems theory: what does it explain, and how does it explain it? Adv. Child Dev. Behav. 44, 65–94.

Hebert, P.D.N., Gregory, T.R., 2005. The promise of DNA barcoding for taxonomy. Syst. Biol. 54, 852–859.

Hull, D.L., 1976. Are species really individuals? Syst. Zool. 25, 174–191.

Inglis, W.G., 1991. Characters: the central mystery of taxonomy and systematics. Biol. J. Linn. Soc. 44, 121–139. https://doi.org/10.1111/j.1095-8312.1991.tb00611.x.

Kapoor, A., Simmonds, P., Lipkin, W.I., et al., 2010. Use of nucleotide composition analysis to infer hosts for three novel picorna-like viruses. J. Virol. 84, 10322–10328.

Kettler, G.C., Martiny, A.C., Huang, K., et al., 2007. Patterns and implications of gene gain and loss in the evolution of *Prochlorococcus*. PLoS Genet. 3. e231.

King, A., 2012. Comments to Proposed Modification to Code Rule 3.21 (Defining Virus Species). ICTV Discussions, http://talk.ictvonline.org/discussions/ictv1/f/63/t/3930. aspx/. Accessed 22 May 2017.

King, A., Adams, M., Lefkowitz, E., Carstens, E., 2012. ICTV Proposal 2011.002sg. in: 2011.002auG.A.v9.statute_and_code_changes.pdf (page 15), http://talk.ictvonline.org/ files/ictv_official_taxonomy_updates_since_the_8th_report/m/general-2008/4444.aspx. Accessed 22 May 2017.

Koonin, E.V., Dolja, V.V., 2013. A virocentric perspective on the evolution of life. Curr. Opin. Virol. 3, 546–557.

Kuhn, J.H., Jahrling, P.B., 2010. Clarification and guidance on the proper usage of virus and virus species names. Arch. Virol. 145, 445–453.

Kuhn, J.H., Dürrwald, R., Bao, Y., et al., 2015. Taxonomic reorganization of the family Bornaviridae. Arch. Virol. 160, 621–632.

Mahner, M., Bunge, M., 1997. Foundations of Biophilosophy. Springer-Verlag, Berlin.

Matthews, R.E.F., 1971. Plant Virology. Academic Press, San Diego.

Matthews, R.E.F., 1979. Classification and nomenclature. Third report of the International Committee on Taxonomy of Viruses. Intervirology 7, 1–115.

Matthews, R.E.F., 1982. Classification and nomenclature of virusesFourth report of the International Committee on Taxonomy of Viruses. Intervirology 17, 1–200.

Matthews, R.E.F., 1983. The history of viral taxonomy. In: Matthews, R.E.F. (Ed.), A Critical Appraisal of Viral Taxonomy. CRC Press, Boca Raton, Florida, pp. 1–35.

Matthews, R.E.F., 1985. Viral taxonomy. Microbiol. Sci. 2, 74–75.

Mayden, R.L., 1997. A hierarchy of species concepts: the denouement in the saga of the species problem. In: Claridge, M.F., Dawah, H.A., Wilson, M.R. (Eds.), Species: The Units of Biodiversity. Chapman and Hall, London, pp. 381–424.

Mayo, M.A., 2002. ICTV at the Paris ICV: results of the plenary session and the binomial ballot. Arch. Virol. 147, 2254–2260.

Mayo, M.A., Horzinek, M., 1998. A revised version of the international code of virus classification and nomenclature. Arch. Virol. 143, 1645–1654.

Mayr, E., 1970. Populations, Species and Evolution. Harvard University Press, Cambridge, MA.

Mayr, E., 1982. The Growth of Biological Thought. Diversity, Evolution and Inheritance. Harvard University Press, Cambridge, MA.

Milavetz, B.I., Balakrishnan, L., 2015. Viral epigenetics. Methods Mol. Biol. 1238, 569–596.

Milne, R.G., 1984. The species problem in plant virology. Microbiol. Sci. 1, 113–122.

Mishler, B.D., 2010. Species are not uniquely real biological entities. In: Ayala, F.J., Arp, R. (Eds.), Contemporary Debates in Philosophy of Biology. Wiley-Blackwell, Chichester, UK, pp. 110–122.

Ovchinnikov, S., Park, H., Varghese, N., Huang, P.S., Pavlopoulos, G.A., Kim, D.E., Kamisetty, H., Kyrpides, N.C., Baker, D., 2017. Protein structure determination using metagenome sequence data. Science 355, 294–298.

Pigliucci, M., 2003. Species as family resemblance concepts: the (dis-) solution of the species problem? Bioessays 25, 596–602.

Pringle, C.R., 1991. The 20th meeting of the executive committee of the ICTV. Virus species, higher taxa, a universal database and other matters. Arch. Virol. 119, 303–304.

Quine, W.V., 1990. Classes versus properties. In: Quiddities: An Intermittently Philosophical Dictionary. Penguin Books, London, pp. 22–24.

Quine, W.V., Ullian, J.S., 1978. The Web of Belief. McGraw-Hill, New York, p. 44.

Simmonds, P., 2015. Methods for virus classification and the challenge of incorporating metagenomic sequence data. J. Gen. Virol. 96, 1193–1206.

Simmonds, P., Adams, M.J., Benkő, M., et al., 2017. Virus taxonomy in the age of metagenomics. Nat. Rev. Microbiol. 15, 161–168.

Stamos, D.N., 2003. The Species Problem. Biological Species, Ontology and the Metaphysics of Biology. Lexington Books, Oxford.

Van Regenmortel, M.H.V., 2003. Viruses are real, virus species are man-made taxonomic constructions. Arch. Virol. 148, 2483–2490.

Van Regenmortel, M.H.V., 2007. Virus species and virus identification: past and current controversies. Infect. Genet. Evol. 7, 133–144.

Van Regenmortel, M.H.V., 2010. Logical puzzles and scientific controversies: the nature of species, viruses and living organisms. Syst. Appl. Microbiol. 33, 1–6.

Van Regenmortel, M.H.V., 2011. Virus species. In: Tibayrenc, M. (Ed.), Genetics and Evolution of Infectious Diseases. Elsevier, London, Burlington, pp. 3–19.

Van Regenmortel, M.H.V., 2016a. The metaphor that viruses are living is alive and well, but it is no more than a metaphor. Stud. Hist. Phil. Biol. Biomed. Sci. 59, 117–124.

Van Regenmortel, M.H.V., 2016b. Classes, taxa and categories in hierarchical virus classification: a review of current debates on definitions and names of virus species. Bionomina 10, 1–21.

Van Regenmortel, M.H.V., 2016c. Only viruses, but not their genome sequences, can be classified into hierarchical species and genus classes. Curr. Top. Virol. 13, 59–68.

Van Regenmortel, M.H.V., Fauquet, C.M., 2002. Only italicized species names of viruses have a taxonomic meaning. Arch. Virol. 147, 2247–2250.

Van Regenmortel, M.H.V., Ackermann, H.-W., Calisher, C.H., et al., 2013. Virus species polemics: 14 senior virologists oppose a proposed change to the ICTV definition of virus species. Arch. Virol. 158, 1115–1119.

Van Rijsbergen, K., 1979. Information Retrieval, second ed. Butterworths, London.

Wildy, P., 1971. Classification and nomenclature of First Report of the International Committee on Nomenclature of Viruses. In: Monographs in Virology. Karger, Basel, p. 5.

FURTHER READING

Brito, A.F., Braconi, C.T., Weidmann, M., et al., 2016. The pangenome of the *Anticarsia gemmatalis* multiple nucleopolyhedrovirus (AgMNPV). Genome Biol. Evol. 8, 94–108.

CHAPTER TWO

The Role of Immune Responses in HIV Mother-to-Child Transmission

Caitlin Milligan[*,†,1], **Jennifer A. Slyker**[‡], **Julie Overbaugh**[*,†]

[*]Division of Human Biology, Fred Hutchinson Cancer Research Center, Seattle, WA, United States
[†]Medical Scientist Training Program, University of Washington School of Medicine, Seattle, WA, United States
[‡]University of Washington, Seattle, WA, United States
[1]Corresponding author: e-mail address: cem26@uw.edu

Contents

Abstract

HIV mother-to-child transmission (MTCT) represents a success story in the HIV/AIDS field given the significant reduction in number of transmission events with the scale-up of antiretroviral treatment and other prevention methods. Nevertheless, MTCT still occurs and better understanding of the basic biology and immunology of transmission will aid in future prevention and treatment efforts. MTCT is a unique setting given that the transmission pair is known and the infant receives passively transferred HIV-specific antibodies from the mother while in utero. Thus, infant exposure to HIV occurs in the

Advances in Virus Research, Volume 100
ISSN 0065-3527
https://doi.org/10.1016/bs.aivir.2017.10.001

face of HIV-specific antibodies, especially during delivery and breastfeeding. This review highlights the immune correlates of protection in HIV MTCT including humoral (neutralizing antibodies, antibody-dependent cellular cytotoxicity, and binding epitopes), cellular, and innate immune factors. We further discuss the future implications of this research as it pertains to opportunities for passive and active vaccination with the ultimate goal of eliminating HIV MTCT.

1. INTRODUCTION

While significant progress has been made in addressing the HIV/AIDS epidemic, over 36 million people were living with the virus in 2015, including over 2 million newly infected individuals (UNAIDS, 2016a). These numbers include 1.8 million children infected with HIV, the majority of whom acquired the virus through HIV mother-to-child transmission (MTCT) (UNAIDS, 2016a). Infants born to HIV-infected mothers are exposed to the virus in the setting of passively acquired maternal HIV-specific antibodies. Thus, MTCT provides distinct insight into the role of preexisting HIV-specific antibodies in HIV transmission. In this review, we will highlight this unique role that HIV MTCT plays in understanding the immune correlates of protection and provide an overview of key aspects of MTCT including the epidemiology, transmission, and current prevention methods. We will also describe the impact of cellular and innate immunity on MTCT and highlight the prospect for new immune-based prevention methods.

2. EPIDEMIOLOGY OF HIV MTCT

Overall, HIV MTCT represents a success in the HIV/AIDS field. The number of new infections among children have decreased 70% since 2000, with approximately 150,000 new infections occurring in 2015 (UNAIDS, 2016b). This success is largely due to the rapid scale-up of antiretroviral (ARV) treatment and prophylaxis for MTCT (detailed later). While in the absence of any intervention approximately 30%–45% of infants born to HIV-infected mothers become infected, with ARVs and other prevention methods transmission is <1% in many resource-rich countries (European Collaborative Study, 2005; Lehman and Farquhar, 2007; Townsend et al., 2014). Furthermore, four countries (Cuba, Armenia, Belarus, and Thailand) have eliminated MTCT as certified by the WHO (WHO, 2016a).

Nevertheless, HIV MTCT continues to occur as women of childbearing age are disproportionately infected by the virus and often do not know their HIV status or have access to prevention measures. For example, in 2015, women aged 15–24 accounted for 20% of new HIV infections, despite representing 11% of the adult population (UNAIDS, 2016b). Similarly, over 300,000 women did not receive ARV treatment for prevention of MTCT (UNAIDS, 2016b). These high infection rates in young women and lack of ARV treatment represent a continued challenge, both in reducing HIV-associated morbidity and mortality in this group as well as in the elimination of MTCT.

3. MODES AND MECHANISMS OF TRANSMISSION

The risk of HIV MTCT depends on a number of factors. However, maternal viral load has been consistently associated with transmission risk (Dickover et al., 1996; John et al., 2001; Mofenson et al., 1999). Maternal virus has been detected in a number of fluids including blood, cervicovaginal fluid, and breast milk (Hénin et al., 1993; Lewis et al., 1998). As such, infant oral, gastrointestinal, and respiratory mucosa are in contact with infected maternal fluids during gestation, delivery, and early childhood.

Given this prolonged exposure to maternal virus, infant infection may occur while in utero, during labor/delivery, or via breastfeeding (Fig. 1). In utero transmission has been documented as early as 8 weeks gestation, but the majority of in utero transmissions occur late in the third trimester (Ehrnst et al., 1991; Lewis et al., 1990; Rouzioux et al., 1995). During labor and delivery, transmission occurs as infants are exposed to infected cervicovaginal secretions and blood. And finally, after delivery infants remain at risk of infection during the breastfeeding period. Breastfeeding transmission occurs when virus infects susceptible cells (e.g., lymphocytes) within or underneath epithelial barriers in the gastrointestinal tract, and may be aided by breaks in infant mucosa. Breast milk HIV RNA levels correlate with those of plasma but are typically 100-fold lower (Lewis et al., 1998; Van de Perre et al., 2012). Despite these lower viral loads, prolonged daily exposure to breast milk over many months results in breastfeeding accounting for up to 40% of all transmissions (BHITS et al., 2004; Nduati et al., 2000).

As viral load is the major risk factor for HIV MTCT, understanding what form of the virus is responsible for infection is relevant to delineating what types of immune responses may be most effective for future prevention

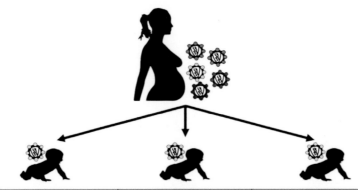

In utero	Labor/delivery	Breastfeeding
Risk factors for transmission		
Maternal viral load	Maternal viral load Prolonged labor/membrane rupture Cervical/vaginal lacerations	Maternal viral load (including breast milk viral load) Duration of breastfeeding
Prevention methods		
Maternal ARVs	Maternal/infant ARVs Minimizing invasive deliveries (e.g., fetal scalp electrodes) Elective cesarean section	Maternal/infant ARVs Formula feeding

Fig. 1 HIV MTCT risk factors and prevention methods. HIV MTCT may occur while the infant is in utero, during delivery, or via breastfeeding. This figure outlines the major risk factors for transmission and current prevention methods.

efforts. Both cell-free and cell-associated virus have been suggested to contribute to HIV MTCT (reviewed in Milligan and Overbaugh, 2014). Cell-associated virus (e.g., infected cells) may be relatively more infectious as cells may aid in crossing mucosal barriers, avoiding detection by host antiviral factors, and by promoting direct cell-to-cell transmission through virologic synapses. These ideas are supported by in vitro studies suggesting that cell-associated HIV is more efficient and infectious across polarized epithelial cell layers such as placental trophoblasts (Arias et al., 2003; Lagaye et al., 2001; Vidricaire et al., 2004). Furthermore, many epidemiologic studies suggest that cell-associated virus contributes to MTCT more than cell-free virus (John et al., 2001; Koulinska et al., 2006; Rousseau et al., 2004; Tuomala et al., 2003). However, nonhuman primate studies have shown that cell-free virus can result in infection (Fazely et al., 1993; Ochs et al., 1993; Van Rompay et al., 2005). Similarly, cell-free virus (as measured by HIV RNA levels) drops after ARV treatment and is associated with a reduction in infant infection risk (Chuachoowong et al., 2000; Graham et al., 2007; Lehman et al., 2008; Shapiro et al., 2005;

Slyker et al., 2012). Elucidating the relative contribution of cell-free and cell-associated virus in HIV MTCT is an active area of research that may further prevention and treatment efforts.

4. CURRENT APPROACHES TO PREVENTION OF MTCT

As maternal viral load is the major risk factor for MTCT, the mainstay of current prevention efforts is ARV treatment to reduce viral loads. ARVs were first shown to be effective in preventing MTCT in the Pediatric AIDS Clinical Trials Group (PACTG) 076 trial. This trial demonstrated that single-drug zidovudine treatment provided to the mother during labor/delivery and to the infant after birth could reduce MTCT by up to 70% (Connor et al., 1994). Over time these ARV regimens have evolved to now consisting of multidrug therapy provided to both the mother and infant. As of 2015, the WHO recommended lifelong treatment for pregnant women (Option B+), with the goals of lowering maternal viral loads to decrease maternal morbidity, reduce MTCT, and retain mothers in care (WHO, 2016b).

Treating HIV-positive women reduces MTCT by reducing maternal viral load and by acting as prophylaxis in the infant. The idea of prophylaxis as prevention was further strengthened by multiple studies demonstrating a reduction in infection when ARVs were provided only to the infant (Chasela et al., 2010; Kumwenda et al., 2008). This concept of ARVs for prophylaxis has been extrapolated to other HIV transmission settings. Preexposure prophylaxis (PrEP) has been shown to be efficacious and is now recommended for those individuals at high risk of HIV infection including serodiscordant couples, men who have sex with men, and intravenous drug users (Celum and Baeten, 2012; WHO, 2016b).

Additionally, a number of nonpharmacologic interventions that reduce the duration of fetal/infant exposure to virus have been associated with reduction of MTCT (Fig. 1). These recommendations include avoiding invasive instruments (e.g., fetal scalp electrodes) and promoting Cesarean sections (C-sections) for mothers with high viral loads (ACOG, 2001). C-sections decrease the time and amount of virus exposure during delivery, however, they also depend on safe access and are not currently recommended by the WHO in resource-limited countries (WHO, 2016b). Similarly, the recommendation on breastfeeding differs between resource-limited and resource-rich countries. While formula feeding is recommended in resource-rich countries where access to clean water and formula is readily available, breastfeeding is still recommended in many countries with the highest MTCT burden. In these resource-limited settings, breastfeeding is associated with reduction in infant mortality from other infectious diseases and malnutrition (Kuhn and Aldrovandi, 2010; WHO, 2016b). Furthermore, the risk of HIV transmission with breastfeeding is considerably lower in the setting of ARVs (Chasela et al., 2010; Kumwenda et al., 2008; Peltier et al., 2009).

5. HARNESSING THE IMMUNE RESPONSE FOR PREVENTION OF MTCT: HUMORAL IMMUNE CORRELATES OF HIV MTCT

In addition to demonstrating the efficacy of ARV therapy for prevention, HIV MTCT has also provided a unique setting in which to study the immune correlates of protection from infection. As described earlier, in the absence of any ARV therapy, fewer than half of infants born to HIV-infected mothers become infected. This relative protection is impressive given that infants face long-term exposure to high viral loads while in utero, during delivery, and via breastfeeding. HIV MTCT is also unique because the transmission pair is known. As HIV-infected mothers are generally diagnosed in pregnancy, it is possible to follow a mother and her infant over time to determine transmission. This close monitoring in the pre- and postnatal periods allows for accurate determination of timing of infection and relevant immune and viral correlates present around transmission. Thus, MTCT represents a setting in which to study the immune correlates of protection from infection as known pairs with high rates of exposure can be closely studied over time.

5.1 Passive Transfer of Antibodies

Of particular interest in HIV MTCT is the role of HIV-specific antibodies in prevention. IgG is passively transferred across the placenta from mother to fetus, with the majority of transfer occurring during the third trimester (Palmeira et al., 2012). Thus, infants born to HIV-infected mothers have HIV-specific antibodies present in circulation at birth, at levels similar to those found in the chronically infected mother (Broliden et al., 1993; Omenda et al., 2013). These antibodies decay over time, but have been detected in infants up to 2 years of age (Gutierrez et al., 2012). Therefore, passive antibodies may provide protection against HIV infection during critical periods of infant exposure in utero, during delivery, and while breastfeeding. Indeed, maternal antibodies have been implicated in infant protection from other viruses including respiratory syncytial virus and influenza (Benowitz et al., 2010; Ochola et al., 2009).

This setting is also similar to that of a vaccine, whereby virus-specific antibodies are present prior to and at the time of virus exposure. Therefore, studying HIV-specific antibody responses in infants who become infected and those who remain uninfected despite ample virus exposure may be useful in defining immune responses important for preventing infection. Understanding if antibodies play a protective role in MTCT, and if so, what functions are important for protection, can help guide rational vaccine research to elicit protective responses.

5.2 Neutralizing Antibodies

Antibodies can have many functions, one of which is neutralization. Neutralizing antibodies (NAbs) are often considered the gold standard of sterilizing immunity as they can bind to and prevent free virus from infecting cells (Fig. 2). Indeed, the majority of viral vaccines work in part by pathogen neutralization (Plotkin, 2010). Thus, the development of an HIV-specific NAb response remains a major goal of HIV vaccine research. As proof of concept, NAbs have been shown to protect nonhuman primates against

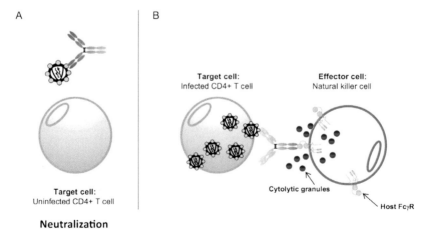

Fig. 2 Neutralizing and ADCC antibodies. (A) HIV-specific neutralizing antibodies bind to free HIV virions, preventing infection of host target cells (CD4 T cells). (B) ADCC-specific antibodies bind envelope displayed on the surface HIV-infected target cells. Subsequent cross-linking (via binding Fc gamma receptors (FcγRs)) to effector cells, such as natural killer cells, results in the release of cytolytic granules and death of the target cell.

simian/human immunodeficiency virus challenge (reviewed in Evans and Silvestri, 2013; Sharma et al., 2015). In the majority of these studies, however, the challenge virus was known to be readily neutralized by the antibodies given to the animals and high doses of antibodies were often used.

In humans, where HIV antigenic diversity is extensive, NAbs must be able to recognize a wide range of diverse circulating strains. There are limited data on the role of preexisting NAbs in preventing human infection, and in the only vaccine trial to show some efficacy in humans (the RV144 trial), NAb titers did not correlate with protection from HIV infection (Haynes et al., 2012; Rerks-Ngarm et al., 2009). As there have been limited numbers of vaccine studies in humans, understanding if NAbs present at the time of exposure are protective in other populations, such as MTCT, is therefore important. MTCT is, however, somewhat distinct in that the maternal virus is continually undergoing escape from her own antibody responses. Thus, an infected mother may harbor a mixture of viruses that range in sensitivity to the passively acquired antibodies in her infant, including viruses that have escaped neutralization.

In MTCT, there is evidence that NAbs contribute to an observed genetic bottleneck in the virus population during transmission. Infants are typically infected with a single viral variant and these variants have been shown to be more resistant to maternal plasma neutralization than maternal virus variants in a number of studies (Dickover et al., 2006; Kliks et al., 1994; Wu et al., 2006; Zhang et al., 2010). These studies suggest that antibodies may limit transmission of the most neutralization-sensitive variants, but do not directly address whether they can prevent infection.

The role of maternal NAbs in the risk of infant infection has been directly assayed with varying results. NAbs in the mother have been associated with protection from transmission in some studies (Barin et al., 2006; Bongertz et al., 2001, 2002; Chaillon et al., 2012; Dickover et al., 2006; Diomede et al., 2012; Kliks et al., 1994; Lathey et al., 1999; Louisirirotchanakul et al., 1999; Permar et al., 2015; Samleerat et al., 2009; Scarlatti et al., 1993a,b; Ugen et al., 1992), while no association has been observed in others (Bal et al., 1996; Broliden et al., 1993; Hengel et al., 1998; Husson et al., 1995; Kittinunvorakoon et al., 2009; Mabondzo et al., 1998; Milligan et al., 2016; Russell et al., 2011). Only one study has directly assayed the association between passively transferred HIV NAbs in infants, which is a more relevant measure of what is in the infant at the time of exposure. In this study, there was no evidence for a protective effect of NAb breadth or potency and infant infection

(Lynch et al., 2011). The differences in outcome observed in the maternal NAb studies may be due to methodological differences including small sample sizes in some studies, the viruses tested in assays, and/or timing of antibody sampling. For example, many studies used lab adapted or heterologous viruses, which may not represent the viruses present in the mother (to which the infant was exposed). With regard to sample timing, the most relevant time to analyze antibody responses is around the time of estimated transmission, however, studies have varied in the time at which they analyzed maternal antibodies. Because NAbs drive viral escape, which in turn leads to new antibody responses, sampling maternal virus and/or antibodies outside the transmission window may not be predictive of immune responses present at transmission. Recent work from our lab testing maternal NAbs against autologous viruses from near the time of transmission showed no association between maternal NAb titer and transmission risk (Milligan et al., 2016). Overall, the studies of NAbs in MTCT suggest that while NAbs may contribute to the genetic bottleneck associated with transmission there is limited evidence to suggest they play a major role in protection from infection at the population level. These studies, nonetheless, do not preclude the possibility of NAbs contributing to protection in a small fraction of cases, which would be hard to detect with the limited sample size of most studies conducted to date.

5.3 Antibody-Dependent Cellular Cytotoxicity

As cell-associated virus has been implicated in MTCT (discussed earlier), NAbs may not be effective at preventing initial infection. Thus, antibodies that kill infected cells, such as those that mediate antibody-dependent cellular cytotoxicity (ADCC), may be important. In ADCC, pathogen-specific antibodies bind to antigen present on the surface of infected cells and to receptors on a variety of effector cells (including natural killer (NK) cells, monocytes, and macrophages) (Fig. 2). This cross-linking results in the release of cytolytic granules (containing perforin and granzyme) and/or antiviral cytokines and subsequent killing of the infected cell. ADCC may, therefore, prevent infection by killing cell-associated virus transmitted by the HIV-infected individual or by eliminating newly infected cells in the exposed person before systemic spread occurs.

In MTCT, ADCC has been implicated in protection. In one study of mothers with high viral loads, higher levels of ADCC in breast milk were associated with lower breastfeeding transmission risk (Mabuka et al., 2012).

A number of other studies, however, have shown no significant association between maternal or infant plasma ADCC and risk of infection (Broliden et al., 1993; Jenkins et al., 1994; Ljunggren et al., 1990; Mabondzo et al., 1995; Milligan et al., 2015; Permar et al., 2015; Pugatch et al., 1997). However, one recent study does suggest there may be a therapeutic effect of ADCC antibodies—in a study of HIV-infected infants, preexisting HIV-specific ADCC activity correlated with increased infant survival (Milligan et al., 2015). In this study, nontransmitting mothers also had higher levels of ADCC antibodies than those who transmitted, but the difference was not significant, suggesting larger studies are needed. Further support for ADCC comes from studies of NK cells; in one study of cord blood, infants who became HIV-infected had a trend toward lower levels of CD16+ NK cells (that are capable of mediating ADCC) compared to those infants who remained uninfected (Gasper et al., 2014). Overall, these data suggest that preexisting ADCC may act early in disease to help control initial infection and may be an important component to consider in an HIV vaccine.

5.4 Identification of Protective Antibody Epitopes

MTCT studies have also focused on identifying the epitope targets of protective maternal HIV-specific antibodies. Such studies give insight into epitopes that should be targeted by a vaccine or immunotherapy. Recent studies suggest that maternal antibodies that recognize and bind the CD4 binding site and V3 of gp120 are protective (Martinez et al., 2017; Permar et al., 2015), however, a number of older studies do not corroborate this finding (Halsey et al., 1992; Parekh et al., 1991; Robertson et al., 1992). Gp41-specific maternal antibodies have also been assayed and have had similarly varying results in MTCT cohorts (Diomede et al., 2012; Tranchat et al., 1999; Ugen et al., 1992, 1997). Similar to NAb studies, these diverging results may be due to a number of methodological differences. Thus, further studies delineating what antibody epitopes are protective in MTCT are needed to inform what epitopes should be targeted in future immune-based prevention efforts.

6. THE ROLE OF CELLULAR AND INNATE IMMUNITY IN HIV MTCT

6.1 T Cells in MTCT

While a significant amount of literature has focused on humoral immune responses in HIV MTCT, T cells have also been implicated in protection. Early in the HIV epidemic, HIV-specific CD4 and CD8 T cells were identified in HIV-exposed uninfected infants (Kuhn et al., 2002; Rowland-Jones et al., 1993) and highly exposed persistently seronegative adults (reviewed in Shen and Smith, 2014). Furthermore, several host genetic polymorphisms in maternal/infant genes related to HIV-specific CD8 T cell responses (e.g., HLA genes) have been associated with reduced risk of transmission (reviewed in Singh and Spector, 2009). These studies suggested a potential role for T cells in MTCT.

HIV-specific CD4 and CD8 T cell responses can be detected in cord and peripheral blood of infants born to HIV-infected mothers, suggesting virus exposure has stimulated infant responses. These HIV-specific cellular responses have been associated with a lower risk of MTCT (John-Stewart et al., 2009; Kuhn et al., 2001). However, how these HIV-specific T cells are generated in the absence of productive infection is not well understood. It is possible that the presence of T cell responses in uninfected infants is merely a marker of exposure and correlates with other protective mechanisms (Lederman et al., 2011).

HIV-specific T cells are also found in breast milk (Sabbaj et al., 2002), suggesting they could provide protection at mucosal sites. In one study, HIV-specific IFNγ CD8 T cell responses in breast milk were associated with a 70% reduction in early breastfeeding transmission (Lohman-Payne et al., 2012). Additionally, higher breast milk levels of CCL4/MIP-beta, a chemokine made by T cells, have been associated with lower transmission risk (Farquhar et al., 2005; Lohman-Payne et al., 2012). Breast milk HIV-specific T cell responses could offer infants protection though a variety of mechanisms including removal of infected cells via T cell-mediated cytolysis or via production of cytokines/chemokines.

6.2 Innate Immune Factors

Innate immune responses provide critical first-line defenses, particularly at mucosal sites. Such innate factors may help activate the adaptive immune system (discussed earlier) to ultimately decrease MTCT risk. Indeed, within MTCT, polymorphisms in receptors important for linking the innate and adaptive arms of the immune system (KIRs and TLRs) have been associated with decreased transmission risk (Beima-Sofie et al., 2013; Hong et al., 2013; Ricci et al., 2010). Alternatively, innate factors may act directly on the virus to prevent infection.

Maternal breast milk contains many known innate factors, several of which have been associated with decreased risk of MTCT. Alpha defensins, mannose-binding lectins, and IL-15 have all been found in breast milk and associated with reduced risk of MTCT in some studies (Ji et al., 2005; Kuhn et al., 2005; Walter et al., 2009), but not others (Bosire et al., 2007; Israëls et al., 2012). Furthermore, studies have suggested that human milk oligosaccharides and lactoferrin can block HIV binding to host cells (Groot et al., 2005; Harmsen et al., 1995; Naarding et al., 2005), and have been associated with reduction of MTCT (Bode et al., 2012). More recently, tenascin-C, a protein involved in fetal development and wound healing, was found in breast milk and shown to bind an HIV epitope critical for binding host cells and initiating infection (Fouda et al., 2013a). While these data suggest that tenascin-C may contribute to virus neutralization, the protein has not been associated with protection in MTCT cohorts to date.

Innate inhibitory molecules have also been described in saliva. For example, secretory leukocyte protease inhibitor has been shown to inhibit HIV infection in vitro (McNeely et al., 1995), and high concentrations in infant saliva have been associated with decreased risk of MTCT (Farquhar et al., 2002). Other factors in saliva include defensins, cathelicidins, mucins, and thrombospondin (Shugars, 1999; Wiesner and Vilcinskas, 2010), however, their role in MTCT has been less extensively studied. Overall, there are limited data on the role of innate immune factors in HIV MTCT, with single studies often providing the only evidence for association. Thus, more research needs to be conducted to clearly delineate the importance of innate immunity in prevention of MTCT.

7. THE WAY FORWARD: THE FUTURE OF PREVENTION OF HIV MTCT

While ARV therapy has resulted in significant reduction of HIV MTCT, transmission continues to occur for a variety of reasons. These reasons include limited access to diagnosis, treatment, and prevention strategies, poor adherence, medication side effects, and drug resistance. Additionally, although combination regimens for prevention of HIV MTCT have been associated with reduced transmission, they are not without potential toxic effects for the mother and fetus. Many ARVs have limited data in pregnant women and children, and have been associated with adverse events including preterm birth and low birth weight (Mofenson, 2016; Santini-Oliveira and Grinsztejn, 2014). Therefore, it is important to consider other therapeutic options including passive immunization and active vaccination, with an ultimate goal of developing a cure for HIV.

7.1 Preventative and Therapeutic Passive Immunization

Passive immunization, whereby pathogen-specific antibodies are directly administered to an individual, has potential benefits over standard ARV therapy. First, passively transferred antibodies have longer half-lives than most current ARVs, therefore allowing for the possibility of decreased dosing and improved therapeutic adherence. Furthermore, the short- and long-term toxicities of passively transferred HIV-specific antibodies may be reduced compared to ARVs. Indeed, passive immunization is safe and effective at preventing MTCT of other diseases such as cytomegalovirus and hepatitis B (Adler and Nigro, 2013; Ma et al., 2014). With regards to HIV, as proof of concept, passive immunization of infant nonhuman primates has been shown to protect against oral challenge with simian–human immunodeficiency virus (Baba et al., 2000; Hofmann-Lehmann et al., 2001). Interestingly, in a recent infant macaque study by Hessell et al. (2016), a combination of neutralizing monoclonal antibodies administered 24 h after oral inoculation of virus was shown to protect against systemic disease even though there was evidence of replicating virus and infected cells in multiple tissues at 24 h. These data suggest that passive immunization after infection may eliminate early virus foci and provide protection from systemic disease.

Passive immunization has also been directly assayed in human MTCT. Initial studies of passive immunization of HIV-infected mothers and their infants with HIV immunoglobulin showed no decrease in HIV-transmission rates compared to control groups who received standard ARVs (Onyango-Makumbi et al., 2011; Stiehm et al., 1999). However, these polyclonal antibody preparations contained many nonneutralizing/non-ADCC antibodies that may have contributed to the lack of efficacy. Nevertheless, the studies did show that the passive immunization approach is safe, and thus, newer studies are currently underway to evaluate the role of broadly NAbs in HIV MTCT. There is an ongoing study in HIV-exposed infants assessing the safety of VRC01, the prototype broadly NAb directed at the CD4 binding site (clinicaltrials.gov ID: NCT02256631). Such broadly NAbs have been shown to neutralize the majority of circulating HIV variants, including those transmitted from mothers to infants (Fouda et al., 2013b; Mabuka et al., 2013; Nakamura et al., 2013; Russell et al., 2013). Individually, these monoclonal antibodies do not provide the same breadth of coverage across viral strains as most ARVs, but may be combined to increase breadth. Studies using passive monoclonal antibodies to protect exposed infants will likely be a major focus of MTCT prevention in upcoming years and may be used in conjunction with other prevention methods including ARVs.

7.2 Active Vaccination to Prevent HIV MTCT

There is also interest in developing vaccination strategies for HIV MTCT. This strategy could involve vaccinating the mother or infant. In HIV-infected women, immunization before, during, or after pregnancy may result in lower viral loads and development of vaccine-induced antibodies that can be transferred to the infant via placental transfer and breast milk. These immune responses may result in reduced risk of MTCT. Alternatively, immunization of an infant shortly after birth may result in development of protective immune responses. There is evidence that infants can mount early, broad NAb responses in natural infection, and thus, there is hope that such responses could be elicited with a vaccine (Goo et al., 2014; Muenchhoff et al., 2016; Simonich et al., 2016). Nonetheless, while immunization of mothers and/or infants has been shown to protect against other viruses, there have been no efficacy studies of neonatal/maternal HIV vaccines in humans. A number of phase I/II trials, however, have shown that vaccination is safe and may produce limited vaccine-specific immune responses (Afolabi et al., 2013; Cunningham et al., 2001; McFarland et al., 2001; Njuguna et al., 2014). Going forward, it remains to be seen if protective broad and potent HIV-specific responses can be elicited with a maternal or infant vaccine.

7.3 The HIV Reservoir and Potential for a Cure

Within HIV MTCT, there is also discussion about the potential for a cure. This excitement stems in large part from the case of the "Mississippi Baby" who was treated very early (within 30 h) and showed no evidence of infection when she/he came off therapy (Persaud et al., 2013). The infant remained without evidence of infection for 2 years before viral rebound occurred (Luzuriaga et al., 2015). The authors hypothesized that early ARV treatment may have restricted/reduced the reservoir of latently infected CD4 T cells that make virus eradication so difficult. Additional studies in HIV-infected infants support this hypothesis that early treatment is associated with a smaller and less diverse reservoir (Ananworanich et al., 2014; Bitnun et al., 2014; Luzuriaga et al., 2014; Palma et al., 2016; Persaud et al., 2012, 2014; Uprety et al., 2015). Nevertheless, other studies suggest viral rebound may occur very quickly after ARVs are discontinued, even when treatment is started early (Ananworanich and Robb, 2014; Giacomet et al., 2014; Wamalwa et al., 2016). These findings are consistent with studies showing the viral reservoir is seeded extremely early (reviewed in

Ronen et al., 2015). Thus, treatment starting at the time HIV infection is detected in blood may be too late to clear or substantially diminish the viral reservoir. However, there is recent evidence in a study of infant macaques that passive immunization 24 h after virus challenge can provide protection from systemic infection and clear early foci of replicating virus which likely contribute to the viral reservoir (Hessell et al., 2016). Overall, these studies of viral reservoir dynamics in infants not only support the concept of early diagnosis and treatment, but also highlight the need for more sensitive methods to detect the HIV reservoir, and, more excitingly, the prospect for a cure.

8. CONCLUSIONS

Since the initial description of pediatric HIV infections in the early 1980s, we have come a long way in the diagnosis, prevention, and treatment of HIV MTCT. While great strides have been made in prevention with ARVs, especially with the scale-up of Option B+, many challenges remain. These challenges highlight the need for new prevention and treatment methods.

HIV MTCT research has not only demonstrated the efficacy of ARVs in PrEP, but has also provided insight into the role of preexisting humoral immune responses in protection from HIV infection. Further research on the basic biology of transmission and immunity will help inform future therapeutic and preventative efforts. These efforts include the exciting prospects of active/passive immunization and a cure for HIV, which combined with current effective prevention methods and improved diagnosis, may ultimately eliminate pediatric HIV infections.

ACKNOWLEDGMENTS

This manuscript was supported in part by the National Institutes of Health (R01 AI076105). The authors would like to thank Dr. Dara Lehman and Dr. Grace John-Stewart for reading and commenting on this manuscript.

REFERENCES

ACOG, 2001. ACOG committee opinion scheduled cesarean delivery and the prevention of vertical transmission of HIV infection. Number 234, May 2000. Int. J. Gynaecol. Obstet. 73 (3), 279–281.
Adler, S.P., Nigro, G., 2013. Prevention of maternal-fetal transmission of cytomegalovirus. Clin. Infect. Dis. 57 (Suppl. 4), S189–92.
Afolabi, M.O., et al., 2013. A phase I randomized clinical trial of candidate human immunodeficiency virus type 1 vaccine MVA.HIVA administered to Gambian infants. PLoS One 8 (10), e78289.
Ananworanich, J., Robb, M.L., 2014. The transient HIV remission in the Mississippi baby: why is this good news? J. Int. AIDS Soc. 17 (1), 19859.

Ananworanich, J., et al., 2014. Reduced markers of HIV persistence and restricted HIV-specific immune responses after early antiretroviral therapy in children. AIDS 28 (7), 1015–1020.

Arias, R.A., Muñoz, L.D., Muñoz-Fernández, M.A., 2003. Transmission of HIV-1 infection between trophoblast placental cells and T-cells take place via an LFA-1-mediated cell to cell contact. Virology 307 (2), 266–277.

Baba, T.W., et al., 2000. Human neutralizing monoclonal antibodies of the IgG1 subtype protect against mucosal simian–human immunodeficiency virus infection. Nat. Med. 6 (2), 200–206.

Bal, A.K., et al., 1996. Syncytium-inhibiting and neutralizing activity in maternal sera fail to prevent vertical transmission of human immunodeficiency virus type 1. Pediatr. Infect. Dis. J. 15 (4), 315–320.

Barin, F., et al., 2006. Revisiting the role of neutralizing antibodies in mother-to-child transmission of HIV-1. JID 193 (11), 1504–1511.

Beima-Sofie, K.M., et al., 2013. Toll-like receptor variants are associated with infant HIV-1 acquisition and peak plasma HIV-1 RNA level. AIDS 27 (15), 2431–2439.

Benowitz, I., et al., 2010. Influenza vaccine given to pregnant women reduces hospitalization due to influenza in their infants. Clin. Infect. Dis. 51 (12), 1355–1361.

BHITS (Breastfeeding and HIV International Transmission Study Group), et al., 2004. Late postnatal transmission of HIV-1 in breast-fed children: an individual patient data meta-analysis. JID 189 (12), 2154–2166.

Bitnun, A., et al., 2014. Early initiation of combination antiretroviral therapy in HIV-1-infected newborns can achieve sustained virologic suppression with low frequency of CD4+ T cells carrying HIV in peripheral blood. Clin. Infect. Dis. 59 (7), 1012–1019.

Bode, L., et al., 2012. Human milk oligosaccharide concentration and risk of postnatal transmission of HIV through breastfeeding. Am. J. Clin. Nutr. 96 (4), 831–839.

Bongertz, V., et al., 2001. Vertical HIV-1 transmission: importance of neutralizing antibody titer and specificity. Scand. J. Immunol. 53 (3), 302–309.

Bongertz, V., et al., 2002. Neutralization titres and vertical HIV-1 transmission. Scand. J. Immunol. 56 (6), 642–644.

Bosire, R., et al., 2007. Breast milk alpha-defensins are associated with HIV type 1 RNA and CC chemokines in breast milk but not vertical HIV type 1 transmission. AIDS Res. Hum. Retroviruses 23 (2), 198–203.

Broliden, K., et al., 1993. Antibody-dependent cellular cytotoxicity and neutralizing activity in sera of HIV-1-infected mothers and their children. Clin. Exp. Immunol. 93 (1), 56–64.

Celum, C., Baeten, J.M., 2012. Antiretroviral-based HIV-1 prevention: antiretroviral treatment and pre-exposure prophylaxis. Antivir. Ther. 17 (8), 1483–1493.

Chaillon, A., et al., 2012. The breadth and titer of maternal HIV-1-specific heterologous neutralizing antibodies are not associated with a lower rate of mother-to-child transmission of HIV-1. J. Virol. 86 (19), 10540–10546.

Chasela, C.S., et al., 2010. Maternal or infant antiretroviral drugs to reduce HIV-1 transmission. NEJM 362 (24), 2271–2281.

Chuachoowong, R., et al., 2000. Short-course antenatal zidovudine reduces both cervicovaginal human immunodeficiency virus type 1 RNA levels and risk of perinatal transmission. JID 181 (1), 99–106.

Connor, E.M., et al., 1994. Reduction of maternal-infant transmission of human immunodeficiency virus type 1 with zidovudine treatment. NEJM 331 (18), 1173–1180.

Cunningham, C.K., et al., 2001. Safety of 2 recombinant HIV-1 envelope vaccines in neonates born to HIV-1-infected women. Clin. Infect. Dis. 32 (5), 801–807.

Dickover, R.E., et al., 1996. Identification of levels of maternal HIV-1 RNA associated with risk of perinatal transmission: effect of maternal zidovudine treatment on viral load. JAMA 275 (8), 599–605.

Dickover, R., et al., 2006. Role of maternal autologous neutralizing antibody in selective perinatal transmission of human immunodeficiency virus type 1 escape variants. J. Virol. 80 (13), 6525–6533.

Diomede, L., et al., 2012. Passively transmitted gp41 antibodies in babies born from HIV-1 subtype C-seropositive women: correlation between fine specificity and protection. J. Virol. 86 (8), 4129–4138.

Ehrnst, A., et al., 1991. HIV in pregnant women and their offspring: evidence for late transmission. Lancet 338 (8761), 203–207.

European Collaborative Study, 2005. Mother-to-child transmission of HIV infection in the era of highly active antiretroviral therapy. Clin. Infect. Dis. 40 (3), 458–465.

Evans, D.T., Silvestri, G., 2013. Nonhuman primate models in AIDS research. Curr. Opin. HIV AIDS 8 (4), 255–261.

Farquhar, C., et al., 2002. Salivary secretory leukocyte protease inhibitor is associated with reduced transmission of human immunodeficiency virus type 1 through breast milk. JID 186 (8), 1173–1176.

Farquhar, C., et al., 2005. CC and CXC chemokines in breastmilk are associated with mother-to-child HIV-1 transmission. Curr. HIV Res. 3 (4), 361–369.

Fazely, F., et al., 1993. Simian immunodeficiency virus infection via amniotic fluid: a model to study fetal immunopathogenesis and prophylaxis. JAIDS 6 (2), 107–114.

Fouda, G.G., et al., 2013a. Tenascin-C is an innate broad-spectrum, HIV-1-neutralizing protein in breast milk. PNAS 110 (45), 18220–18225.

Fouda, G.G., et al., 2013b. Postnatally-transmitted HIV-1 Envelope variants have similar neutralization-sensitivity and function to that of nontransmitted breast milk variants. Retrovirology 10 (1), 3.

Gasper, M.A., et al., 2014. Natural killer cell and T-cell subset distributions and activation influence susceptibility to perinatal HIV-1 infection. AIDS 28 (8), 1115–1124.

Giacomet, V., et al., 2014. No cure of HIV infection in a child despite early treatment and apparent viral clearance. Lancet 384 (9950), 1320.

Goo, L., et al., 2014. Early development of broadly neutralizing antibodies in HIV-1-infected infants. Nat. Med. 20 (6), 655–658.

Graham, S.M., et al., 2007. Initiation of antiretroviral therapy leads to a rapid decline in cervical and vaginal HIV-1 shedding. AIDS 21 (4), 501–507.

Groot, F., et al., 2005. Lactoferrin prevents dendritic cell-mediated human immunodeficiency virus type 1 transmission by blocking the DC-SIGN–gp120 interaction. J. Virol. 79 (5), 3009–3015.

Gutierrez, M., et al., 2012. Has highly active antiretroviral therapy increased the time to seroreversion in HIV exposed but uninfected children? Clin. Infect. Dis. 55 (9), 1255–1261.

Halsey, N.A., et al., 1992. Lack of association between maternal antibodies to V3 loop peptides and maternal-infant HIV-1 transmission. JAIDS 5 (2), 153–157.

Harmsen, M.C., et al., 1995. Antiviral effects of plasma and milk proteins: lactoferrin shows potent activity against both human immunodeficiency virus and human cytomegalovirus replication in vitro. JID 172 (2), 380–388.

Haynes, B.F., et al., 2012. Immune-correlates analysis of an HIV-1 vaccine efficacy trial. NEJM 366 (14), 1275–1286.

Hengel, R.L., et al., 1998. Neutralizing antibody and perinatal transmission of human immunodeficiency virus type 1. AIDS Res. Hum. Retroviruses 14 (6), 475–481.

Hénin, Y., et al., 1993. Virus excretion in the cervicovaginal secretions of pregnant and nonpregnant HIV-infected women. JAIDS 6 (1), 72–75.

Hessell, A.J., et al., 2016. Early short-term treatment with neutralizing human monoclonal antibodies halts SHIV infection in infant macaques. Nat. Med. 22 (4), 362–368.

Hofmann-Lehmann, R., et al., 2001. Passive immunization against oral AIDS virus transmission: an approach to prevent mother-to-infant HIV-1 transmission? J. Med. Primatol. 30 (4), 190–196.

Hong, H.A., et al., 2013. KIR2DS4 allelic variants: differential effects on in utero and intra-partum HIV-1 mother-to-child transmission. Clin. Immunol. 149 (3), 498–508.

Husson, R.N., et al., 1995. Vertical transmission of human immunodeficiency virus type 1: autologous neutralizing antibody, virus load, and virus phenotype. J. Pediatr. 126 (6), 865–871.

Israëls, J., et al., 2012. Mannose-binding lectin and the risk of HIV transmission and disease progression in children: a systematic review. Pediatr. Infect. Dis. J. 31 (12), 1272–1278.

Jenkins, M., et al., 1994. Association between anti-human immunodeficiency virus type 1 (HIV-1) antibody-dependent cellular cytotoxicity antibody titers at birth and vertical transmission of HIV-1. JID 170 (2), 308–312.

Ji, X., Gewurz, H., Spear, G.T., 2005. Mannose binding lectin (MBL) and HIV. Mol. Immunol. 42 (2), 145–152.

John, G.C., et al., 2001. Correlates of mother-to-child human immunodeficiency virus type 1 (HIV-1) transmission: association with maternal plasma HIV-1 RNA load, genital HIV-1 DNA shedding, and breast infections. JID 183 (2), 206–212.

John-Stewart, G.C., et al., 2009. HV-1-specific cytotoxic T lymphocytes and breast milk HIV-1 transmission. JID 199 (6), 889–898.

Kittinunvorakoon, C., et al., 2009. Mother to child transmission of HIV-1 in a Thai population: role of virus characteristics and maternal humoral immune response. J. Med. Virol. 81 (5), 768–778.

Kliks, S.C., et al., 1994. Features of HIV-1 that could influence maternal-child transmission. JAMA 272 (6), 467–474.

Koulinska, I.N., et al., 2006. Transmission of cell-free and cell-associated HIV-1 through breast-feeding. JAIDS 41 (1), 93–99.

Kuhn, L., Aldrovandi, G., 2010. Survival and health benefits of breastfeeding versus artificial feeding in infants of HIV-infected women: developing versus developed world. Clin. Perinatol. 37 (4), 843–862.

Kuhn, L., et al., 2001. T-helper cell responses to HIV envelope peptides in cord blood: protection against intrapartum and breast-feeding transmission. AIDS 15 (1), 1–9.

Kuhn, L., et al., 2002. HIV-specific cellular immune responses in newborns exposed to HIV in utero. Clin. Infect. Dis. 34 (2), 267–276.

Kuhn, L., et al., 2005. Alpha-defensins in the prevention of HIV transmission among breastfed infants. JAIDS 39 (2), 138–142.

Kumwenda, N.I., et al., 2008. Extended antiretroviral prophylaxis to reduce breast-milk HIV-1 transmission. NEJM 359 (2), 119–129.

Lagaye, S., et al., 2001. Cell-to-cell contact results in a selective translocation of maternal human immunodeficiency virus type 1 quasispecies across a trophoblastic barrier by both transcytosis and infection. J. Virol. 75 (10), 4780–4791.

Lathey, J.L., et al., 1999. Lack of autologous neutralizing antibody to HIV-1 and macrophage tropism are associated with mother-to-infant transmission. JID 180 (2), 344–350.

Lederman, M.M., et al., 2011. Immunologic failure despite suppressive antiretroviral therapy is related to activation and turnover of memory CD4 cells. JID 204 (8), 1217–1226.

Lehman, D.A., Farquhar, C., 2007. Biological mechanisms of vertical HIV-1 transmission. Rev. Med. Virol. 17 (6), 381–403.

Lehman, D.A., et al., 2008. HIV-1 persists in breast milk cells despite antiretroviral treatment to prevent mother-to-child transmission. AIDS 22 (12), 1475–1485.

Lewis, S.H., et al., 1990. HIV-1 in trophoblastic and villous Hofbauer cells, and haematological precursors in eight-week fetuses. Lancet 335 (8689), 565–568.

Lewis, P., et al., 1998. Cell-free human immunodeficiency virus type 1 in breast milk. JID 177 (1), 34–39.

Ljunggren, K., et al., 1990. Antibodies mediating cellular cytotoxicity and neutralization correlate with a better clinical stage in children born to human immunodeficiency virus-infected mothers. JID 161 (2), 198–202.

Lohman-Payne, B., et al., 2012. Breast milk cellular HIV-specific interferon γ responses are associated with protection from peripartum HIV transmission. AIDS 26 (16), 2007–2016.

Louisirirotchanakul, S., et al., 1999. Role of maternal humoral immunity in vertical transmission of HIV-1 subtype E in Thailand. JAIDS 21 (4), 259–265.

Luzuriaga, K., et al., 2014. HIV-1 proviral reservoirs decay continuously under sustained virologic control in HIV-1-infected children who received early treatment. JID 210 (10), 1529–1538.

Luzuriaga, K., et al., 2015. Viremic relapse after HIV-1 remission in a perinatally infected child. NEJM 372 (8), 786–788.

Lynch, J.B., et al., 2011. The breadth and potency of passively acquired human immunodeficiency virus type 1-specific neutralizing antibodies do not correlate with the risk of infant infection. J. Virol. 85 (11), 5252–5261.

Ma, L., et al., 2014. Mother-to-child transmission of HBV: review of current clinical management and prevention strategies. Rev. Med. Virol. 24 (6), 396–406.

Mabondzo, A., et al., 1995. Relationships between humoral factors in HIV-1-infected mothers and the occurrence of HIV infection in their infants. Clin. Exp. Immunol. 102 (3), 476–480.

Mabondzo, A., et al., 1998. Lack of correlation between vertical transmission of HIV-1 and maternal antibody titers against autologous virus in human monocyte-derived macrophages. J. Acquir. Immune Defic. Syndr. Hum. Retrovirol. 17 (1), 92–94.

Mabuka, J., et al., 2012. HIV-specific antibodies capable of ADCC are common in breastmilk and are associated with reduced risk of transmission in women with high viral loads. PLoS Pathog. 8 (6), e1002739.

Mabuka, J., et al., 2013. HIV-1 maternal and infant variants show similar sensitivity to broadly neutralizing antibodies, but sensitivity varies by subtype. AIDS 27 (10), 1535–1544.

Martinez, D.R., et al., 2017. Maternal binding and neutralizing IgG responses targeting the C terminal region of the V3 loop are predictive of reduced peripartum HIV-1 transmission risk. J. Virol. 91 (9), pii: e02422-16.

McFarland, E.J., et al., 2001. HIV-1 gp120-specific antibodies in neonates receiving an HIV-1 recombinant gp120 vaccine. JID 184 (10), 1331–1335.

McNeely, T.B., et al., 1995. Secretory leukocyte protease inhibitor: a human saliva protein exhibiting anti-human immunodeficiency virus 1 activity in vitro. J. Clin. Invest. 96 (1), 456–464.

Milligan, C., Overbaugh, J., 2014. The role of cell-associated virus in mother-to-child HIV transmission. JID 210 (Suppl. 3), S631–40.

Milligan, C., et al., 2015. Passively acquired antibody-dependent cellular cytotoxicity (ADCC) activity in HIV-infected infants is associated with reduced mortality. Cell Host Microbe 17 (4), 500–506.

Milligan, C., et al., 2016. Maternal neutralization-resistant virus variants do not predict infant HIV infection risk. MBio 7 (1), e02221–15.

Mofenson, L.M., 2016. Antiretroviral therapy and adverse pregnancy outcome: the elephant in the room? JID 213 (7), 1051–1054.

Mofenson, L.M., et al., 1999. Risk factors for perinatal transmission of human immunodeficiency virus type 1 in women treated with zidovudine. NEJM 341 (6), 385–393.

Muenchhoff, M., et al., 2016. Nonprogressing HIV-infected children share fundamental immunological features of nonpathogenic SIV infection. Sci. Transl. Med. 8 (358), 358ra125.

Naarding, M.A., et al., 2005. Lewis X component in human milk binds DC-SIGN and inhibits HIV-1 transfer to CD4 + T lymphocytes. J. Clin. Invest. 115 (11), 3256–3264.

Nakamura, K.J., et al., 2013. Coverage of primary mother-to-child HIV transmission isolates by second-generation broadly neutralizing antibodies. AIDS 27 (3), 337–346.

Nduati, R., et al., 2000. Effect of breastfeeding and formula feeding on transmission of HIV-1: a randomized clinical trial. JAMA 283 (9), 1167–1174.

Njuguna, I.N., et al., 2014. PedVacc 002: a phase I/II randomized clinical trial of MVA. HIVA vaccine administered to infants born to human immunodeficiency virus type 1-positive mothers in Nairobi. Vaccine 32 (44), 5801–5808.

Ochola, R., et al., 2009. The level and duration of RSV-specific maternal IgG in infants in Kilifi Kenya. In: Ng, L.F.P. (Ed.), PLoS One, 4(12), p. e8088.

Ochs, H.D., et al., 1993. Intra-amniotic inoculation of pigtailed macaque (Macaca Nemestrina) fetuses with SIV and HIV-1. J. Med. Primatol. 22 (2–3), 162–168.

Omenda, M.M., et al., 2013. Evidence for efficient vertical transfer of maternal HIV-1 envelope-specific neutralizing antibodies but no association of such antibodies with reduced infant infection. JAIDS 64 (2), 163–166.

Onyango-Makumbi, C., et al., 2011. Safety and efficacy of HIV hyperimmune globulin for prevention of mother-to-child HIV transmission in HIV-1-infected pregnant women and their infants in Kampala, Uganda. JAIDS 58 (4), 399–407.

Palma, P., et al., 2016. Early antiretroviral treatment (eART) limits viral diversity over time in a long-term HIV viral suppressed perinatally infected child. BMC Infect. Dis. 16 (1), 742.

Palmeira, P., et al., 2012. IgG placental transfer in healthy and pathological pregnancies. Clin. Dev. Immunol. 2012 (3), 985646–13.

Parekh, B.S., et al., 1991. Lack of correlation between maternal antibodies to V3 loop peptides of gp120 and perinatal HIV-1 transmission. The NYC perinatal HIV transmission collaborative study. AIDS 5 (10), 1179–1184.

Peltier, C.A., et al., 2009. Breastfeeding with maternal antiretroviral therapy or formula feeding to prevent HIV postnatal mother-to-child transmission in Rwanda. AIDS 23 (18), 2415–2423.

Permar, S.R., et al., 2015. Maternal HIV-1 envelope-specific antibody responses and reduced risk of perinatal transmission. J. Clin. Invest. 125 (7), 2702–2706.

Persaud, D., et al., 2012. Dynamics of the resting CD4(+) T-cell latent HIV reservoir in infants initiating HAART less than 6 months of age. AIDS 26 (12), 1483–1490.

Persaud, D., et al., 2013. Absence of detectable HIV-1 viremia after treatment cessation in an infant. NEJM 369 (19), 1828–1835.

Persaud, D., et al., 2014. Influence of age at virologic control on peripheral blood human immunodeficiency virus reservoir size and serostatus in perinatally infected adolescents. JAMA Pediatr. 168 (12), 1138–1146.

Plotkin, S.A., 2010. Correlates of protection induced by vaccination. Clin. Vaccine Immunol. 17 (7), 1055–1065.

Pugatch, D., et al., 1997. Delayed generation of antibodies mediating human immunodeficiency virus type 1-specific antibody-dependent cellular cytotoxicity in vertically infected infants. JID 176 (3), 643–648.

Rerks-Ngarm, S., et al., 2009. Vaccination with ALVAC and AIDSVAX to prevent HIV-1 infection in Thailand. NEJM 361 (23), 2209–2220.

Ricci, E., et al., 2010. Toll-like receptor 9 polymorphisms influence mother-to-child transmission of human immunodeficiency virus type 1. J. Transl. Med. 8 (1), 49.

Robertson, C.A., et al., 1992. Maternal antibodies to gp120 V3 sequence do not correlate with protection against vertical transmission of human immunodeficiency virus. JID 166 (4), 704–709.

Ronen, K., Sharma, A., Overbaugh, J., 2015. HIV transmission biology: translation for HIV prevention. AIDS 29 (17), 2219–2227.

Rousseau, C.M., et al., 2004. Association of levels of HIV-1-infected breast milk cells and risk of mother-to-child transmission. JID 190 (10), 1880–1888.

Rouzioux, C., et al., 1995. Estimated timing of mother-to-child HIV-1 transmission by use of a Markov model. Am. J. Epidemiol. 142 (12), 1330–1337.

Rowland-Jones, S.L., et al., 1993. HIV-specific cytotoxic T-cell activity in an HIV-exposed but uninfected infant. Lancet 341 (8849), 860–861.

Russell, E.S., et al., 2011. The genetic bottleneck in vertical transmission of subtype C HIV-1 is not driven by selection of especially neutralization-resistant virus from the maternal viral population. J. Virol. 85 (16), 8253–8262.

Russell, E.S., et al., 2013. HIV type 1 subtype C variants transmitted through the bottleneck of breastfeeding are sensitive to new generation broadly neutralizing antibodies directed against quaternary and CD4-binding site epitopes. AIDS Res. Hum. Retroviruses 29 (3), 511–515.

Sabbaj, S., et al., 2002. Human immunodeficiency virus-specific CD8(+) T cells in human breast milk. J. Virol. 76 (15), 7365–7373.

Samleerat, T., et al., 2009. Maternal neutralizing antibodies against a CRF01_AE primary isolate are associated with a low rate of intrapartum HIV-1 transmission. Virology 387 (2), 388–394.

Santini-Oliveira, M., Grinsztejn, B., 2014. Adverse drug reactions associated with antiretroviral therapy during pregnancy. Expert Opin. Drug Saf. 13 (12), 1623–1652.

Scarlatti, G., et al., 1993a. Mother-to-child transmission of human immunodeficiency virus type 1: correlation with neutralizing antibodies against primary isolates. JID 168 (1), 207–210.

Scarlatti, G., et al., 1993b. Neutralizing antibodies and viral characteristics in mother-to-child transmission of HIV-1. AIDS 7 (Suppl. 2), S45–S48.

Shapiro, R.L., et al., 2005. Highly active antiretroviral therapy started during pregnancy or postpartum suppresses HIV-1 RNA, but not DNA, in breast milk. JID 192 (5), 713–719.

Sharma, A., Boyd, D.F., Overbaugh, J., 2015. Development of SHIVs with circulating, transmitted HIV-1 variants. J. Med. Primatol. 44 (5), 296–300.

Shen, R., Smith, P.D., 2014. Mucosal correlates of protection in HIV-1-exposed sero-negative persons. Am. J. Reprod. Immunol. 72 (2), 219–227.

Shugars, D.C., 1999. Endogenous mucosal antiviral factors of the oral cavity. JID 179 (Suppl. 3), S431–5.

Simonich, C.A., et al., 2016. HIV-1 neutralizing antibodies with limited hypermutation from an infant. Cell 166 (1), 77–87.

Singh, K.K., Spector, S.A., 2009. Host genetic determinants of human immunodeficiency virus infection and disease progression in children. Pediatr. Res. 65 (5 Pt. 2), 55R–63R.

Slyker, J.A. et al., 2012. Incidence and correlates of HIV-1 RNA detection in the breast milk of women receiving HAART for the prevention of HIV-1 transmission. L. Myer, ed. PLoS One, 7(1), p. e29777.

Stiehm, E.R., et al., 1999. Efficacy of zidovudine and human immunodeficiency virus (HIV) hyperimmune immunoglobulin for reducing perinatal HIV transmission from HIV-infected women with advanced disease: results of pediatric AIDS Clinical Trials Group protocol 185. JID 179 (3), 567–575.

Townsend, C.L., et al., 2014. Earlier initiation of ART and further decline in mother-to-child HIV transmission rates, 2000–2011. AIDS 28 (7), 1049–1057.

Tranchat, C., et al., 1999. Maternal humoral factors associated with perinatal human immunodeficiency virus type-1 transmission in a cohort from Kigali, Rwanda, 1988–1994. J. Infect. 39 (3), 213–220.

Tuomala, R.E., et al., 2003. Cell-associated genital tract virus and vertical transmission of human immunodeficiency virus type 1 in antiretroviral-experienced women. JID 187 (3), 375–384.

Ugen, K.E., et al., 1992. Vertical transmission of HIV infection: reactivity of maternal sera with glycoprotein 120 and 41 peptides from HIV type 1. J. Clin. Invest. 89 (6), 1923–1930.

Ugen, K.E., et al., 1997. Vertical transmission of human immunodeficiency virus type 1: ser-oreactivity by maternal antibodies to the carboxy region of the gp41 envelope glycopro-tein. JID 175 (1), 63–69.

UNAIDS, 2016a. AIDS by the Numbers. Available at: http://www.unaids.org/sites/default/files/media_asset/AIDS-by-the-numbers-2016_en.pdf. [Accessed April 10, 2017].

UNAIDS, 2016b. Prevention Gap Report. Available at: http://www.unaids.org/sites/default/files/media_asset/2016-prevention-gap-report_en.pdf. [Accessed April 10, 2017].

Uprety, P., et al., 2015. Cell-associated HIV-1 DNA and RNA decay dynamics during early combination antiretroviral therapy in HIV-1-infected infants. Clin. Infect. Dis. 61 (12), 1862–1870.

Van de Perre, P., et al., 2012. HIV-1 reservoirs in breast milk and challenges to elimination of breast-feeding transmission of HIV-1. Sci. Transl. Med. 4 (143), 143sr3.

Van Rompay, K.K.A., et al., 2005. Attenuated poxvirus-based SIV vaccines given in infancy partially protect infant and juvenile macaques against repeated oral challenge with viru-lent SIV. JAIDS 38 (2), 124–134.

Vidricaire, G., Imbeault, M., Tremblay, M.J., 2004. Endocytic host cell machinery plays a dominant role in intracellular trafficking of incoming human immunodeficiency virus type 1 in human placental trophoblasts. J. Virol. 78 (21), 11904–11915.

Walter, J., et al., 2009. High concentrations of interleukin 15 in breast milk are associated with protection against postnatal HIV transmission. JID 200 (10), 1498–1502.

Wamalwa, D., et al., 2016. Treatment interruption after 2-year antiretroviral treatment initiated during acute/early HIV in infancy. AIDS 30 (15), 2303–2313.

WHO, 2016a. WHO Validates Countries' Elimination of Mother-to-Child Transmission of HIV and syphilis. WHO. Available at: http://www.who.int/mediacentre/news/statements/2016/mother-child-hiv-syphilis/en/. [Accessed April 10, 2017].

WHO, 2016b. Consolidated Guidelines on the Use of Antiretroviral Drugs for Treating and Preventing HIV Infection: Recommendations for a Public Health Approach. Available at: http://www.who.int/hiv/pub/arv/arv-2016/en/. [Accessed April 10, 2017].

Wiesner, J., Vilcinskas, A., 2010. Antimicrobial peptides: the ancient arm of the human immune system. Virulence 1 (5), 440–464.

Wu, X., et al., 2006. Neutralization escape variants of human immunodeficiency virus type 1 are transmitted from mother to infant. J. Virol. 80 (2), 835–844.

Zhang, H., et al., 2010. Functional properties of the HIV-1 subtype C envelope glycoprotein associated with mother-to-child transmission. Virology 400 (2), 164–174.

CHAPTER THREE

African Swine Fever Virus Biology and Vaccine Approaches

Yolanda Revilla*, Daniel Pérez-Núñez*, Juergen A. Richt[†,1]

*Centro Biología Molecular Severo Ochoa, CSIC-UAM, Madrid, Spain
†Diagnostic Medicine/Pathobiology, Center of Excellence for Emerging and Zoonotic Animal Diseases (CEEZAD), College of Veterinary Medicine, Kansas State University, Manhattan, KS, United States
[1]Corresponding author: e-mail address: jricht@vet.k-state.edu

Contents

Abstract

African swine fever (ASF) is an acute and often fatal disease affecting domestic pigs and wild boar, with severe economic consequences for affected countries. ASF is endemic in sub-Saharan Africa and the island of Sardinia, Italy. Since 2007, the virus emerged in the republic of Georgia, and since then spread throughout the Caucasus region and Russia. Outbreaks have also been reported in Belarus, Ukraine, Lithuania, Latvia, Estonia, Romania, Moldova, Czech Republic, and Poland, threatening neighboring West European countries. The causative agent, the African swine fever virus (ASFV), is a large, enveloped, double-stranded DNA virus that enters the cell by macropinocytosis and a clathrin-dependent mechanism. African Swine Fever Virus is able to interfere with various cellular signaling pathways resulting in immunomodulation, thus making the development of an efficacious vaccine very challenging. Inactivated preparations of African Swine Fever Virus do not confer protection, and the role of antibodies in protection remains unclear. The use of live-attenuated vaccines, although rendering suitable levels

Advances in Virus Research, Volume 100
ISSN 0065-3527
https://doi.org/10.1016/bs.aivir.2017.10.002

of protection, presents difficulties due to safety and side effects in the vaccinated animals. Several African Swine Fever Virus proteins have been reported to induce neutralizing antibodies in immunized pigs, and vaccination strategies based on DNA vaccines and recombinant proteins have also been explored, however, without being very successful. The complexity of the virus particle and the ability of the virus to modulate host immune responses are most likely the reason for this failure. Furthermore, no permanent cell lines able to sustain productive virus infection by both virulent and naturally attenuated African Swine Fever Virus strains exist so far, thus impairing basic research and the commercial production of attenuated vaccine candidates.

 ## 1. EMERGENCE AND HOST RANGE OF AFRICAN SWINE FEVER VIRUS

African swine fever virus (ASFV), believed to be one of the most dangerous infectious diseases of pigs, causes hemorrhagic fever in domestic and feral pigs (Costard et al., 2013; Vinuela, 1985). Depending on the virulence of the 23 characterized genotypes of the virus, the course of ASF infection causes a range of clinical syndromes (OIE, 2012), ranging from highly acute disease with 100% mortality, to long-term persistent infection. Upon infection with highly virulent strains, clinical signs involve pulmonary oedema, serious depression, high fever, anorexia, spotty skin, cyanosis, thrombocytopenia, lymphopenia, and hemorrhagic lesions (Blome et al., 2013; Karalyan et al., 2012a; Zakaryan et al., 2014). Conversely, African wild pigs (bushpigs, warthogs) are usually asymptomatically infected and constitute the reservoir hosts of African Swine Fever Virus in Africa (Penrith et al., 2013).

In the past, African Swine Fever Virus affected domestic pigs in European countries, including Spain, Portugal, Italy, and France. Nevertheless, the disease was eradicated from these countries by the mid-1990s, with the exception of Sardinia, where it is still endemic (Iglesias et al., 2017; Martinez-Lopez et al., 2015; Sanchez-Vizcaino et al., 2013).

ASF was reintroduced in 2007 to Eastern Europe via the Transcaucasus, especially Georgia, from which it spread to Armenia, Belarus, Ukraine, the Russian Federation, and in very recent times, to Estonia, Lithuania, Latvia, Romania, Moldova, Czech Republic, and Poland (ESFA AHAW Panel, 2015; Gallardo et al., 2014; Sanchez-Vizcaino et al., 2013; Wozniakowski et al., 2016) causing numerous outbreaks within domestic pigs and/or wild boar populations (Gogin et al., 2013; Sanchez-Vizcaino et al., 2013). A considerable risk of African Swine Fever Virus introduction into central Europe exists, since this region offers a growing population of wild boar (Massei et al., 2015), abundant road transportation of pigs (Eurostat, 2013), and transient traffic and shipments through large seaports and airports

(Costard et al., 2013; De la Torre et al., 2015; Mur et al., 2012a,b). Further-more, an ASF outbreak indeed occurred in Belgium in 1985 after the illegal introduction of infected pork products, which was rapidly eradicated (Biront et al., 1987).

2. VIRUS TRANSMISSION AND SPREAD

Transmission of African Swine Fever Virus occurs via contact among infected animals, intake of infected material, and/or soft tick vectors (Ornithodoros) (Boinas et al., 2004; European Food Safety Authority Panel on Animal Health and Welfare, 2010; European Food Safety Authority, 2014; Sanchez-Vizcaino et al., 2012). Three transmission cycles have been reported in endemic areas: (i) a domestic pig/pig cycle, which does not involve other vertebrate or invertebrate hosts, (ii) a domestic pig/tick/wild pig cycle, and (iii) a domestic pig/tick cycle without warthog involvement (Gallardo et al., 2011). Persistence of the virus may occur for many months and some of the infected animals may not show clinical signs, and may even mimic other diseases (Botija, 1982; Penrith and Vosloo, 2009; Thomson et al., 1979). Persistently infected pigs seem to be involved in the spread of African Swine Fever Virus, producing sporadic outbreaks in formerly African Swine Fever Virus-free zones. This hypothesis has been supported by the fact that— under experimental conditions—pigs which survive with subacute infections shed virus for at least 70 days (de Carvalho Ferreira et al., 2013a,b). The disease, whose notification to the World Organization for Animal Health (OIE) is mandatory, produces important socioeconomic consequences (De la Torre et al., 2015; European Food Safety Authority, 2014) and presents a severe risk of spread to many countries worldwide.

3. MOLECULAR BIOLOGY OF THE VIRUS

African Swine Fever Virus is a large, cytoplasmic, double-stranded DNA virus that replicates in cells of the mononuclear phagocyte system, mainly monocytes and macrophages, although other cell types can be infected, especially later during the infection; the activation of target cells by African Swine Fever Virus replication plays a key role during African Swine Fever Virus infection, being a modulating element of virus pathogenesis (Carrasco et al., 1996; Carrascosa et al., 1999; Gomez-Villamandos et al., 2013; Vinuela, 1985).

African Swine Fever Virus virions are icosahedral structures of approximately 200 nm, which are formed by concentric layers (Fig. 1): the internal

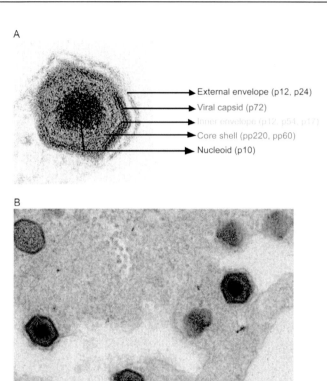

Fig. 1 Structure of the extracellular African Swine Fever Virus and virion egress from cells. (A) Electron microscopy image of the extracellular African Swine Fever Virus particle. The African Swine Fever Virus virion is composed of different concentric layers: the external envelope (*red*), the viral capsid (*green*), the inner envelope (*yellow*), the core shell (*blue*), and the nucleoid (*purple*). Examples of proteins present in each layer are shown in *brackets* (reviewed in Salas and Andres, 2013). (B) Electron microscopy image of African Swine Fever Virus virions emerging from infected cells.

core, the core shell, the inner membrane, the capsid, and, in the extracellular virions, the external envelope (Andres et al., 1997; Breese and DeBoer, 1967; Carrascosa et al., 1984).

The internal core is formed by the nucleoid, containing the viral genome and some nucleoproteins such as the DNA-binding protein p10 (Munoz et al., 1993). Furthermore, this layer organizes all the elements necessary for the synthesis of the early messenger RNAs (mRNAs): the transcriptional machinery, the poly(A) polymerase, and the capping enzyme (Salas and Andres, 2013). The core shell is a wide protein layer surrounding the core, mostly composed by the polyproteins pp220 and pp62 (Andres et al., 1997, 2002a,b). Both polyproteins are successively processed by a viral protease (S273R gene) (Alejo et al., 2003). The inner envelope is next to the core shell and appears as a single lipid membrane by electron microscopy (Salas and Andres, 2013). This layer is derived from the endoplasmic reticulum (ER) (Andres et al., 1998) and contains the viral proteins p54, p17, and p12 (Rodriguez et al., 2004; Salas and Andres, 2013; Suarez et al., 2010). The capsid is the furthest layer of the intracellular virions and is composed of about 2000 hexagonal capsomers. The p72 protein is the major component of the capsomers and constitutes 33% of the total mass of the virion (Carrascosa et al., 1984; Garcia-Escudero et al., 1998). The outer envelope of the extracellular viral particles is taken from the cellular plasma membrane during the budding process by which African Swine Fever Virus egresses from the cell (Breese and DeBoer, 1967; Carrascosa et al., 1984). The outer envelope contains one of the viral proteins with a molecular weight of about 12 kDa, which has been identified as the viral factor needed for the attachment of the virus to host cells (Carrascosa et al., 1991). Other proteins described to be localized within the virus particle are the homologue of the cellular CD2 protein, called CD2v (D. Pérez-Núñez, M.L. Nogal, and Y. Revilla, personal communication), which mediates the hemadsorption to infected cells (Borca et al., 1998; Rodriguez et al., 1993). African Swine Fever Virus morphogenesis occurs in specialized areas of the cytoplasm, named viral factories, which develop in infected cells near the nucleus and the microtubule organization centre. Viral factories essentially exclude host proteins but are surrounded by ER membranes and vimentin boxes (Heath et al., 2001). In addition to ER membranes, mitochondria are also recruited to the periphery of viral factories (Rojo et al., 1998).

The African Swine Fever Virus genome is a linear double-stranded DNA molecule which varies in length from 170 to 190 kbp among different African Swine Fever Virus strains (Chapman et al., 2008; Portugal et al., 2015; Yanez et al., 1995). This is due to the size variability of several ORFs, especially in the multigene families, and to the variation of short tandem repeats within genes and intergenic regions (Lubisi et al., 2007). African Swine Fever Virus genes are closely distributed, codified in both DNA strands without introns. Genome termini are hairpin loops covalently cross-linked, being present in two possible forms, inverted and complementary to each other (Almazan et al., 1992; Almendral et al., 1990; Dixon et al., 2013).

African Swine Fever Virus mRNAs are structurally similar to the corresponding mRNA molecules of the cellular machinery. In vitro transcribed viral mRNAs possess a cap structure in its 5′ UTR and a poly(A) tail of 33 nucleotides in its 3′ UTR (Salas et al., 1981). The cap structure is mostly of the m7G (5′) pppAm type, suggesting that an enzymatic activity for viral RNA capping is required. In this regard, African Swine Fever Virus encodes a guanylyltransferase (ORF NP868R) able to exert triphosphatase and guanylyltransferase activities (Pena et al., 1993; Yanez et al., 1995). In addition to the capping enzyme, the African Swine Fever Virus genome encodes a gene (ORF C475L) with similarity to other poly(A) polymerases, suggesting that the virus also possesses its own viral poly(A) polymerase (Rodriguez and Salas, 2013; Yutin et al., 2009).

African Swine Fever Virus is independent from the host cell machinery to carry out transcriptional processes and encodes about 20 genes considered to be important for mRNA modification and translation (Rodriguez and Salas, 2013). Indeed, the African Swine Fever Virus virion contains a DNA-dependent RNA polymerase consisting of several subunits, which is able to control the expression of viral genes (Rodriguez and Salas, 2013) in a time-dependent manner (Fig. 2). Early transcription uses virus-encoded transcription enzymes enclosed in the core (Kuznar et al., 1980; Salas et al., 1983). Most of immediate early and early genes belong to the multigene families, which are believed to be involved in the control of host responses to African Swine Fever Virus infection (Afonso et al., 2004) and in virus DNA replication (Rodriguez and Salas, 2013). The mechanism used by African Swine Fever Virus to temporally express its genes has been reported to be similar to the mechanism displayed by poxviruses (Broyles, 2003; Rodriguez and Salas, 2013).

4. VIRUS ENTRY, INTRACELLULAR TRAFFIC, AND VIRAL MACHINERY OF TRANSLATION

The mechanism by which African Swine Fever Virus enters host cells has been a controversial matter. Viral entry into host cells is also a key target for inhibiting African Swine Fever Virus infection and for potential vaccine development. Early studies described African Swine Fever Virus cell entry as a temperature, energy, cholesterol, and low-pH-dependent procedure, which involves receptor-mediated endocytosis (Alcami et al., 1989a,b; Carrascosa et al., 1999; Valdeira et al., 1998). Other, more recent studies determined that viral entry requires dynamin and is a clathrin-dependent process (Galindo et al., 2015; Hernaez and Alonso, 2010). Through the application of various pharmacological inhibitors and specific protein constructions inducing a dominant negative effect against key protein players in virus entry, it has been demonstrated that African Swine Fever Virus entry in

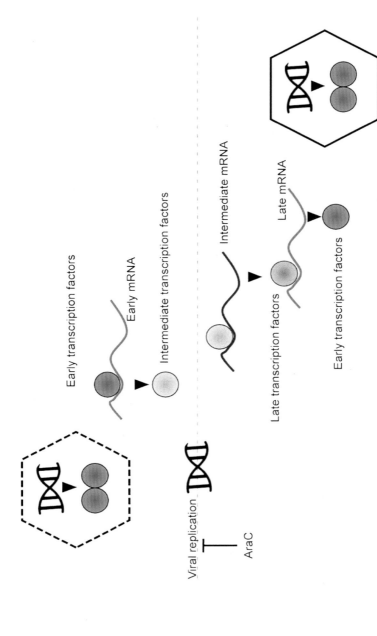

Fig. 2 Schematic representation of the transcriptional cascade mechanism proposed for African Swine Fever Virus. After viral entry, immediate early and early genes are expressed, while after viral replication intermediate- and late gene synthesis takes place. AraC is an inhibitor of viral replication.

Vero and porcine IPAM cells is mainly achieved by macropinocytosis, in a process that requires sodium/proton exchangers (Na^+/H^+), activation of EGFR, phosphorylation of PI3K and Pak1 kinases, together with the activation of the small Rho-GTPase Rac1, resulting in actin-dependent blebbing/ruffling perturbations of the cell membrane, allowing virions to get access to the host cell (Fig. 3). Inhibition of macropinocytosis regulators, as well as treatment with the drug EIPA (5-(N-ethyl-N-isopropyl) amiloride), results in a marked decrease in African Swine Fever Virus entry and infectious virus (Sanchez et al., 2012).

4.1 African Swine Fever Virus Entry and Traffic

It has been recently described that the mechanism of African Swine Fever Virus entry includes outer envelope disruption, capsid disassembly, and inner envelope fusion before the viral core can be released from endosomes (Andres, 2017; Hernaez et al., 2016). Linking of African Swine Fever Virus entry with the endosomal pathway (Alcami et al., 1989a,b, 1990; Valdeira and Geraldes, 1985), virus progression throughout the endocytic pathway and the role of Rab GTPases have been also described (Cuesta-Geijo et al., 2012).

Many viruses alter the cellular trafficking machinery by encoding specific viral proteins able to interact with key functional cytoplasm proteins, in order to induce novel membrane structures that constitute centers where viruses replicate and viral morphogenesis is achieved (Cruz and Buchkovich, 2017). These structures, named viral factories (or virosomes), consist of replicase proteins, virus genomes, and host proteins and are able to recruit host factors associated with cellular stress and defense mechanisms, suggesting that

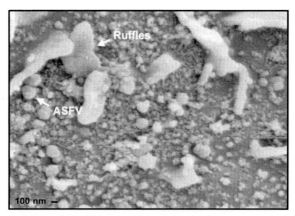

Fig. 3 Ruffles and Blebs formation at the cellular surface after 10 min of African Swine Fever Virus addition to cells. Scanning electronic microscopy image showing African Swine Fever Virus-Ba71V strain after 10 min of virus addition to Vero cells.

cell defense routes are subverted by pathogens to create sites of replication (Netherton et al., 2007).

African Swine Fever Virus has also been shown to induce the collapse of endoplasmic reticulum cisternae, and this collapse is dependent on the viral protein p54, an inner envelope protein targeting the ER (Rodriguez et al., 2004; Windsor et al., 2012; reviewed in Munoz-Moreno et al., 2015).

The adaptor protein 1 (AP-1) is a heterotetramer involved in the transport of proteins from the *trans*-Golgi network (TGN) to endosomes (Nakatsu and Ohno, 2003). AP-1 engages clathrin to form clathrin-coated vesicles that select their cargo by recognizing sorting signals in the cytoplasmic tail of integral membrane proteins. Two sorting signals, selectively recognized by AP-1, have been identified so far: the tyrosine (YXXF) and the dileucine ([D/E]XXXL[L/I]) motifs (Canagarajah et al., 2013). Several viruses are able to bind AP-1; for instance, HIV-Nef binds to AP-1 through a well-characterized dileucine (di-Leu) motif (Bresnahan et al., 1998; Madrid et al., 2005) leading to the stabilization of AP-1 and resulting in an alteration of the endocytic pathway and increase in HIV virulence. The E6 protein from bovine papillomavirus type 1 (BPV-1) also binds AP-1 (Tong et al., 1998), and AP-1 has been associated with viral spread in human herpes virus 6 infection (Mori et al., 2008).

It has been proposed by Perez-Nunez et al. (2015), that binding of ASF viral proteins to AP-1 might induce reorganization of the Golgi and reorganization of cellular traffic during African Swine Fever Virus infection, with the aim of facilitating viral replication, encapsulation and/or viral progression. The CD2v African Swine Fever Virus-protein shares significant similarity to that of the CD2 protein in T cells and is responsible for hemadsorption. It was identified as the viral protein binding to AP-1, and localizing around the viral factory during African Swine Fever Virus infection (see Fig. 4). Furthermore, it was shown that after

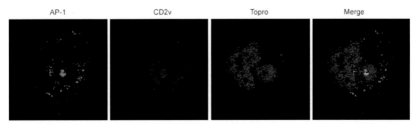

Fig. 4 Subcellular localization of CD2v during African Swine Fever Virus infection. COS cells infected with African Swine Fever Virus-E70 strain after 16 h were stained with specific antibodies against the adaptor protein 1 (AP-1) (in *green*) and CD2v protein (*red*). Nucleic acids were stained with Topro3.

BFA treatment, a drug that targets AP-1 delocalization from membranes to cytoplasm (Stamnes and Rothman, 1993), AP-1 was dispersed into the cytoplasm in African Swine Fever Virus-infected cells; in contrast, CD2v localization was not affected by BFA and remained attached to the membranes surrounding the viral factories (Perez-Nunez et al., 2015). Interestingly, sequence analysis of CD2v identified a di-Leu motif predicted to mediate binding to AP-1, but Perez-Nunez et al. (2015) demonstrated that this di-Leu motif in CD2v was neither involved in colocalization nor in interaction between CD2v and AP-1. These results are in contrast to the above described mechanism for HIV-Nef. In addition, a region within the cytoplasmic tail of CD2v was identified, which does not contain the di-Leu motif, but interacts with AP-1, suggesting that this region could represent an as yet uncharacterized novel viral AP-1-binding motif with vital consequences for cellular traffic and virus infectivity (Perez-Nunez et al., 2015).

4.2 African Swine Fever Virus Control of Cellular Protein Synthesis

It is well known that viruses depend on the cellular machinery to replicate and synthesize viral proteins, as they display limited genomes that cannot encode the whole functions required to accomplish these complex processes. Therefore, several viruses have developed complicated mechanisms to hijack the cellular translation machinery in order to use it for their own protein synthesis. The majority of these strategies are based on switching on/off the activity of the eukaryotic initiation factors (eIFs), which play key roles in protein synthesis. Frequently, viruses target two important steps in eukaryotic translation initiation: (i) the phosphorylation of eIF2 and (ii) the recruitment of ribosomal subunits to the mRNA by targeting eIF4F and eukaryotic translation factor 4E-binding proteins (4E-BPs). Phosphorylation of eIF2α (P-eIF2α) by PKR is an important host defense mechanisms against viral infections. Many viruses have developed mechanisms to evade PKR activation. Among them, Epstein–Barr virus encodes double-stranded (ds) RNAs that bind PKR but do not trigger the activation of the kinase (Schneider and Mohr, 2003; Walsh and Mohr, 2011). Vaccinia Virus (VV), herpes simplex virus-1 (HSV-1), influenza, and reovirus encode dsRNA-binding proteins that mask or sequester dsRNA, preventing the activation of PKR (Beattie et al., 1995; Khoo et al., 2002; Lloyd and Shatkin, 1992; Mulvey et al., 1999; Salvatore et al., 2002). Frequently, viruses use redundant mechanisms to guarantee the inhibition of antiviral pathways. For instance HSV-1, in addition to inhibiting PKR activation, encodes for proteins that avoid P-eIF2α by activating specific phosphatases (Mulvey et al., 2003). Another regulation mechanism is the recruitment of ribosomes and eIF4F formation. eIF4F is a complex formed by three proteins: eIF4A, eIF4E, and eIF4G (Prevot et al., 2003) and, as central part of the cap-dependent translation machinery, is tightly regulated to protect against stress and viral infections. Complex DNA viruses, in contrast to nearly all other viruses studied so far, allow the formation of eIF4F but still are able to inhibit cellular protein synthesis (Walsh and Mohr, 2004; Walsh et al., 2005, 2008).

African Swine Fever Virus, in analogy to other complex DNA viruses, has developed a sophisticated mechanism to hijack the cellular translation machinery by not only altering the activity of the translation initiation factors but also their cellular localization. It has been described that, similar to VV infections, P-eIF2α level diminished at early time points post-African Swine Fever Virus infection (Castello et al., 2009b). African Swine Fever Virus encodes a protein, called DP71L (also called l14L or 23NL, depending on the viral strain), which possesses a characteristic binding protein phosphatase 1 (PP1) motif (VxF) (Rivera et al., 2007). Furthermore, it possesses an N-terminal sequence of basic residues and its C-terminal domain is similar to the HSV-1-encoded neurovirulence factor ICP34.5 (Goatley et al., 1999). Importantly, DP71L interacts with PP1 in vitro (Rivera et al., 2007) and in vivo (Zhang et al., 2010). Transfection of DP71L induces a decrease of phosphorylated eIF2α and enhances the expression of cotransfected reporter molecules, suggesting that DP71L plays a role in keeping the cellular translation machinery active in order to allow viral protein synthesis (Zhang et al., 2010). Deletion of the l14L gene (the DP71L gene of African Swine Fever Virus strain E70) from the genome of the virulent Spanish African Swine Fever Virus isolate E70, reduced virulence of the E70 virus for domestic pigs (Zsak et al., 1996), whereas deletion of the gene from the virulent Malawi LIL 20/1 isolate did not reduce its virulence, suggesting that the Malawi isolate may encode another viral gene, which can compensate for the loss of l14L/DP71L (Afonso et al., 1998).

eIF4G is a substrate for caspase-3 (Bushell et al., 1999; Prevot et al., 2003), during apoptosis activation (Marissen and Lloyd, 1998). However, it was reported that eIF4G was resistant to caspase-3 cleavage in African Swine Fever Virus-infected cells (Castello et al., 2009b). In addition, it was previously described that African Swine Fever Virus encodes for an inhibitor of apoptosis –like protein (IAP) called A224L, which functions as an inhibitor of caspase 3 (Nogal et al., 2001). The possibility that the African Swine Fever Virus protein A224L protects the cellular translation machinery from caspase 3-mediated degradation needs to be explored in the future. Furthermore, ASVF induces mTOR-mediated phosphorylation of eIF4G at Ser1108 (Castello et al., 2009b), which has been associated with "translational activation" (Kimball et al., 2000; Raught et al., 2000), and triggers the phosphorylation of eIF4E at Ser209 by Mnk-1. eIF4E phosphorylation reaches its maximum levels at 16-h postinfection and is suppressed in the presence of Mnk-1 inhibitors, suggesting that Mnk-1 activation is critical during African Swine Fever Virus infection, as reported before in other systems (Pyronnet, 2000; Pyronnet et al., 1999). Similar to VV and other DNA viruses (Buchkovich et al., 2008), African Swine Fever Virus infection promotes 4E-BP1-hyperphosphorylation at early time points postinfection allowing activation of translation, whereas it is hypophosphorylated at later time points postinfection; this step results in cap-dependent translation inhibition. The differential phosphorylation stages of 4E-BP1 probably reflect an African Swine Fever Virus-mediated mechanism to support viral protein synthesis during early African Swine Fever Virus replication stages and stop viral protein synthesis during the late morphogenesis, a time at which viral proteins have been already synthesized, and cell energy should be used for virion particle assembly and egress. Furthermore, many of the components of the translation machinery (eIF4G, eIF4E, eIF2, eIF3b, and the eukaryotic elongation factor 2), ribosomes, and mitochondria are relocated from a diffused distribution throughout the cytoplasm to the viral factories (Castello et al., 2009b). Since viral RNAs localize at the periphery of the viral factories, it is likely that active translation of viral mRNAs is limited to these foci in African Swine Fever Virus-infected cells.

During infection, many viruses modify the distribution and quantity of cellular mRNAs by using different strategies, for example, by interfering with the efficiency of translation. In this regard, HSV-1 accumulates cellular mRNAs at the nucleus of infected cells (Sandri-Goldin, 2011), whereas adenovirus (Yatherajam et al., 2011), vesicular stomatitis virus (von Kobbe et al., 2000), poliovirus (Castello et al., 2009a; Park et al., 2008), and influenza virus (Satterly et al., 2007) impair host mRNAs export from the nucleus to the cytoplasm. HSV-1 (Cheng and Deutscher, 2005) and gammaherpesviruses (Covarrubias et al., 2011; Richner et al., 2011) stimulate cellular mRNA degradation. VV also induces mRNA degradation, probably via viral-encoded decapping enzymes (Parrish and Moss, 2007; Parrish et al., 2007). A decrease in the amount of cytoplasmically located polyadenylated mRNAs, together with an increase of nuclear RNAs, was described during African Swine Fever Virus infection (Castello et al., 2009b), indicating that poly(A) mRNA stability and nuclear RNA export are targeted during African Swine Fever Virus infection. Finally, the African

Swine Fever Virus genome encodes for a protein called g5R/African Swine Fever Virus-DP, which displays the Nudix motif, which is present in the host decapping enzyme 2 (Dcp2) or the VV viral proteins D9 and D10 (McLennan, 2007). g5R has in vitro decapping activity (Parrish et al., 2009), localizes around viral factories, and is able to bind mRNA during African Swine Fever Virus infection, among other functions (Quintas et al., 2017). Therefore, this viral enzyme represents a candidate to be the viral factor involved in the degradation of cellular mRNAs, probably contributing to the cellular shutoff.

In summary, African Swine Fever Virus cell entry is a temperature, energy, cholesterol, and low-pH-dependent procedure, requiring dynamin and clathrin (Galindo et al., 2015; Hernaez and Alonso, 2010). African Swine Fever Virus entry in Vero and porcine IPAM cells is mainly achieved by macropinocytosis, in a process that requires Na^+/H^+, activation of EGFR, phosphorylation of PI3K and Pak1 kinases, together with the activation of the small Rho-GTPase Rac1, resulting in actin-dependent blebbing/ruffling perturbations of the cell membrane, allowing virions to get access to the host cell. African Swine Fever Virus, in analogy to other complex DNA viruses, has developed a sophisticated mechanism to hijack the cellular translation machinery in order to use it for its own protein synthesis. The majority of these strategies are based on African Swine Fever Virus-induced switching on/off the activity of the eIFs, together with alterations of their subcellular distribution during African Swine Fever Virus infection.

5. AFRICAN SWINE FEVER VIRUS GENES MODULATING HOST RESPONSES

When the complete 170–190 kbp DNA sequence of African Swine Fever Virus (Boinas et al., 2004; Chapman et al., 2008; de Villiers et al., 2010; Granberg et al., 2016; Rodriguez et al., 2015; Yanez et al., 1995) was analyzed, genes coding for structural proteins, for enzymes with functions related to DNA replication, for DNA repair, gene transcription, and protein modification (Yanez et al., 1995) as well as for proteins involved in virus–host interactions were identified (Borca et al., 1998; Miskin et al., 1998; Nogal et al., 2001; Rodriguez et al., 2002). Among them, gene products involved in DNA replication and repair, including a DNA polymerase (G1211R) and a proliferating cell nuclear antigen-like protein (E301R) (Yanez et al., 1995), have been reported. African Swine Fever Virus also encodes enzymes involved in DNA repair, such as a DNA polymerase (O174L), an ATP-dependent DNA ligase (NP419L), and an endonuclease (E296R) (Garcia-Escudero et al., 2003; Jezewska et al., 2006; Redrejo-Rodriguez et al., 2006). It is also assumed that African Swine Fever Virus encodes enzymes and factors required to transcribe and process mRNAs, since ASF viral transcription does not require the host RNA polymerase II and virions are transcriptionally active (Salas et al., 1981, 1986; Santaren and Vinuela, 1986).

African Swine Fever Virus manipulates cellular mechanisms and the host defense by encoding a variety of immunomodulatory proteins that efficiently interfere with host immune responses (reviewed in Munoz-Moreno et al., 2015). Actually, the ability of African Swine Fever Virus to evade immune surveillance is via the modulation of the expression of proinflammatory molecules and cytokines. In this regard, it has been shown that ORF A238L contains ankyrin repeats which are homologous to those described in the IκB family, and binds the transcription factor p65-NFκB to act as a bona fide IκB-α viral homologue (Revilla et al., 1998); this results in the modulation of genes depending on NFκB in infected cells. This was first demonstrated by ectopic expression of A238L and by analysis of the expression of genes under the control of NFκB, showing that the observed NFκB inhibition was specific (Powell et al., 1996; Revilla et al., 1998). Interestingly, the A238L sequence does not contain motifs phosphorylated by IκB kinase, suggesting that the viral protein A238L is a natural, constitutive, and irreversible suppressor of NFκB activity (Tait et al., 2000). It is largely known that monocytes and macrophages play a central role in antigen presentation and secretion of bioactive molecules, e.g. prostaglandin E2 (PGE2), whose synthesis is firmly controlled by cyclooxigenase-2 (COX-2) (Janelle et al., 2002). Several viruses regulate COX-2 expression in order to modulate, among other things, the synthesis of PGE2 (Fang et al., 2012; Janelle et al., 2002; Murono et al., 2001; Pollara et al., 2012; Steer et al., 2003; Tung et al., 2011). African Swine Fever Virus has been shown to modulate not only the expression of COX-2 but also other two important inflammatory factors, such as TNF-α and iNOS (Granja et al., 2006a,b), through the regulation of the transcriptional coactivator proteins CBP and p300 (Granja et al., 2008, 2009). CBP/p300 interacts with numerous transcription factors to coordinate the expression of specific sets of genes in response to diverse physiological stimuli (Goodman and Smolik, 2000; Vo and Goodman, 2001; reviewed in Sanchez et al., 2013).

In addition, viral proteins homologous to host apoptosis inhibitory proteins have been described: (i) ORF A179L, structurally and functionally similar to Bcl2 (Banjara et al., 2017; Revilla et al., 1997) and ORF A224L, an

IAP homologue that inhibits caspase activation and also promotes survival through NFκB activation (Nogal et al., 2001; Rodriguez et al., 2002). Other reported African Swine Fever Virus proteins interfering with host immune responses include the DP71L protein, which putatively prevents the shutoff of protein synthesis induced by phosphorylation of PKR (Rivera et al., 2007; Zhang et al., 2010), the I329L protein, which acts as an inhibitor of Toll-like receptor pathways, and several members of the multigene families 360 and 530, which have been implicated in inhibiting type I interferon induction (Afonso et al., 2004; de Oliveira et al., 2011). Finally, it is important to note that African Swine Fever Virus also encodes adhesion proteins, such as EP153R (a lectin-like protein) which is involved in apoptosis and MHC presentation (Hurtado et al., 2004, 2011), and the ORF EP402R/CD2v, whose N-terminal domain shares high homology with the host CD2 protein. This viral protein is essential for the binding of erythrocytes to infected macrophages, a phenomenon called hemadsorption (Rodriguez et al., 1993), whose role in viral pathogenesis is not clearly understood so far (Borca et al., 1998). The CD2v intracellular domain has a role in binding to cytoplasmic adaptor protein SH3P7 (Kay-Jackson et al., 2004) and to AP-1, a cellular factor involved in cellular traffic (see earlier) and regulated by CD2v (Perez-Nunez et al., 2015).

6. AFRICAN SWINE FEVER VIRUS VACCINES

Pigs surviving African Swine Fever Virus infection develop a strong and protective immunity, indicating that an effective vaccine against African Swine Fever Virus might be possible. Attenuated African Swine Fever Virus strains induce immune responses which afford long-term resistance to homologous but not to heterologous African Swine Fever Virus challenge (Leitao et al., 2001; Mulumba-Mfumu et al., 2016), and the correlate of protection seem to be virus-specific T-cell responses (King et al., 2011; Revilla et al., 1992). Nevertheless, attenuated African Swine Fever Virus vaccine candidates produce several side effects such as chronic lesions, fever, viremia, hypergammaglobulemia, and/or joint swelling (King et al., 2011; Leitao et al., 2001; Revilla et al., 1992). Despite the fact that several research groups during the past few years have developed novel vaccine technologies, ranging from inactivated viruses, recombinant proteins/peptides, and DNA vaccines to live-attenuated vaccine (LAV) candidates, an efficacious, safe African Swine Fever Virus vaccine does currently not exist.

6.1 Modulation of the Host Immune System by African Swine Fever Virus

Animals surviving African Swine Fever Virus infection develop a protective immune response. Therefore, naturally or genetically attenuated or moderately virulent African Swine Fever Virus strains have been used as LAV candidates. These attenuated African Swine Fever Virus strains induced a long-term resistance to homologous but not to heterologous virus challenge (King et al., 2011; Leitao et al., 2001; Mulumba-Mfumu et al., 2016), and the protection was found to correlate with virus-specific T-cell responses and cytokine production (King et al., 2011; Revilla et al., 1992). However, the correlates of protective immunity to African Swine Fever Virus infection are weakly characterized yet, although questions about viral antigen presentation and MHC modulation in the context of African Swine Fever Virus-infected porcine macrophages have been partially answered (Gonzalez Juarrero et al., 1992; reviewed in Alvarez et al., 2013).

There are conflicting reports on the role of cytokines and IFN during African Swine Fever Virus infection. Replication of virulent African Swine Fever Virus strains in porcine macrophages pretreated with bovine IFNα (Esparza et al., 1998) and of cell culture-adapted African Swine Fever Virus-Ba71V in Vero cells pretreated with human IFNα was reduced (Paez et al., 1990). In contrast, induction of IFN in porcine macrophages by polyI:C did not affect the replication of either the virulent Kirawira or the attenuated Uganda strain of African Swine Fever Virus (Wardley et al., 1979). Older studies from Revilla and coworkers described that African Swine Fever Virus infection induced the modulation of IFNγ production by T lymphocytes (Revilla et al., 1992). More recently, it has been reported that nonvirulent African Swine Fever Virus strains, which do not encode genes from multigene family (MGF)360 and MGF505 (Chapman et al., 2008; Portugal et al., 2015), induce moderate amounts of IFN after in vitro infection of pig macrophages, in comparison to virulent African Swine Fever Virus strains, which produce lower amounts of IFNs and other regulatory cytokines (Afonso et al., 2004; Gil et al., 2008; Zhang et al., 2006). In this context, it is noteworthy to mention that IFNα and IFNβ expression occurred in animals during infection with African Swine Fever Virus Georgia2007/1 (Karalyan et al., 2012b) and other virulent African Swine Fever Virus strains. The most relevant source of IFN production in vivo after African Swine Fever Virus virulent infection are most likely dendritic cells (DCs) (Golding et al., 2016), which had been previously demonstrated to produce significant amounts of IFN in response to other types of viral infections (O'keeffe et al., 2012). However, African Swine Fever Virus infection of DCs has not been clearly demonstrated so far, neither in vitro nor in vivo, posing the interesting question whether IFN production by DCs is indirect due to factors secreted by African Swine Fever Virus-infected macrophages or by direct infection of this subset of cells.

6.2 Cells Susceptible to African Swine Fever Virus Infection

In infected animals, pig monocytes and alveolar macrophages are the major target cells for African Swine Fever Virus replication (Gomez-Villamandos et al., 2013); this has important consequences for the pathogenesis of African Swine Fever Virus, as these cells play key roles in the immune response through phagocytosis, antigen presentation, or cytokine secretion (Gordon et al., 1995; Van Furth et al., 1972). Porcine alveolar macrophages (PAM) express CD14, SLAII, CD163, CD169, CD203, and CD16 receptors (Ezquerra et al., 2009). CD163 is a scavenger receptor whose expression is restricted to the monocyte/macrophage lineage and is normally used as a marker for monocytic differentiation and maturation (Law et al., 1993; Sanchez et al., 1999); it acts as the high-affinity scavenger receptor for the hemoglobin/haptoglobin complex and activates a signaling pathway that induces pro- and antiinflammatory cytokines (Poderoso et al., 2011).

The susceptibility to African Swine Fever Virus is linked to the maturation status of monocyte–macrophage cells that correlates with an upregulation of CD163 (Mccullough et al., 1999; Sanchez-Torres et al., 2003). Yet, the role of CD163 as an African Swine Fever Virus receptor is controversial, as its presence is not enough to increase susceptibility of nonpermissive cells to the virus (Lithgow et al., 2014). Furthermore, pigs lacking CD163 are not resistant to Georgia 2007/1 African Swine Fever Virus strain (Popescu et al., 2017).

Due to the difficulty to obtain reproducible results, the lot-to-lot variations, the costly cell preparations, and animal welfare reasons, freshly made PAM are not an ideal cell population to produce African Swine Fever Virus. These problems were partially overcome several years ago by the adaptation of the Ba71 (virulent) African Swine Fever Virus strain to Vero cells (Ba71V) (Enjuanes et al., 1976) and recently, by the finding that COS-7 cells (an SV40 T-antigen-transformed epithelial green monkey cell line), allow productive African Swine Fever Virus infection (Granja et al., 2006a; Hurtado et al., 2010). However, the generation of LAV still requires porcine cell lines able to sustain a productive African Swine Fever Virus infection. We have recently characterized four different permanent porcine cell lines—IPAM WT (Weingartl et al., 2002) (CRL-2845), IPAM-CD163 (Lee and Lee, 2010), WSL (Keil et al., 2014), and CΔ2+ (Chitko-Mckown et al., 2013)—regarding their ability to sustain productive infections with virulent

African Swine Fever Virus isolates Armenia/07 and E70, and the attenuated NH/P68 African Swine Fever Virus isolate; we also determined their virus production capacity (Sanchez et al., 2017). Our results indicate that these porcine cell lines do not show a mature macrophage phenotype and that the level of infection and viral production in IPAM-WT, IPAM-CD163, and CΔ2+ are much lower than those obtained in PAM, with the exception of WSL; the latter cell line is able to sustain the growth of the attenuated, but not virulent, African Swine Fever Virus strains. Thus, a permanent porcine cell line able to allow the study of African Swine Fever Virus–macrophage interaction and to sustain the productive infection both of attenuated and virulent African Swine Fever Virus strains is not available so far. This fact seriously compromises the production of putative LAVs for ASF, since such cells are the basis for the commercial production of these vaccines.

6.3 Live-Attenuated African Swine Fever Virus Vaccines

During the period of ASF outbreaks in Spain and Portugal which lasted from 1962 to 1995, natural African Swine Fever Virus isolates were obtained and attenuated by cell passages (Ribeiro, 1982); cell-attenuated African Swine Fever Virus strains were used to vaccinate an indeterminate number of pigs in the field. It has been reported that attenuated African Swine Fever Virus strains OURT88/3 and NH/P68 protect pigs against challenge with homologous virulent strains (Leitao et al., 2001; Malogolovkin et al., 2015; Mulumba-Mfumu et al., 2016), although only partial crossprotection was shown against heterologous viruses. Furthermore, these naturally attenuated strains induced various side effects, depending on the dose, and postvaccination reactions including petechiae, necrotic foci, joint swelling, and pneumonia were noted. Partial protection against a heterologous African Swine Fever Virus strain, apparently related to virus-specific IFNγ production, was observed with the attenuated African Swine Fever Virus strain OURT88/3 (King et al., 2011). Strategies focused on reducing the side effects of LAVs have been unsuccessful so far, since the deletion of virulence genes such as DP71L and DP96R reduced the ability of the attenuated virus to protect against homologous challenge (Abrams et al., 2013). The generation of genetically modified variants derived from naturally attenuated African Swine Fever Virus strains has been approached (see Fig. 5). The recombinant NH/P68 variants, lacking several genes involved in virus–cell interaction (e.g., A224L, A238L, A276R), showed various degree of protection (60%–100%), both against homologous and heterologous (Armenia 2007) African Swine Fever Virus strains (C. Gallardo and Y. Revilla, personal communication). However, the NH/P68-based vaccine candidate's

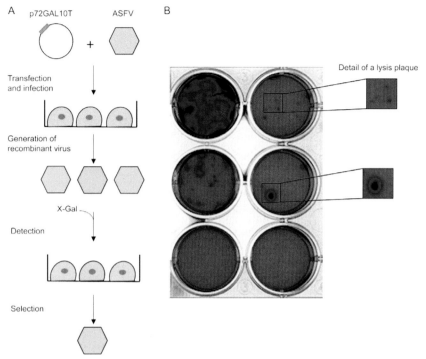

Fig. 5 Method to construct recombinant ASF viruses lacking specific genes. (A) Schematic representation of the experimental procedures. The flanking sequences of the gene of interest are cloned into the p72-BetaGAL10T vector. Cells are transfected with these constructions and African Swine Fever Virus-infected, to allow homologous recombination. Positive recombinant viruses carry a copy of beta-GAL instead of the targeted gene, allowing the selection of recombinant virus by titration in the presence of X-GAL. (B) Examples of *blue plaques* representing recombinant ASF viruses.

still induced (low) viremia and side effects such as arthritis and necrotic foci in most of the vaccinated pigs which most likely prevents their commercial use. We believe that some degree of virus replication is needed to induce protective immunity, and it might be difficult to eliminate some of the observed side effects. The genetic manipulation of the virulent Georgia 2007 isolate by deleting the 9GL and the MGF360/505 genes has been shown to attenuate the virus, but vaccination with the attenuated deletion mutant did not confer protection against parental virus challenge in pigs (O'donnell et al., 2016).

Lately, several groups have develop attenuated African Swine Fever Virus vaccines by using either virulent strains (e.g., Benin, Georgia, OUR/88/1, and Ba71), which, after genetic manipulation and deletion of genes regulating type I IFN responses, or deletion of the CD2v gene, are attenuated and confer protection against homologous and heterologous African Swine Fever Virus strains (López-Monteagudo et al., 2016; Reis et al., 2016). Interestingly, vaccination experiments using recombinant viruses revealed several key characteristics of the immune response against African Swine Fever Virus, namely, that deletion of genes downregulating IFNβ is a key factor in the mechanism of attenuation and that deletion of genes such as DP148R or A276R, both of them involved in IFNβ modulation, produces attenuated viruses which are efficacious against African Swine Fever Virus challenge (Reis et al., 2016; Revilla et al., manuscript in preparation). As discussed earlier, it is clear that novel innovative technology and new approaches are needed to produce an efficacious and safe African Swine Fever Virus vaccine. It is pertinent to state that the identification of virulence genes and the correlate of protective immune responses to African Swine Fever Virus infection can only be elucidated through detailed studies on the molecular mechanisms used by the virus to modulate host immune responses and the contribution of the innate and adaptive immune systems to protection; only after this critical information is obtained, rationally designed vaccines against ASF can be constructed.

6.4 Subunit Vaccines

Studies carried out many years ago showed that vaccination of pigs with different amounts of percoll-purified, UV-inactivated African Swine Fever Virus-Ba71V did not confer protection against live virus, either homologous or heterologous (Forman et al., 1982; Mebus and Dardiri, 1980; Revilla, Y., personal communication; Stone and Hess, 1967). Recently, these results have been confirmed, showing that inactivated African Swine Fever Virus does not confer protection, even in the presence of various adjuvants (Blome et al., 2014), suggesting that antibodies induced by African Swine Fever Virus structural protein might not be sufficient to protect pigs against virulent African Swine Fever Virus challenge. In contrast, transfer of antibodies derived from African Swine Fever Virus-infected pigs was reported to protect pigs against a lethal African Swine Fever Virus challenge (Onisk et al., 1994). Several African Swine Fever Virus proteins are able to induce neutralizing antibodies in immunized pigs. Among these proteins, p54 and p30 (Gomez-Puertas et al., 1996, 1998) were shown to be involved in various steps of virus attachment and internalization. Nevertheless, immunization of pigs with recombinant p54 and p30 proteins expressed in baculovirus did not protect against virulent African Swine Fever Virus challenge. Similarly, a vaccine based on African Swine Fever Virus proteins p30, p54, p22, and p72 produced in baculovirus failed to protect pigs against a virulent

African Swine Fever Virus challenge, despite producing neutralizing antibodies (Neilan et al., 2004); the above discussed results added to the controversy about the role of antibody-mediated neutralization of African Swine Fever Virus in protection against ASF (Escribano et al., 2013). On the other hand, vaccination with baculovirus-expressed African Swine Fever Virus proteins EP402R/CD2v revealed a considerable degree of protection against homologous African Swine Fever Virus challenge (Ruiz-Gonzalvo et al., 1996).

Several protocols using specific African Swine Fever Virus DNA vaccines have been also developed. In one of those attempts, the African Swine Fever Virus genes p30 and p54 were cloned in-frame with a fragment encoding for the single variable chain of a specific antibody recognizing swine leukocyte antigen II, in order to target the viral proteins to cells bearing SLA-II. Following this strategy, specific T cells against African Swine Fever Virus proteins could be detected; however, neither neutralizing antibodies nor protection against a virulent challenge was achieved (Argilaguet et al., 2011). Others generated constructs expressing the extracellular domain of HA fused to viral p30 and p54 proteins, showing that this modification significantly enhanced both humoral and cellular immune responses in pigs, however, without conferring protection against virulent African Swine Fever Virus challenge. In another attempt, cDNA constructs encoding various African Swine Fever Virus genes, further fused to ubiquitin, conferred partial protection against challenge in the absence of African Swine Fever Virus-specific antibodies; protection correlated with robust CTL response, mainly with antigen-specific CD8+ T cells (Argilaguet et al., 2012; Lacasta et al., 2014). These results reinforce the role of virus-specific T-cell responses in African Swine Fever Virus protection and suggest the existence of multiple African Swine Fever Virus antigens with potential protective capacity.

Our recent approach using a combination of a variety of African Swine Fever Virus-specific proteins and cDNAs (heterologous prime-boost vaccine) was able to induce a robust immune response in terms of neutralizing antibodies and IFNγ production; however, vaccinated pigs were not protected against virulent challenge with the Armenia 2007 strain (Y. Revilla and J.A. Richt, personal communication).

In conclusion, DNA- and peptide-based vaccines have been shown to induce specific antiviral immune responses based on either neutralizing antibodies or virus-specific T-cells, but either no protection or only partial protection was afforded when vaccinated pigs were challenged with virulent African Swine Fever Virus.

6.5 The Future of African Swine Fever Virus Vaccinology

While an effective vaccine for ASF is not currently available, several vaccine approaches—as discussed in detail earlier—have demonstrated varying levels of protection. LAVs are the best hope for a protective ASF vaccine but some of them still do not offer good heterologous protection and suffer from side effects and safety issues (reversal to virulence). Detailed studies on the molecular mechanisms used by African Swine Fever Virus to modulate host immune responses and deleting respective virulence genes from the viral genome will most likely allow scientists in the near future to make safer LAVs without the above described negative effects. Producing LAVs, which afford heterologous protection against a variety of African Swine Fever Virus genotypes, will be much harder. In order to do this, crossprotective epitopes on African Swine Fever Virus-specific proteins have to be identified, and the role of cellular and humoral immune responses in protection against ASF needs to be elucidated. In contrast to LAVs, subunit protein/DNA ASF vaccines are safe and do not cause serious side effects, but only offer partial protection. This might be due to the delivery method or the requirement of different protective African Swine Fever Virus antigens in the vaccine mix. Since the role of the humoral and cellular arm of the adaptive immune system in protection against ASF is still not clear and the protective African Swine Fever Virus antigens are not defined, this approach at this time seems more a trial-and-error than a rationally designed approach. In addition to the open questions regarding the protective African Swine Fever Virus antigens, some of the viral proteins might induce antibodies which might enhance uptake of the virus into cells. Such an antibody-dependent enhancement could occur when virus-specific antibodies facilitate virus entry into host cells which carry Fc receptors on their surface. This could lead to a more rapid and severe disease after African Swine Fever Virus challenge of vaccinated animals. There is some evidence that immunopathological mechanisms are part of the ASF pathogenesis. Therefore, in order to rationally design future efficacious and safe LAVs and subunit vaccines, the detailed identification of virulence genes and the correlate of protective immune responses to African Swine Fever Virus infection need to be achieved. Molecular mechanisms used by the virus to modulate host immune responses, the role of African Swine Fever Virus protein in protection, and immunopathology, as well as the contribution of the innate and adaptive immune systems to protection need to be studied in detail. Only a significant investment into basic African Swine Fever Virus research will translate into a mitigation tool, i.e., vaccine, which can be safely used to avoid severe economic hardship for pig farmers around the world.

ACKNOWLEDGMENTS

The authors would like to acknowledge the DHS Center of Excellence for Emerging and Zoonotic Animal Diseases (CEEZAD) and Kansas State NBAF Transition Funds, provided by the State of Kansas, for supporting this work. This work was further supported by Kansas State University-CBMSO Contract #868 and by Ministerio de Ciencia e Innovación of Spain, BIO2013-46605.

REFERENCES

Abrams, C.C., Goatley, l., Fishbourne, E., Chapman, D., Cooke, l., Oura, C.A., Netherton, C.L., Takamatsu, H.H., Dixon, l.K., 2013. Deletion of virulence associated genes from attenuated African swine fever virus isolate OUR T88/3 decreases its ability to protect against challenge with virulent virus. Virology 443, 99–105.

Afonso, C.L., Zsak, L., Carrillo, C., Borca, M.V., Rock, D.L., 1998. African swine fever virus NL gene is not required for virus virulence. J. Gen. Virol. 79 (Pt. 10), 2543–2547.

Afonso, C.L., Piccone, M.E., Zaffuto, K.M., Neilan, J., Kutish, G.F., Lu, Z., Balinsky, C.A., Gibb, T.R., Bean, T.J., Zsak, L., Rock, D.L., 2004. African swine fever virus multigene family 360 and 530 genes affect host interferon response. J. Virol. 78, 1858–1864.

Alcami, A., Carrascosa, A.L., Vinuela, E., 1989a. The entry of African swine fever virus into Vero cells. Virology 171, 68–75.

Alcami, A., Carrascosa, A.L., Vinuela, E., 1989b. Saturable binding sites mediate the entry of African swine fever virus into Vero cells. Virology 168, 393–398.

Alcami, A., Carrascosa, A.L., Vinuela, E., 1990. Interaction of African swine fever virus with macrophages. Virus Res. 17, 93–104.

Alejo, A., Andres, G., Salas, M.L., 2003. African swine fever virus proteinase is essential for core maturation and infectivity. J. Virol. 77, 5571–5577.

Almazan, F., Rodriguez, J.M., Andres, G., Perez, R., Vinuela, E., Rodriguez, J.F., 1992. Transcriptional analysis of multigene family 110 of African swine fever virus. J. Virol. 66, 6655–6667.

Almendral, J.M., Almazan, F., Blasco, R., Vinuela, E., 1990. Multigene families in African swine fever virus: family 110. J. Virol. 64, 2064–2072.

Alvarez, B., Poderoso, T., Alonso, F., Ezquerra, A., Dominguez, J., Revilla, C., 2013. Antigen targeting to APC: from mice to veterinary species. Dev. Comp. Immunol. 41, 153–163.

Andres, G., 2017. African swine fever virus gets undressed: new insights on the entry pathway. J. Virol. 91, pii: e01906-16.

Andres, G., Simon-Mateo, C., Vinuela, E., 1997. Assembly of African swine fever virus: role of polyprotein pp220. J. Virol. 71, 2331–2341.

Andres, G., Garcia-Escudero, R., Simon-Mateo, C., Vinuela, E., 1998. African swine fever virus is enveloped by a two-membraned collapsed cisterna derived from the endoplasmic reticulum. J. Virol. 72, 8988–9001.

Andres, G., Alejo, A., Salas, J., Salas, M.L., 2002a. African swine fever virus polyproteins pp220 and pp62 assemble into the core shell. J. Virol. 76, 12473–12482.

Andres, G., Garcia-Escudero, R., Salas, M.L., Rodriguez, J.M., 2002b. Repression of African swine fever virus polyprotein pp220-encoding gene leads to the assembly of icosahedral core-less particles. J. Virol. 76, 2654–2666.

Argilaguet, J.M., Perez-Martin, E., Gallardo, C., Salguero, F.J., Borrego, B., Lacasta, A., Accensi, F., Diaz, I., Nofrarias, M., Pujols, J., Blanco, E., Perez-Filgueira, M., Escribano, J.M., Rodriguez, F., 2011. Enhancing DNA immunization by targeting African Swine Fever Virus antigens to SLA-II bearing cells. Vaccine 29, 5379–5385.

Argilaguet, J.M., Perez-Martin, E., Nofrarias, M., Gallardo, C., Accensi, F., Lacasta, A., Mora, M., Ballester, M., Galindo-Cardiel, I., Lopez-Soria, S., Escribano, J.M., Reche, P.A., Rodriguez, F., 2012. DNA vaccination partially protects against

African swine fever virus lethal challenge in the absence of antibodies. PLoS One 7, e40942.

Banjara, S., Caria, S., Dixon, L.K., Hinds, M.G., Kvansakul, M., 2017. Structural insight into African swine fever virus A179L-mediated inhibition of apoptosis. J. Virol. 91, pii: e02228-16.

Beattie, E., Denzler, K.L., Tartaglia, J., Perkus, M.E., Paoletti, E., Jacobs, B.L., 1995. Reversal of the interferon-sensitive phenotype of a vaccinia virus lacking E3L by expression of the reovirus S4 gene. J. Virol. 69, 499–505.

Biront, P., Castryck, F., Leunen, J., 1987. An epizootic of African swine fever in Belgium and its eradication. Vet. Rec. 120, 432–434.

Blome, S., Gabriel, C., Beer, M., 2013. Pathogenesis of African swine fever in domestic pigs and European wild boar. Virus Res. 173, 122–130.

Blome, S., Gabriel, C., Beer, M., 2014. Modern adjuvants do not enhance the efficacy of an inactivated African swine fever virus vaccine preparation. Vaccine 32, 3879–3882.

Boinas, F.S., Hutchings, G.H., Dixon, L.K., Wilkinson, P.J., 2004. Characterization of pathogenic and non-pathogenic African swine fever virus isolates from Ornithodoros erraticus inhabiting pig premises in Portugal. J. Gen. Virol. 85, 2177–2187.

Borca, M.V., Carrillo, C., Zsak, L., Laegreid, W.W., Kutish, G.F., Neilan, J.G., Burrage, T.G., Rock, D.L., 1998. Deletion of a CD2-like gene, 8-DR, from African swine fever virus affects viral infection in domestic swine. J. Virol. 72, 2881–2889.

Botija, C.S., 1982. African swine fever. New developments. Rev. Sci. Tech. 1, 1065–1094.

Breese Jr., S.S., Deboer, C.J., 1967. Chemical structure of African swine fever virus investigated by electron microscopy. J. Gen. Virol. 1, 251–252.

Bresnahan, P.A., Yonemoto, W., Ferrell, S., Williams-Herman, D., Geleziunas, R., Greene, W.C., 1998. A dileucine motif in HIV-1 Nef acts as an internalization signal for CD4 downregulation and binds the AP-1 clathrin adaptor. Curr. Biol. 8, 1235–1238.

Broyles, S.S., 2003. Vaccinia virus transcription. J. Gen. Virol. 84, 2293–2303.

Buchkovich, N.J., Yu, Y., Zampieri, C.A., Alwine, J.C., 2008. The TORrid affairs of viruses: effects of mammalian DNA viruses on the PI3K-Akt-mTOR signalling pathway. Nat. Rev. Microbiol. 6, 266–275.

Bushell, M., Mckendrick, L., Janicke, R.U., Clemens, M.J., Morley, S.J., 1999. Caspase-3 is necessary and sufficient for cleavage of protein synthesis eukaryotic initiation factor 4G during apoptosis. FEBS Lett. 451, 332–336.

Canagarajah, B.J., Ren, X., Bonifacino, J.S., Hurley, J.H., 2013. The clathrin adaptor complexes as a paradigm for membrane-associated allostery. Protein Sci. 22, 517–529.

Carrasco, L., De Lara, F.C., Martin De Las Mulas, J., Gomez-Villamandos, J.C., Hervas, J., Wilkinson, P.J., Sierra, M.A., 1996. Virus association with lymphocytes in acute African swine fever. Vet. Res. 27, 305–312.

Carrascosa, J.L., Carazo, J.M., Carrascosa, A.L., Garcia, N., Santisteban, A., Vinuela, E., 1984. General morphology and capsid fine structure of African swine fever virus particles. Virology 132, 160–172.

Carrascosa, A.L., Sastre, I., Vinuela, E., 1991. African swine fever virus attachment protein. J. Virol. 65, 2283–2289.

Carrascosa, A.L., Bustos, M.J., Galindo, I., Vinuela, E., 1999. Virus-specific cell receptors are necessary, but not sufficient, to confer cell susceptibility to African swine fever virus. Arch. Virol. 144, 1309–1321.

Castello, A., Izquierdo, J.M., Welnowska, E., Carrasco, L., 2009a. RNA nuclear export is blocked by poliovirus 2A protease and is concomitant with nucleoporin cleavage. J. Cell Sci. 122, 3799–3809.

Castello, A., Quintas, A., Sanchez, E.G., Sabina, P., Nogal, M., Carrasco, L., Revilla, Y., 2009b. Regulation of host translational machinery by African swine fever virus. PLoS Pathog. 5, e1000562.

Chapman, D.A., Tcherepanov, V., Upton, C., Dixon, L.K., 2008. Comparison of the genome sequences of non-pathogenic and pathogenic African swine fever virus isolates. J. Gen. Virol. 89, 397–408.

Cheng, Z.F., Deutscher, M.P., 2005. An important role for RNase R in mRNA decay. Mol. Cell 17, 313–318.

Chitko-Mckown, C.G., Chapes, S.K., Miller, L.C., Riggs, P.K., Ortega, M.T., Green, B.T., Mckown, R.D., 2013. Development and characterization of two porcine monocyte-derived macrophage cell lines. Res. Immunol. 3, 26–32.

Costard, S., Mur, L., Lubroth, J., Sanchez-Vizcaino, J.M., Pfeiffer, D.U., 2013. Epidemiology of African swine fever virus. Virus Res. 173, 191–197.

Covarrubias, S., Gaglia, M.M., Kumar, G.R., Wong, W., Jackson, A.O., Glaunsinger, B.A., 2011. Coordinated destruction of cellular messages in translation complexes by the gammaherpesvirus host shutoff factor and the mammalian exonuclease Xrn1. PLoS Pathog. 7, e1002339.

Cruz, L., Buchkovich, N.J., 2017. Rerouting the traffic from a virus perspective. Front. Biol. 22, 1845–1866.

Cuesta-Geijo, M.A., Galindo, I., Hernaez, B., Quetglas, J.I., Dalmau-Mena, I., Alonso, C., 2012. Endosomal maturation, Rab7 GTPase and phosphoinositides in African swine fever virus entry. PLoS One 7, e48853.

De Carvalho Ferreira, H.C., Backer, J.A., Weesendorp, E., Klinkenberg, D., Stegeman, J.A., Loeffen, W.L., 2013a. Transmission rate of African swine fever virus under experimental conditions. Vet. Microbiol. 165, 296–304.

De Carvalho Ferreira, H.C., Weesendorp, E., Quak, S., Stegeman, J.A., Loeffen, W.L., 2013b. Quantification of airborne African swine fever virus after experimental infection. Vet. Microbiol. 165, 243–251.

De la Torre, A., Bosch, J., Iglesias, I., Muñoz, M.J., Mur, L., Martínez-López, B., Martínez, M., Sánchez-Vizcaíno, J.M., 2015. Assessing the risk of African swine fever introduction into the European Union by wild boar. Transbound Emerg. Dis. 62 (3), 272–279. https://doi.org/10.1111/tbed.12129.

De Oliveira, V.L., Almeida, S.C., Soares, H.R., Crespo, A., Marshall-Clarke, S., Parkhouse, R.M., 2011. A novel TLR3 inhibitor encoded by African swine fever virus (ASFV). Arch. Virol. 156, 597–609.

De Villiers, E.P., Gallardo, C., Arias, M., Da Silva, M., Upton, C., Martin, R., Bishop, R.P., 2010. Phylogenomic analysis of 11 complete African swine fever virus genome sequences. Virology 400, 128–136.

Dixon, L.K., Chapman, D.A., Netherton, C.L., Upton, C., 2013. African swine fever virus replication and genomics. Virus Res. 173, 3–14.

European Food Safety Authority Panel on Animal Health and Welfare, 2010. Scientific opinion on African swine fever. EFSA J. 8 (3), 149 pp. https://doi.org/10.2903/j.efsa.2010.1556.

European Food Safety Authority, 2014. Evaluation of possible mitigation measures to prevent introduction and spread of African swine fever virus through wild boar. EFSA J. 12 (3), 3616, 23 pp. https://doi.org/10.2903/j.efsa.2014.3616.

ESFA AHAW Panel (EFSA Panel on Animal Health and Welfare), 2015. Scientific opinion on African swine fever. EFSA J. 13 (7), 4163, 92 pp. https://doi.org/10.2903/j.efsa.2015.41632015.

Enjuanes, L., Carrascosa, A.L., Moreno, M.A., Vinuela, E., 1976. Titration of African swine fever (ASF) virus. J. Gen. Virol. 32, 471–477.

Escribano, J.M., Galindo, I., Alonso, C., 2013. Antibody-mediated neutralization of African swine fever virus: myths and facts. Virus Res. 173, 101–109.

Esparza, I., González, J.C., Viñuela, E., 1998. Effect of interferon-alpha, interferon-gamma and tumour necrosis factor on African swine fever virus replication in porcine monocytes and macrophages. J. Gen. Virol. 69, 2973–2980.

Eurostat, 2013. Pig Population—Annual Data.

Ezquerra, A., Revilla, C., Alvarez, B., Perez, C., Alonso, F., Dominguez, J., 2009. Porcine myelomonocytic markers and cell populations. Dev. Comp. Immunol. 33, 284–298.

Fang, J., Hao, Q., Liu, L., Li, Y., Wu, J., Huo, X., Zhu, Y., 2012. Epigenetic changes mediated by microRNA miR29 activate cyclooxygenase 2 and lambda-1 interferon production during viral infection. J. Virol. 86, 1010–1020.

Forman, A.J., Wardley, R.C., Wilkinson, P.J., 1982. The immunological response of pigs and guinea pigs to antigens of African swine fever virus. Arch. Virol. 74, 91–100.

Galindo, I., Cuesta-Geijo, M.A., Hlavova, K., Munoz-Moreno, R., Barrado-gil, L., Dominguez, J., Alonso, C., 2015. African swine fever virus infects macrophages, the natural host cells, via clathrin- and cholesterol-dependent endocytosis. Virus Res. 200, 45–55.

Gallardo, C., Okoth, E., Pelayo, V., Anchuelo, R., Martin, E., Simon, A., Llorente, A., Nieto, R., Soler, A., Martin, R., Arias, M., Bishop, R.P., 2011. African swine fever viruses with two different genotypes, both of which occur in domestic pigs, are associated with ticks and adult warthogs, respectively, at a single geographical site. J. Gen. Virol. 92, 432–444.

Gallardo, C., Fernandez-Pinero, J., Pelayo, V., Gazaev, I., Markowska-Daniel, I., Pridotkas, G., Nieto, R., Fernandez-Pacheco, P., Bokhan, S., Nevolko, O., Drozhzhe, Z., Perez, C., Soler, A., Kolvasov, D., Arias, M., 2014. Genetic variation among African swine fever genotype II viruses, eastern and central Europe. Emerg. Infect. Dis. 20, 1544–1547.

Garcia-Escudero, R., Andres, G., Almazan, F., Vinuela, E., 1998. Inducible gene expression from African swine fever virus recombinants: analysis of the major capsid protein p72. J. Virol. 72, 3185–3195.

Garcia-Escudero, R., Garcia-Diaz, M., Salas, M.L., Blanco, L., Salas, J., 2003. DNA polymerase X of African swine fever virus: insertion fidelity on gapped DNA substrates and AP lyase activity support a role in base excision repair of viral DNA. J. Mol. Biol. 326, 1403–1412.

Gil, S., Sepulveda, N., Albina, E., Leitao, A., Martins, C., 2008. The low-virulent African swine fever virus (ASFV/NH/P68) induces enhanced expression and production of relevant regulatory cytokines (IFNalpha, TNFalpha and IL12p40) on porcine macrophages in comparison to the highly virulent African Swine Fever Virus/L60. Arch. Virol. 153, 1845–1854.

Goatley, L.C., Marron, M.B., Jacobs, S.C., Hammond, J.M., Miskin, J.E., Abrams, C.C., Smith, G.L., Dixon, L.K., 1999. Nuclear and nucleolar localization of an African swine fever virus protein, I14L, that is similar to the herpes simplex virus-encoded virulence factor ICP34.5. J. Gen. Virol. 80 (Pt. 3), 525–535.

Gogin, A., Gerasimov, V., Malogolovkin, A., Kolbasov, D., 2013. African swine fever in the North Caucasus region and the Russian Federation in years 2007-2012. Virus Res. 173, 198–203.

Golding, J.P., Goatley, L., Goodbourn, S., Dixon, L.K., Taylor, G., Netherton, C.L., 2016. Sensitivity of African swine fever virus to type I interferon is linked to genes within multigene families 360 and 505. Virology 493, 154–161.

Gomez-Puertas, P., Rodriguez, F., Oviedo, J.M., Ramiro-Ibanez, F., Ruiz-Gonzalvo, F., Alonso, C., Escribano, J.M., 1996. Neutralizing antibodies to different proteins of African swine fever virus inhibit both virus attachment and internalization. J. Virol. 70, 5689–5694.

Gomez-Puertas, P., Rodriguez, F., Oviedo, J.M., Brun, A., Alonso, C., Escribano, J.M., 1998. The African swine fever virus proteins p54 and p30 are involved in two distinct steps of virus attachment and both contribute to the antibody-mediated protective immune response. Virology 243, 461–471.

Gomez-Villamandos, J.C., Bautista, M.J., Sanchez-Cordon, P.J., Carrasco, L., 2013. Pathology of African swine fever: the role of monocyte-macrophage. Virus Res. 173, 140–149.

Gonzalez Juarrero, M., Mebus, C.A., Pan, R., Revilla, Y., Alonso, J.M., Lunney, J.K., 1992. Swine leukocyte antigen and macrophage marker expression on both African swine fever virus-infected and non-infected primary porcine macrophage cultures. Vet. Immunol. Immunopathol. 32, 243–259.

Goodman, R.H., Smolik, S., 2000. CBP/p300 in cell growth, transformation, and development. Genes Dev. 14, 1553–1577.

Gordon, S., Clarke, S., Greaves, D., Doyle, A., 1995. Molecular immunobiology of macrophages: recent progress. Curr. Opin. Immunol. 7, 24–33.

Granberg, F., Torresi, C., Oggiano, A., Malmberg, M., Iscaro, C., De Mia, G.M., Belak, S., 2016. Complete genome sequence of an African swine fever virus isolate from Sardinia, Italy. Genome Announc. 4, pii: e01220-16.

Granja, A.G., Nogal, M.L., Hurtado, C., Del Aguila, C., Carrascosa, A.L., Salas, M.L., Fresno, M., Revilla, Y., 2006a. The viral protein A238L inhibits TNF-alpha expression through a CBP/p300 transcriptional coactivators pathway. J. Immunol. 176, 451–462.

Granja, A.G., Sabina, P., Salas, M.L., Fresno, M., Revilla, Y., 2006b. Regulation of inducible nitric oxide synthase expression by viral A238L-mediated inhibition of p65/RelA acetylation and p300 transactivation. J. Virol. 80, 10487–10496.

Granja, A.G., Perkins, N.D., Revilla, Y., 2008. A238L inhibits NF-ATc2, NF-kappa B, and c-Jun activation through a novel mechanism involving protein kinase C-theta-mediated up-regulation of the amino-terminal transactivation domain of p300. J. Immunol. 180, 2429–2442.

Granja, A.G., Sanchez, E.G., Sabina, P., Fresno, M., Revilla, Y., 2009. African swine fever virus blocks the host cell antiviral inflammatory response through a direct inhibition of PKC-theta-mediated p300 transactivation. J. Virol. 83, 969–980.

Heath, C.M., Windsor, M., Wileman, T., 2001. Aggresomes resemble sites specialized for virus assembly. J. Cell Biol. 153, 449–455.

Hernaez, B., Alonso, C., 2010. Dynamin- and clathrin-dependent endocytosis in African swine fever virus entry. J. Virol. 84, 2100–2109.

Hernaez, B., Guerra, M., Salas, M.L., Andres, G., 2016. African swine fever virus undergoes outer envelope disruption, capsid disassembly and inner envelope fusion before core release from multivesicular endosomes. PLoS Pathog. 12, e1005595.

Hurtado, C., Granja, A.G., Bustos, M.J., Nogal, M.L., Gonzalez De Buitrago, G., De Yebenes, V.G., Salas, M.L., Revilla, Y., Carrascosa, A.L., 2004. The C-type lectin homologue gene (EP153R) of African swine fever virus inhibits apoptosis both in virus infection and in heterologous expression. Virology 326, 160–170.

Hurtado, C., Bustos, M.J., Carrascosa, A.L., 2010. The use of COS-1 cells for studies of field and laboratory African swine fever virus samples. J. Virol. Methods 164, 131–134.

Hurtado, C., Bustos, M.J., Granja, A.G., De Leon, P., Sabina, P., Lopez-Vinas, E., Gomez-Puertas, P., Revilla, Y., Carrascosa, A.L., 2011. The African swine fever virus lectin EP153R modulates the surface membrane expression of MHC class I antigens. Arch. Virol. 156, 219–234.

Iglesias, I., Rodriguez, A., Feliziani, F., Rolesu, S., De La Torre, A., 2017. Spatio-temporal analysis of African swine fever in Sardinia (2012-2014): trends in domestic pigs and wild boar. Transbound. Emerg. Dis. 64, 656–662.

Janelle, M.E., Gravel, A., Gosselin, J., Tremblay, M.J., Flamand, L., 2002. Activation of monocyte cyclooxygenase-2 gene expression by human herpesvirus 6. Role for cyclic AMP-responsive element-binding protein and activator protein-1. J. Biol. Chem. 277, 30665–30674.

Jezewska, M.J., Marcinowicz, A., Lucius, A.L., Bujalowski, W., 2006. DNA polymerase X from African swine fever virus: quantitative analysis of the enzyme-ssDNA interactions and the functional structure of the complex. J. Mol. Biol. 356, 121–141.

Karalyan, Z., Zakaryan, H., Arzumanyan, H., Sargsyan, K., Voskanyan, H., Hakobyan, L., Abroyan, L., Avetisyan, A., Karalova, E., 2012a. Pathology of porcine peripheral white blood cells during infection with African swine fever virus. BMC Vet. Res. 8, 18.

Karalyan, Z., Zakaryan, H., Sargsyan, K., Voskanyan, H., Arzumanyan, H., Avagyan, H., Karalova, E., 2012b. Interferon status and white blood cells during infection with African swine fever virus in vivo. Vet. Immunol. Immunopathol. 145, 551–555.

Kay-Jackson, P.C., Goatley, L.C., Cox, L., Miskin, J.E., Parkhouse, R.M., Wienands, J., Dixon, L.K., 2004. The CD2v protein of African swine fever virus interacts with the actin-binding adaptor protein SH3P7. J. Gen. Virol. 85, 119–130.

Keil, G.M., Giesow, K., Portugal, R., 2014. A novel bromodeoxyuridine-resistant wild boar lung cell line facilitates generation of African swine fever virus recombinants. Arch. Virol. 159, 2421–2428.

Khoo, D., Perez, C., Mohr, I., 2002. Characterization of RNA determinants recognized by the arginine- and proline-rich region of Us11, a herpes simplex virus type 1-encoded double-stranded RNA binding protein that prevents PKR activation. J. Virol. 76, 11971–11981.

Kimball, S.R., Jefferson, L.S., Nguyen, H.V., Suryawan, A., Bush, J.A., Davis, T.A., 2000. Feeding stimulates protein synthesis in muscle and liver of neonatal pigs through an mTOR-dependent process. Am. J. Physiol. Endocrinol. Metab. 279, E1080–7.

King, K., Chapman, D., Argilaguet, J.M., Fishbourne, E., Hutet, E., Cariolet, R., Hutchings, G., Oura, C.A., Netherton, C.L., Moffat, K., Taylor, G., Le Potier, M.F., Dixon, L.K., Takamatsu, H.H., 2011. Protection of European domestic pigs from virulent African isolates of African swine fever virus by experimental immunisation. Vaccine 29, 4593–4600.

Kuznar, J., Salas, M.L., Vinuela, E., 1980. DNA-dependent RNA polymerase in African swine fever virus. Virology 101, 169–175.

Lacasta, A., Ballester, M., Monteagudo, P.L., Rodriguez, J.M., Salas, M.L., Accensi, F., Pina-Pedrero, S., Bensaid, A., Argilaguet, J., Lopez-Soria, S., Hutet, E., Le Potier, M.F., Rodriguez, F., 2014. Expression library immunization can confer protection against lethal challenge with African swine fever virus. J. Virol. 88, 13322–13332.

Law, S.K., Micklem, K.J., Shaw, J.M., Zhang, X.P., Dong, Y., Willis, A.C., Mason, D.Y., 1993. A new macrophage differentiation antigen which is a member of the scavenger receptor superfamily. Eur. J. Immunol. 23, 2320–2325.

Lee, Y.J., Lee, C., 2010. Deletion of the cytoplasmic domain of CD163 enhances porcine reproductive and respiratory syndrome virus replication. Arch. Virol. 155, 1319–1323.

Leitao, A., Cartaxeiro, C., Coelho, R., Cruz, B., Parkhouse, R.M., Portugal, F., Vigario, J.D., Martins, C.L., 2001. The non-haemadsorbing African swine fever virus isolate ASFV/NH/P68 provides a model for defining the protective anti-virus immune response. J. Gen. Virol. 82, 513–523.

Lithgow, P., Takamatsu, H., Werling, D., Dixon, L., Chapman, D., 2014. Correlation of cell surface marker expression with African swine fever virus infection. Vet. Microbiol. 168, 413–419.

Lloyd, R.M., Shatkin, A.J., 1992. Translational stimulation by reovirus polypeptide sigma 3: substitution for VAI RNA and inhibition of phosphorylation of the alpha subunit of eukaryotic initiation factor 2. J. Virol. 66, 6878–6884.

López-Monteagudo, P.L.A., Gallei, A., Veljko, N., Rodriguez, J., López, E., Pina, S., Acensi, F., Navas, M.J., Collado, J., Correa-Fiz, M.F., Bosch, L., Salas, M.L., Rodriguez, F., 2016. In: Experimental Characterization of a Recombinant Live Attenuated African Swine Fever Virus with Crossprotective Capabilities. Epizone 10th Annual Meeting. Madrid.

Lubisi, B.A., Bastos, A.D., Dwarka, R.M., Vosloo, W., 2007. Intra-genotypic resolution of African swine fever viruses from an East African domestic pig cycle: a combined p72-CVR approach. Virus Genes 35, 729–735.

Madrid, R., Janvier, K., Hitchin, D., Day, J., Coleman, S., Noviello, C., Bouchet, J., Benmerah, A., Guatelli, J., Benichou, S., 2005. Nef-induced alteration of the early/recycling endosomal compartment correlates with enhancement of HIV-1 infectivity. J. Biol. Chem. 280, 5032–5044.

Malogolovkin, A., Burmakina, G., Tulman, E.R., Delhon, G., Diel, D.G., Salnikov, N., Kutish, G.F., Kolbasov, D., Rock, D.L., 2015. African swine fever virus CD2v and C-type lectin gene loci mediate serological specificity. J. Gen. Virol. 96, 866–873.

Marissen, W.E., Lloyd, R.E., 1998. Eukaryotic translation initiation factor 4G is targeted for proteolytic cleavage by caspase 3 during inhibition of translation in apoptotic cells. Mol. Cell. Biol. 18, 7565–7574.

Martinez-Lopez, B., Perez, A.M., Feliziani, F., Rolesu, S., Mur, L., Sanchez-Vizcaino, J.M., 2015. Evaluation of the risk factors contributing to the African swine fever occurrence in Sardinia, Italy. Front. Microbiol. 6, 314.

Massei, G., Kindberg, J., Licoppe, A., Gacic, D., Sprem, N., Kamler, J., Baubet, E., Hohmann, U., Monaco, A., Ozolins, J., Cellina, S., Podgorski, T., Fonseca, C., Markov, N., Pokorny, B., Rosell, C., Nahlik, A., 2015. Wild boar populations up, numbers of hunters down? A review of trends and implications for Europe. Pest Manag. Sci. 71 (4), 492–500.

Mccullough, K.C., Basta, S., Knotig, S., Gerber, H., Schaffner, R., Kim, Y.B., Saalmuller, A., Summerfield, A., 1999. Intermediate stages in monocyte-macrophage differentiation modulate phenotype and susceptibility to virus infection. Immunology 98, 203–212.

Mclennan, A.G., 2007. Decapitation: poxvirus makes RNA lose its head. Trends Biochem. Sci. 32, 297–299.

Mebus, C.A., Dardiri, A.H., 1980. Western hemisphere isolates of African swine fever virus: asymptomatic carriers and resistance to challenge inoculation. Am. J. Vet. Res. 41, 1867–1869.

Miskin, J.E., Abrams, C.C., Goatley, L.C., Dixon, L.K., 1998. A viral mechanism for inhibition of the cellular phosphatase calcineurin. Science 281, 562–565.

Mori, Y., Koike, M., Moriishi, E., Kawabata, A., Tang, H., Oyaizu, H., Uchiyama, Y., Yamanishi, K., 2008. Human herpesvirus-6 induces MVB formation, and virus egress occurs by an exosomal release pathway. Traffic 9, 1728–1742.

Mulumba-Mfumu, L.K., Goatley, L.C., Saegerman, C., Takamatsu, H.H., Dixon, L.K., 2016. Immunization of African indigenous pigs with attenuated genotype I African swine fever virus OURT88/3 induces protection against challenge with virulent strains of genotype I. Transbound. Emerg. Dis. 63, e323–7.

Mulvey, M., Poppers, J., Ladd, A., Mohr, I., 1999. A herpesvirus ribosome-associated, RNA-binding protein confers a growth advantage upon mutants deficient in a GADD34-related function. J. Virol. 73, 3375–3385.

Mulvey, M., Poppers, J., Sternberg, D., Mohr, I., 2003. Regulation of eIF2alpha phosphorylation by different functions that act during discrete phases in the herpes simplex virus type 1 life cycle. J. Virol. 77, 10917–10928.

Munoz, M., Freije, J.M., Salas, M.L., Vinuela, E., Lopez-Otin, C., 1993. Structure and expression in E. coli of the gene coding for protein p10 of African swine fever virus. Arch. Virol. 130, 93–107.

Munoz-Moreno, R., Galindo, I., Cuesta-Geijo, M.A., Barrado-Gil, L., Alonso, C., 2015. Host cell targets for African swine fever virus. Virus Res. 209, 118–127.

Mur, L., Martinez-Lopez, B., Martinez-Aviles, M., Costard, S., Wieland, B., Pfeiffer, D.U., Sanchez-Vizcaino, J.M., 2012a. Quantitative risk assessment for the introduction of African swine fever virus into the European Union by legal import of live pigs. Transbound. Emerg. Dis. 59, 134–144.

Mur, L., Martinez-Lopez, B., Sanchez-Vizcaino, J.M., 2012b. Risk of African swine fever introduction into the European Union through transport-associated routes: returning trucks and waste from international ships and planes. BMC Vet. Res. 8, 149.

Murono, S., Inoue, H., Tanabe, T., Joab, I., Yoshizaki, T., Furukawa, M., Pagano, J.S., 2001. Induction of cyclooxygenase-2 by Epstein-Barr virus latent membrane protein 1 is involved in vascular endothelial growth factor production in nasopharyngeal carcinoma cells. Proc. Natl. Acad. Sci. U.S.A. 98, 6905–6910.

Nakatsu, F., Ohno, H., 2003. Adaptor protein complexes as the key regulators of protein sorting in the post-Golgi network. Cell Struct. Funct. 28, 419–429.

Neilan, J.G., Zsak, L., Lu, Z., Burrage, T.G., Kutish, G.F., Rock, D.L., 2004. Neutralizing antibodies to African swine fever virus proteins p30, p54, and p72 are not sufficient for antibody-mediated protection. Virology 319, 337–342.

Netherton, C., Moffat, K., Brooks, E., Wileman, T., 2007. A guide to viral inclusions, membrane rearrangements, factories, and viroplasm produced during virus replication. Adv. Virus Res. 70, 101–182.

Nogal, M.L., Gonzalez De Buitrago, G., Rodriguez, C., Cubelos, B., Carrascosa, A.L., Salas, M.L., Revilla, Y., 2001. African swine fever virus Iap homologue inhibits caspase activation and promotes cell survival in mammalian cells. J. Virol. 75, 2535–2543.

O'donnell, V., Holinka, L.G., Sanford, B., Krug, P.W., Carlson, J., Pacheco, J.M., Reese, B., Risatti, G.R., Gladue, D.P., Borca, M.V., 2016. African swine fever virus Georgia isolate harboring deletions of 9GL and MGF360/505 genes is highly attenuated in swine but does not confer protection against parental virus challenge. Virus Res. 221, 8–14.

OIE, 2012. African Swine Fever. Manual of Diagnostic Tests and Vaccines for Terrestrial Animals. www.oie.int/en/internationalstandard-setting/terrestrial-manual/accessonline.

O'keeffe, M., Fancke, B., Suter, M., Ramm, G., Clark, J., Wu, L., Hochrein, H., 2012. Nonplasmacytoid, high IfN-alpha-producing, bone marrow dendritic cells. J. Immunol. 188, 3774–3783.

Onisk, D.V., Borca, M.V., Kutish, G., Kramer, E., Irusta, P., Rock, D.L., 1994. Passively transferred African swine fever virus antibodies protect swine against lethal infection. Virology 198, 350–354.

Paez, E., Garcia, F., Gil Fernandez, C., 1990. Interferon cures cells lytically and persistently infected with African swine fever virus in vitro. Arch. Virol. 112, 115–127.

Park, N., Katikaneni, P., Skern, T., Gustin, K.E., 2008. Differential targeting of nuclear pore complex proteins in poliovirus-infected cells. J. Virol. 82, 1647–1655.

Parrish, S., Moss, B., 2007. Characterization of a second vaccinia virus mRNA-decapping enzyme conserved in poxviruses. J. Virol. 81, 12973–12978.

Parrish, S., Resch, W., Moss, B., 2007. Vaccinia virus D10 protein has mRNA decapping activity, providing a mechanism for control of host and viral gene expression. Proc. Natl. Acad. Sci. U.S.A. 104, 2139–2144.

Parrish, S., Hurchalla, M., Liu, S.W., Moss, B., 2009. The African swine fever virus g5R protein possesses mRNA decapping activity. Virology 393, 177–182.

Pena, L., Yanez, R.J., Revilla, Y., Vinuela, E., Salas, M.L., 1993. African swine fever virus guanylyltransferase. Virology 193, 319–328.

Penrith, M.L., Vosloo, W., 2009. Review of African swine fever: transmission, spread and control. J. S. Afr. Vet. Assoc. 80, 58–62.

Penrith, M.L., Vosloo, W., Jori, F., Bastos, A.D., 2013. African swine fever virus eradication in Africa. Virus Res. 173, 228–246.

Perez-Nunez, D., Garcia-Urdiales, E., Martinez-Bonet, M., Nogal, M.L., Barroso, S., Revilla, Y., Madrid, R., 2015. CD2v interacts with adaptor protein AP-1 during African swine fever infection. PLoS One 10, e0123714.

Poderoso, T., Martinez, P., Alvarez, B., Handler, A., Moreno, S., Alonso, F., Ezquerra, A., Dominguez, J., Revilla, C., 2011. Delivery of antigen to sialoadhesin or CD163 improves the specific immune response in pigs. Vaccine 29, 4813–4820.

Pollara, J.J., Spesock, A.H., Pickup, D.J., Laster, S.M., Petty, I.T., 2012. Production of prostaglandin E(2) in response to infection with modified vaccinia Ankara virus. Virology 428, 146–155.

Popescu, L., Gaudreault, N.N., Whitworth, K.M., Murgia, M.V., Nietfeld, J.C., Mileham, A., Samuel, M., Wells, K.D., Prather, R.S., Rowland, R.R., 2017. Genetically edited pigs lacking CD163 show no resistance following infection with the African swine fever virus isolate, Georgia 2007/1. Virology 501, 102–106.

Portugal, R., Coelho, J., Hoper, D., Little, N.S., Smithson, C., Upton, C., Martins, C., Leitao, A., Keil, G.M., 2015. Related strains of African swine fever virus with different virulence: genome comparison and analysis. J. Gen. Virol. 96, 408–419.

Powell, P.P., Dixon, L.K., Parkhouse, R.M., 1996. An IkappaB homolog encoded by African swine fever virus provides a novel mechanism for downregulation of proinflammatory cytokine responses in host macrophages. J. Virol. 70, 8527–8533.

Prevot, D., Darlix, J.L., Ohlmann, T., 2003. Conducting the initiation of protein synthesis: the role of eif4G. Biol. Cell 95, 141–156.

Pyronnet, S., 2000. Phosphorylation of the cap-binding protein eIF4E by the MAPK-activated protein kinase Mnk1. Biochem. Pharmacol. 60, 1237–1243.

Pyronnet, S., Imataka, H., Gingras, A.C., Fukunaga, R., Hunter, T., Sonenberg, N., 1999. Human eukaryotic translation initiation factor 4G (eIF4G) recruits mnk1 to phosphorylate eIF4E. EMBO J. 18, 270–279.

Quintas, A., Perez-Nunez, D., Sanchez, E.G., Nogal, M.L., Hentze, M.W., Castello, A., Revilla, Y., 2017. Characterization of the African swine fever virus decapping enzyme during infection. J Virol. pii: JVI.00990-17.

Raught, B., Gingras, A.C., Gygi, S.P., Imataka, H., Morino, S., Gradi, A., Aebersold, R., Sonenberg, N., 2000. Serum-stimulated, rapamycin-sensitive phosphorylation sites in the eukaryotic translation initiation factor 4GI. EMBO J. 19, 434–444.

Redrejo-Rodriguez, M., Garcia-Escudero, R., Yanez-Munoz, R.J., Salas, M.L., Salas, J., 2006. African swine fever virus protein pE296R is a DNA repair apurinic/apyrimidinic endonuclease required for virus growth in swine macrophages. J. Virol. 80, 4847–4857.

Reis, A.L., Abrams, C.C., Goatley, L.C., Netherton, C., Chapman, D.G., Sanchez-Cordon, P., Dixon, L.K., 2016. Deletion of African swine fever virus interferon inhibitors from the genome of a virulent isolate reduces virulence in domestic pigs and induces a protective response. Vaccine 34, 4698–4705.

Revilla, Y., Pena, L., Vinuela, E., 1992. Interferon-gamma production by African swine fever virus-specific lymphocytes. Scand. J. Immunol. 35, 225–230.

Revilla, Y., Cebrian, A., Baixeras, E., Martinez, C., Vinuela, E., Salas, M.L., 1997. Inhibition of apoptosis by the African swine fever virus Bcl-2 homologue: role of the BH1 domain. Virology 228, 400–404.

Revilla, Y., Callejo, M., Rodriguez, J.M., Culebras, E., Nogal, M.L., Salas, M.L., Vinuela, E., Fresno, M., 1998. Inhibition of nuclear factor kappaB activation by a virus-encoded IkappaB-like protein. J. Biol. Chem. 273, 5405–5411.

Ribeiro, 1982. Déclaration sur la vaccination contre la Peste Porcine Africaine à la XXXe Session Générale de l'Office International des Epizooties. Bull. Off. Int. Epizoot. 58, 1031–1040.

Richner, J.M., Clyde, K., Pezda, A.C., Cheng, B.Y., Wang, T., Kumar, G.R., Covarrubias, S., Coscoy, L., Glaunsinger, B., 2011. Global mRNA degradation during lytic gammaherpesvirus infection contributes to establishment of viral latency. PLoS Pathog. 7, e1002150.

Rivera, J., Abrams, C., Hernaez, B., Alcazar, A., Escribano, J.M., Dixon, L., Alonso, C., 2007. The MyD116 African swine fever virus homologue interacts with the catalytic subunit of protein phosphatase 1 and activates its phosphatase activity. J. Virol. 81, 2923–2929.

Rodriguez, J.M., Salas, M.L., 2013. African swine fever virus transcription. Virus Res. 173, 15–28.

Rodriguez, J.M., Yanez, R.J., Almazan, F., Vinuela, E., Rodriguez, J.F., 1993. African swine fever virus encodes a CD2 homolog responsible for the adhesion of erythrocytes to infected cells. J. Virol. 67, 5312–5320.

Rodriguez, C.I., Nogal, M.L., Carrascosa, A.L., Salas, M.L., Fresno, M., Revilla, Y., 2002. African swine fever virus IAP-like protein induces the activation of nuclear factor kappa B. J. Virol. 76, 3936–3942.

Rodriguez, J.M., Garcia-Escudero, R., Salas, M.L., Andres, G., 2004. African swine fever virus structural protein p54 is essential for the recruitment of envelope precursors to assembly sites. J. Virol. 78, 4299–4313.

Rodriguez, J.M., Moreno, L.T., Alejo, A., Lacasta, A., Rodriguez, F., Salas, M.L., 2015. Genome sequence of African swine fever virus BA71, the virulent parental strain of the nonpathogenic and tissue-culture adapted BA71V. PLoS One 10, e0142889.

Rojo, G., Chamorro, M., Salas, M.L., Vinuela, E., Cuezva, J.M., Salas, J., 1998. Migration of mitochondria to viral assembly sites in African swine fever virus-infected cells. J. Virol. 72, 7583–7588.

Ruiz-Gonzalvo, F., Rodriguez, F., Escribano, J.M., 1996. Functional and immunological properties of the baculovirus-expressed hemagglutinin of African swine fever virus. Virology 218, 285–289.

Salas, M.L., Andres, G., 2013. African swine fever virus morphogenesis. Virus Res. 173, 29–41.

Salas, M.L., Kuznar, J., Vinuela, E., 1981. Polyadenylation, methylation, and capping of the RNA synthesized in vitro by African swine fever virus. Virology 113, 484–491.

Salas, M.L., Kuznar, J., Vinuela, E., 1983. Effect of rifamycin derivatives and coumermycin A1 on in vitro RNA synthesis by African swine fever virus. Brief report. Arch. Virol. 77, 77–80.

Salas, M.L., Rey-Campos, J., Almendral, J.M., Talavera, A., Vinuela, E., 1986. Transcription and translation maps of African swine fever virus. Virology 152, 228–240.

Salvatore, M., Basler, C.F., Parisien, J.P., Horvath, C.M., Bourmakina, S., Zheng, H., Muster, T., Palese, P., Garcia-Sastre, A., 2002. Effects of influenza A virus NS1 protein on protein expression: the NS1 protein enhances translation and is not required for shut-off of host protein synthesis. J. Virol. 76, 1206–1212.

Sanchez, C., Domenech, N., Vazquez, J., Alonso, F., Ezquerra, A., Dominguez, J., 1999. The porcine 2A10 antigen is homologous to human CD163 and related to macrophage differentiation. J. Immunol. 162, 5230–5237.

Sanchez, E.G., Quintas, A., Perez-Nunez, D., Nogal, M., Barroso, S., Carrascosa, A.L., Revilla, Y., 2012. African swine fever virus uses macropinocytosis to enter host cells. PLoS Pathog. 8, e1002754.

Sanchez, E.G., Quintas, A., Nogal, M., Castello, A., Revilla, Y., 2013. African swine fever virus controls the host transcription and cellular machinery of protein synthesis. Virus Res. 173, 58–75.

Sanchez, E.G., Riera, E., Nogal, M., Gallardo, C., Fernandez, P., Bello-Morales, R., Lopez-Guerrero, J.A., Chitko-McKown, C.G., Richt, J.A., Revilla, Y., 2017. Phenotyping and susceptibility of established porcine cells lines to African Swine Fever Virus infection and viral production. Sci. Rep. 7 (1), 10369.

Sanchez-Torres, C., Gomez-Puertas, P., Gomez-Del-Moral, M., Alonso, F., Escribano, J.M., Ezquerra, A., Dominguez, J., 2003. Expression of porcine CD163 on monocytes/macrophages correlates with permissiveness to African swine fever infection. Arch. Virol. 148, 2307–2323.

Sanchez-Vizcaino, J.M., Mur, L., Martinez-Lopez, B., 2012. African swine fever: an epidemiological update. Transbound. Emerg. Dis. 59 (Suppl. 1), 27–35.

Sanchez-Vizcaino, J.M., Mur, L., Martinez-Lopez, B., 2013. African swine fever (ASF): five years around Europe. Vet. Microbiol. 165, 45–50.

Sandri-Goldin, R.M., 2011. The many roles of the highly interactive HSV protein ICP27, a key regulator of infection. Future Microbiol. 6, 1261–1277.

Santaren, J.F., Vinuela, E., 1986. African swine fever virus-induced polypeptides in Vero cells. Virus Res. 5, 391–405.

Satterly, N., Tsai, P.L., Van Deursen, J., Nussenzveig, D.R., Wang, Y., Faria, P.A., Levay, A., Levy, D.E., Fontoura, B.M., 2007. Influenza virus targets the mRNA export machinery and the nuclear pore complex. Proc. Natl. Acad. Sci. U.S.A. 104, 1853–1858.

Schneider, R.J., Mohr, I., 2003. Translation initiation and viral tricks. Trends Biochem. Sci. 28, 130–136.

Stamnes, M.A., Rothman, J.E., 1993. The binding of Ap-1 clathrin adaptor particles to Golgi membranes requires ADP-ribosylation factor, a small GTP-binding protein. Cell 73, 999–1005.

Steer, S.A., Moran, J.M., Maggi, L.B.J., Buller, R.M., Perlman, H., Corbett, J.A., 2003. Regulation of cyclooxygenase-2 expression by macrophages in response to double-stranded RNA and viral infection. J. Immunol. 170, 1070–1076.

Stone, S.S., Hess, W.R., 1967. Antibody response to inactivated preparations of African swine fever virus in pigs. Am. J. Vet. Res. 28, 475–481.

Suarez, C., Gutierrez-Berzal, J., Andres, G., Salas, M.L., Rodriguez, J.M., 2010. African swine fever virus protein p17 is essential for the progression of viral membrane precursors toward icosahedral intermediates. J. Virol. 84, 7484–7499.

Tait, S.W., Reid, E.B., Greaves, D.R., Wileman, T.E., Powell, P.P., 2000. Mechanism of inactivation of NF-kappa B by a viral homologue of I kappa b alpha. Signal-induced release of I kappa b alpha results in binding of the viral homologue to NF-kappa B. J. Biol. Chem. 275, 34656–34664.

Thomson, G.R., Gainaru, M.D., Van Dellen, A.F., 1979. African swine fever: pathogenicity and immunogenicity of two non-haemadsorbing viruses. Onderstepoort J. Vet. Res. 46, 149–154.

Tong, X., Boll, W., Kirchhausen, T., Howley, P.M., 1998. Interaction of the bovine papillomavirus E6 protein with the clathrin adaptor complex AP-1. J. Virol. 72, 476–482.

Tung, W.H., Hsieh, H.L., Lee, I.T., Yang, C.M., 2011. Enterovirus 71 modulates a COX-2/PGE2/cAMP-dependent viral replication in human neuroblastoma cells: role of the c-Src/EGFR/p42/p44 MAPK/CREB signaling pathway. J. Cell. Biochem. 112, 559–570.

Valdeira, M.L., Geraldes, A., 1985. Morphological study on the entry of African swine fever virus into cells. Biol. Cell 55, 35–40.

Valdeira, M.L., Bernardes, C., Cruz, B., Geraldes, A., 1998. Entry of African swine fever virus into Vero cells and uncoating. Vet. Microbiol. 60, 131–140.

Van Furth, R., Cohn, Z.A., Hirsch, J.G., Humphrey, J.H., Spector, W.G., Langevoort, H.L., 1972. The mononuclear phagocyte system: a new classification of macrophages, monocytes, and their precursor cells. Bull. World Health Organ. 46, 845–852.

Vinuela, E., 1985. African swine fever virus. Curr. Top. Microbiol. Immunol. 116, 151–170.

Vo, N., Goodman, R.H., 2001. CREB-binding protein and p300 in transcriptional regulation. J. Biol. Chem. 276, 13505–13508.

Von Kobbe, C., Van Deursen, J.M., Rodrigues, J.P., Sitterlin, D., Bachi, A., Wu, X., Wilm, M., Carmo-Fonseca, M., Izaurralde, E., 2000. Vesicular stomatitis virus matrix protein inhibits host cell gene expression by targeting the nucleoporin Nup98. Mol. Cell 6, 1243–1252.

Walsh, D., Mohr, I., 2004. Phosphorylation of eif4E by Mnk-1 enhances HSV-1 translation and replication in quiescent cells. Genes Dev. 18, 660–672.

Walsh, D., Mohr, I., 2011. Viral subversion of the host protein synthesis machinery. Nat. Rev. Microbiol. 9, 860–875.

Walsh, D., Perez, C., Notary, J., Mohr, I., 2005. Regulation of the translation initiation factor eIF4F by multiple mechanisms in human cytomegalovirus-infected cells. J. Virol. 79, 8057–8064.

Walsh, D., Arias, C., Perez, C., Halladin, D., Escandon, M., Ueda, T., Watanabe-Fukunaga, R., Fukunaga, R., Mohr, I., 2008. Eukaryotic translation initiation factor 4F architectural alterations accompany translation initiation factor redistribution in poxvirus-infected cells. Mol. Cell. Biol. 28, 2648–2658.

Wardley, R.C., Hamilton, F., Wilkinson, P.J., 1979. The replication of virulent and attenuated strains of African swine fever virus in porcine macrophages. Arch. Virol. 61, 217–225.

Weingartl, H.M., Sabara, M., Pasick, J., Van Moorlehem, E., Babiuk, L., 2002. Continuous porcine cell lines developed from alveolar macrophages: partial characterization and virus susceptibility. J. Virol. Methods 104, 203–216.

Windsor, M., Hawes, P., Monaghan, P., Snapp, E., Salas, M.L., Rodriguez, J.M., Wileman, T., 2012. Mechanism of collapse of endoplasmic reticulum cisternae during African swine fever virus infection. Traffic 13, 30–42.

Wozniakowski, G., Kozak, E., Kowalczyk, A., Lyjak, M., Pomorska-Mol, M., Niemczuk, K., Pejsak, Z., 2016. Current status of African swine fever virus in a population of wild boar in eastern Poland (2014–2015). Arch. Virol. 161, 189–195.

Yanez, R.J., Rodriguez, J.M., Nogal, M.L., Yuste, L., Enriquez, C., Rodriguez, J.F., Vinuela, E., 1995. Analysis of the complete nucleotide sequence of African swine fever virus. Virology 208, 249–278.

Yatherajam, G., Huang, W., Flint, S.J., 2011. Export of adenoviral late mRNA from the nucleus requires the Nxf1/Tap export receptor. J. Virol. 85, 1429–1438.

Yutin, N., Wolf, Y.I., Raoult, D., Koonin, E.V., 2009. Eukaryotic large nucleo-cytoplasmic DNA viruses: clusters of orthologous genes and reconstruction of viral genome evolution. Virol. J. 6, 223.

Zakaryan, H., Karalova, E., Voskanyan, H., Ter-Pogossyan, Z., Nersisyan, N., Hakobyan, A., Saroyan, D., Karalyan, Z., 2014. Evaluation of hemostaseological status of pigs experimentally infected with African swine fever virus. Vet. Microbiol. 174, 223–228.

Zhang, F., Hopwood, P., Abrams, C.C., Downing, A., Murray, F., Talbot, R., Archibald, A., Lowden, S., Dixon, L.K., 2006. Macrophage transcriptional responses following in vitro infection with a highly virulent African swine fever virus isolate. J. Virol. 80, 10514–10521.

Zhang, F., Moon, A., Childs, K., Goodbourn, S., Dixon, L.K., 2010. The African swine fever virus Dp71L protein recruits the protein phosphatase 1 catalytic subunit to dephosphorylate eIF2alpha and inhibits CHOP induction but is dispensable for these activities during virus infection. J. Virol. 84, 10681–10689.

Zsak, L., Lu, Z., Kutish, G.F., Neilan, J.G., Rock, D.L., 1996. An African swine fever virus virulence-associated gene NL-S with similarity to the herpes simplex virus ICP34.5 gene. J. Virol. 70, 8865–8871.

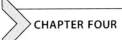

CHAPTER FOUR

Morbillivirus Pathogenesis and Virus–Host Interactions

Kristin Pfeffermann, Mareike Dörr, Florian Zirkel, Veronika von Messling[1]
Paul-Ehrlich-Institut, Langen, Germany
[1]Corresponding author: e-mail address: veronika.vonmessling@pei.de

Contents

Abstract

Despite the availability of safe and effective vaccines against measles and several animal morbilliviruses, they continue to cause regular outbreaks and epidemics in susceptible populations. Morbilliviruses are highly contagious and share a similar pathogenesis in their respective hosts. This review provides an overview of morbillivirus history and the general replication cycle and recapitulates Morbillivirus pathogenesis focusing on common and unique aspects seen in different hosts. It also summarizes the state of knowledge regarding virus–host interactions on the cellular level with an emphasis on viral interference with innate immune response activation, and highlights remaining knowledge gaps.

Advances in Virus Research, Volume 100
ISSN 0065-3527
https://doi.org/10.1016/bs.aivir.2017.12.003

75

1. INTRODUCTION

The morbillivirus genus belongs to the virus family *Paramyxoviridae* in the order *Mononegavirales*, which is characterized by a nonsegmented, single-stranded linear RNA genome of negative polarity. Virions are pleomorphic, but most frequently spherical in shape and around 150 nm in diameter, and consist of a ribonucleoprotein (RNP) surrounded by an envelope fitted with viral proteins (Lamb and Parks, 2013; Wang et al., 2011). Morbilliviruses are highly contagious and cause moderate to severe respiratory and gastrointestinal disease and profound immune suppression in their respective hosts. The latter results in an increased susceptibility to opportunistic infections that can lead to life-threatening complications such as pneumonia (Durrheim et al., 2014; Lamb and Parks, 2013). In previously unexposed populations, morbilliviruses can cause large outbreaks and result in high morbidity and mortality (Appel and Summers, 1995; Shanks et al., 2015). In populations with endemic virus circulation, the epidemiology changes to that of a childhood disease, as survivors normally develop lifelong immunity (Anderson and May, 1985; Blixenkrone-Møller et al., 1993). Measles virus (MeV) is the prototype human pathogenic morbillivirus, and the genus includes several important animal pathogens such as Rinderpest virus (RPV), the second virus worldwide to be eradicated by targeted vaccination (Amarasinghe et al., 2017; de Vries et al., 2015; Njeumi et al., 2012), Peste des petits ruminants virus (PPRV), Canine distemper virus (CDV), Phocine distemper virus (PDV), Cetacean morbillivirus (CeMV), and the recently identified Feline morbillivirus (FeMV) (Fig. 1) (Amarasinghe et al., 2017). Furthermore, the morbillivirus-related sequences discovered in bat and rodent species may lead to redefinition of the genus in the future (Drexler et al., 2012).

2. HISTORY

The first reports of measles are from Rhazes and date back to the 9th century BC (Furuse et al., 2010). Before the isolation of the measles-causing virus in 1954 by John Enders and Thomas Peeples and the subsequent development of the first vaccine in 1963, epidemics occurred every few years, and approximately 90% of the population contracted measles during childhood (Enders and Peebles, 1954; Hilleman, 1992). Even though safe and effective live-attenuated vaccines have since led to a substantial reduction in cases, the disease remains an important cause of childhood morbidity and mortality

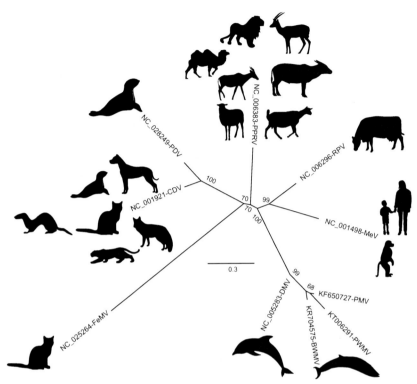

Fig. 1 Morbillivirus genus phylogenetic tree, based on representative phosphoprotein gene sequences. Molecular Evolutionary Genetics Analysis 6 (MEGA6) was used for phylogeny inference according to the maximum likelihood algorithm.

(Durrheim et al., 2014). Because of the high infectivity of the virus, a minimum of 95% herd immunity is required to prevent sporadic outbreaks (Fox, 1983; Nourjah and Frerichs, 1995). This immunization level has not yet been reached or is challenging to maintain in many regions, due to reduced vaccine acceptance, logistical issues, or budget deficits. As a consequence, measles epidemics continue to occur in large parts of the world.

Rinderpest, also referred to as the "cattle plague," is believed to have originated in Asia, reaching Egypt by around 3000 BC, from where it spread to Europe and Africa. Although rinderpest was known in Europe since medieval times, it was first described in 1712 by the Italian professor of medicine Bernardino Ramazzini, who observed several clinical similarities between rinderpest and smallpox (Ramazzini, 1712). In the 1950s, Walter Plowright, a British veterinary pathologist, developed an effective live-attenuated vaccine. In 1961, he also identified RPV as the causative agent of this acute and highly contagious disease (Plowright, 1962). The global effort to eradicate rinderpest officially started in 1994. Toward this, the Food and Agricultural Organization (FAO) in collaboration with the Organization Mondiale de la Santé (Office international des épizooties (OIE)), and International Atomic Energy Agency (IAEA) established the Global Rinderpest Eradication Programme (GREP), which ultimately resulted in the declaration of global RPV eradication in 2011 (de Vries et al., 2015; Njeumi et al., 2012).

The closely related peste des petits ruminants, which affects primarily goats and sheep, was first described in 1942 in West Africa, and the causative agent of this disease was identified in 1979 (Gibbs et al., 1979). However, infections likely have existed before but were underreported due to their similarity with rinderpest (Baron et al., 2016; Gargadennec and Lalanne, 1942). Phylogenetic analyses suggest that PPRV spread to East Africa in the 1980s and to Pakistan and India in 1990s, finally reaching Tibet in 2007 and Mongolia in 2016 (Taylor, 2016; Wang et al., 2009). Nearly, all PPRV outbreaks are due to movement of livestock, and the virus can then spread from livestock to wild ruminants, which serve as reservoir for subsequent livestock reinfections (Arzt et al., 2010; Bao et al., 2011; Munir, 2014). As PPRV not only affects goats and sheep, but can also infect wild small ruminants, cattle, buffalos, camelids, gazelles, Asiatic lions, and even pigs, the eradication of this disease will prove difficult (Abu Elzein et al., 1990; Anderson and McKay, 1994; Balamurugan et al., 2012; Khalafalla et al., 2010; Nawathe and Taylor, 1979).

Canine distemper, which affects a broad range of domestic and wild carnivores, has first been described in the 17th century. CDV is distributed globally, and most domestic carnivores are vaccinated (Deem et al., 2000). However, its high infectivity and considerable mortality may threaten to eradicate endangered species (Harder and Osterhaus, 1997; Martinez-Gutierrez and Ruiz-Saenz, 2016).

In the last decades, several distinct viruses have been found in aquatic mammals and were identified as the primary cause of massive animal strandings (van Bressem et al., 2014; van de Bildt et al., 2000). In 1988, PDV, a distinct but closely CDV-related morbillivirus, was isolated from seal populations in the North Sea during an epidemic with high mortality rates (Kennedy, 1998; Osterhaus and Vedder, 1988). Subsequently, PDV infections were also found in seals at the North American Atlantic coast (Duignan et al., 1993), making PDV the most ecologically significant pathogen of pinnipeds in the Northern hemisphere (Bodewes et al., 2013;

Duignan et al., 1994). Serological data indicate that not only several seal species but also the Atlantic walrus and polar bears may be infected with PDV (Cattet et al., 2004; Daoust et al., 1993; Duignan et al., 1994; Kennedy et al., 1989). In the late 1980s, many of the porpoises found stranded at the coast lines of Europe also displayed distemper-like lesions (Kennedy et al., 1988; Visser et al., 1993), and porpoise morbillivirus was isolated as the causative agent (McCullough et al., 1991; Welsh et al., 1992). Dolphins in the Mediterranean Sea, along the US coast, and more recently in Brazil and Western Australia were affected by a closely related dolphin morbillivirus (Domingo et al., 1990; Groch et al., 2014; Stephens et al., 2014), both belonging to the CeMV species (Barrett et al., 1993; Blixenkrone-Møller et al., 1994; Rima et al., 1995). In recent years, CeMV has also been isolated from stranded pilot whales and beaked whales (Jacob et al., 2016; Taubenberger et al., 2000; West et al., 2015), illustrating its global distribution.

In 2012, the first feline morbillivirus (FeMV) was reported in domestic cats in China (Woo et al., 2012). Since then, FeMV has been found in various countries on different continents (Darold et al., 2017; Lorusso et al., 2015; Sakaguchi et al., 2014; Sharp et al., 2016). FeMV seems to be associated with feline renal disease and can persist in the urinary tract rather than the central nervous system (CNS), the site of persistence of other morbilliviruses (Sharp et al., 2016).

3. GENOME ORGANIZATION

The morbillivirus RNA genomes are between 15.7 and 16 kb in length (Wang et al., 2011), and comply with the "rule of six," indicating that the number of nucleotides in each respective genome is a multiple of six. This probably reflects the precise packing of six nucleotides by a nucleocapsid protein subunit and is a requirement for efficient replication (Calain and Roux, 1993; Sidhu et al., 1995). Genome-size viral RNA is found exclusively encapsidated by nucleocapsid proteins, and together with the viral RNA-dependent RNA polymerase (RdRp) forms the RNP complex (Lamb & Parks, 2013; Sourimant and Plemper, 2016). All morbillivirus genomes encode six structural and two nonstructural proteins in the following order: nucleocapsid (N) protein, phosphoprotein (P), matrix (M), hemagglutinin (H), fusion (F), and large polymerase (L) proteins (Fig. 2). The two accessory proteins C and V are expressed from the P open reading frame and are involved in innate immune response interference and particle infectivity (Lamb and Parks, 2013). The genome is transcribed progressively from

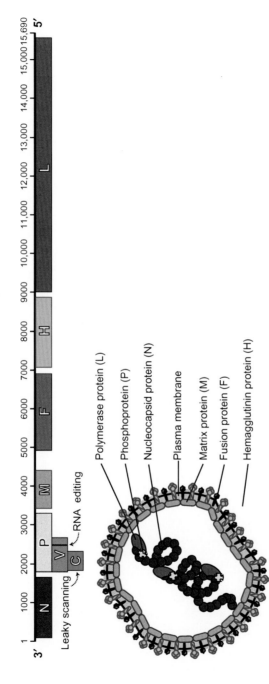

Fig. 2 Morbillivirus genome organization and particle structure. The negative-stranded RNA genome encodes six genes, yielding the structural nucleoprotein (N), phosphoprotein (P), matrix (M), fusion (F), hemagglutinin (H), and polymerase (L) proteins, as well as the accessory V and C proteins transcribed from the P gene. The viral particle is composed of the ribonucleoprotein (RNP) complex including the N protein-encapsidated viral RNA with the associated P and L proteins, and the envelope consisting of the M, F, H proteins.

the 3′-end by the RdRp into six separate, subgenomic positive sense mRNAs, that are capped and possess a poly (A) tail, due to reiterative copying of the polyadenylation site (Wang et al., 2011). The open reading frames are flanked by 3′ and 5′ untranslated regions encoding the necessary transcription initiation and termination signals (Castaneda and Wong, 1990; Horikami and Moyer, 1991; Sidhu et al., 1995). The P open reading frame is transcribed into an exact-copy mRNA that encodes the P mRNA as well as a predominant RNA-edited version in which the RNA transcriptase stutters on the template at an RNA editing motif midway down the element. This leads to the insertion of one pseudo-templated guanine (Cattaneo et al., 1989). The resulting V protein thus shares the amino terminus with the P protein but has a unique carboxy-terminal domain. In contrast, C mRNA transcription is initiated at an alternative start codon.

4. INFECTION CYCLE

Morbilliviruses initiate infection through attachment of the H protein to its cellular receptors CD150 (signaling lymphocyte activation molecule, SLAM-F1) on immune cell subsets (Tatsuo et al., 2000, 2001) or nectin-4 (PVRL4) on epithelial cells (Delpeut et al., 2014; Mühlebach et al., 2011). Conformational changes in the H protein trigger F protein-mediated fusion between the viral and cellular membranes, thereby releasing the RNP into the cytoplasm (Ader-Ebert et al., 2015; Lamb & Parks, 2013). At early infection stages, the RdRp transcriptase activity leads to the linear accumulation of viral mRNAs. At each intergenic junction, a poly (A) signal triggers the termination of transcription and reinitiation at the 3′ leader sequence of the next gene (Cattaneo et al., 1987; Plumet et al., 2005). Once sufficient N protein has been synthetized to ensure encapsidation of newly replicated genomes, the RdRp switches from transcription to replication mode and initiates the generation of positive sense antigenomes that in turn serve as templates for the synthesis of negative sense genomes (Lamb and Parks, 2013).

Upon encapsidation, the RNP interacts with the M protein for efficient transport to the plasma membrane, where it is enveloped by a host cell-derived lipid-bilayer carrying the F and H proteins, and nascent viral particles are subsequently released from the plasmamembrane (Cathomen et al., 1998; Tahara et al., 2007). The trimeric F protein is synthesized as a precursor protein (F0) that is activated following posttranslational cleavage by cellular proteases to yield the mature form consisting of disulfide-linked

F1 and F2 active subunits (Plattet et al., 2016; Watanabe et al., 1995). The H protein forms tetramers consisting of dimers of dimers (Navaratnarajah et al., 2009). It is the primary target of neutralizing antibodies (Tahara et al., 2013, 2016), and in response to this selection pressure, has the highest degree of genetic variability (Ke et al., 2015; Kessler et al., 2011).

5. SIMILARITIES AND DIFFERENCES IN MORBILLIVIRUS DISEASE MANIFESTATION

Each member of the morbillivirus genus has its distinct host range, with some overlap among the ungulate morbilliviruses RPV and PPRV, and the carnivore morbilliviruses CDV and PDV as well as possibly the different marine morbilliviruses (Wang et al., 2011). Even though disease severity varies among susceptible species, they all experience a similar pathogenesis. Infection occurs by inhalation of aerosol droplets or airborne virus particles, by direct contact with body fluids, or through fomites (Black, 2013; de Vries et al., 2017; Furuse et al., 2010). In addition to horizontal transmission, several morbilliviruses have been reported to transmit vertically (Chiba, 2003; Krakowka et al., 1974).

CD150 or SLAM-F1, which is expressed on activated lymphocytes, dendritic cell subsets, and macrophages, acts as common entry receptor for morbilliviruses (Cocks et al., 1995; Tatsuo et al., 2001). Upon infection, dendritic cells throughout the respiratory tract and other CD150-expressing cells in the alveolar lumen and lining the alveolar epithelium have been identified as the first targets (Lemon et al., 2011; Mesman et al., 2012). These cells then carry the virus to secondary lymphoid organs, and as early as 2 days after infection the virus can be found in the bronchus-associated lymphoid tissue (BALT) and trachea-bronchial lymph nodes (Lemon et al., 2011; Pope et al., 2013). The subsequent systemic spread to all immune tissues coincides with a fever spike, which is usually the first clinical sign of morbillivirus infection, and may exceed 40°C (Pope et al., 2013; von Messling et al., 2003). At the same time, a drop in white blood cell counts and an inhibition of the non-specific lymphocyte proliferation activity is observed, which continue to decrease as the virus amplifies in the immune system (Ryon et al., 2002; von Messling et al., 2004). Since the infection levels in peripheral blood mononuclear cells (PBMCs) are still low at this stage of infection, migration to the sites of infection may be an important factor contributing to leukopenia in addition to virus-induced cell death (Okada et al., 2000; Pillet and von Messling, 2009; Richetta et al., 2013). In contrast to the leukopenia, there is a strong correlation between PBMC infection levels and the extent of proliferation inhibition (Delpeut et al., 2017; Svitek and von Messling, 2007). However, while the white blood cell count rapidly recovers after virus clearance, the inability of PBMCs to proliferate upon stimulation may persist for weeks or even months (Griffin et al., 1994). The resulting immune suppression impairs the ability of the immune system to respond to other infections, and opportunistic or secondary infections greatly contribute to morbillivirus morbidity and mortality (de Vries et al., 2012; Mina et al., 2015; Slifka et al., 2003). In patients and terrestrial mammals, bacterial infections of the digestive or respiratory tract are the most frequent complications (Beckford et al., 1985; Durrheim et al., 2014), while parasitic and mycotic coinfections are common in marine mammals (Domingo et al., 1992; Kennedy et al., 1989; Siebert et al., 2010). Since memory T lymphocytes and follicular B lymphocytes are among the depleted immune cell populations, a temporary immune amnesia has recently been proposed for MeV (de Vries et al., 2012; Mina et al., 2015) and can be assumed for other morbilliviruses as well.

After amplification in immune tissues, morbilliviruses spread to epithelia, using nectin-4, which is expressed on the basolateral surface, as cellular receptor (Mühlebach et al., 2011; Noyce et al., 2011). This spread is associated with the onset of clinical signs and occurs 6–10 days after infection. Clinically, respiratory and to a lesser extent gastrointestinal signs are most prominent (Abramson et al., 1995; Appel, 1970; El Harrak et al., 2012; Miller, 1964). Since respiratory infections affect the diving ability of marine mammals, pneumonia is almost always seen in stranded morbillivirus-positive animals (Kennedy et al., 1989; van Bressem et al., 2014). Stomatitis, nasal discharge, cough and in severe cases labored breathing, as well as diarrhea are frequently observed (Kennedy et al., 1989; von Messling et al., 2003). In the absence of bacterial secondary infections, interstitial pneumonia, hyperplasia, edema, and focal epithelial necrosis are characteristic histopathological changes, and cytoplasmic and nuclear acidophilic inclusion bodies are indicative of sites of infection (Appel, 1970; Duignan et al., 1992; Truong et al., 2014).

The characteristic rash, a hallmark of MeV and CDV infection, is less obvious for other morbilliviruses, probably at least in part due to fur and skin color and composition. If detectable, rash consists of erythematous patches with 3–8 mm diameter. It usually appears first on the neck and face, especially around the mouth, and the number of patches increase and they often become confluent as the disease progresses (Suringa et al., 1970; von

Messling et al., 2003). In addition, Koplik spots, small white papules on an erythematous base, appear on mucosal surfaces (Suringa et al., 1970). Histologically, multinucleated syncytia are sometimes seen in the epidermis, and infiltration of mononuclear cells in response to the endothelial viral antigens results in dermal edema and spongioses (Kimura et al., 1975). The rash is also often accompanied by conjunctivitis and abnormal hyper- and parakeratosis (Grone et al., 2004; Kimura et al., 1975). In RPV and PPRV infections, mucosa involvement and conjunctivitis are also common (Baron et al., 2016), and in aquatic mammals, subcutaneous edema and cyanosis of the buccal mucosa, conjunctivitis, and keratosis of flippers, head, trunk, and tail have been reported (Daoust et al., 1993; Duignan et al., 1992; Kennedy et al., 1989).

The pathogenesis of the recently discovered FeMV in cats remains to be characterized in detail. It is most frequently detected in kidney tissue and urine and may be associated with chronic kidney disease in cats, but a clear causal relationship has yet to be established (Park et al., 2016).

6. MORBILLIVIRUS-ASSOCIATED NEUROLOGICAL COMPLICATIONS

Neurological involvement is common for carnivore morbilliviruses, and a rare but devastating complication in MeV, but has not been reported for other morbilliviruses so far (Cosby et al., 2002). In addition to an acute immune-mediated or sometimes virus-induced encephalitis, MeV can also cause measles inclusion body encephalitis, which occurs mainly in immunosuppressed individuals after the systemic infection has been resolved. In children infected during infancy when the immune system is still immature, the virus can establish a persistent infection in the CNS, leading to subacute sclerosing panencephalitis years later (Fisher et al., 2015). Carnivore morbilliviruses readily invade the CNS, and during the acute disease-infected neurons, astrocytes and glia cells are found in the gray and sometimes also the white matter (Rudd et al., 2006; Summers et al., 1979). With resolution of the infection-induced immune suppression, immune-mediated demyelination is observed, reproducing many aspects of measles inclusion body encephalitis (Summers and Appel, 1994; Summers et al., 1979). Old dog encephalitis, which occurs months or years after recovery from CDV, shares clinical and pathological similarities with MeV subacute sclerosing panencephalitis, but the underlying mechanism remains to be characterized (Headley et al., 2009).

7. MORBILLIVIRUS–HOST INTERACTIONS

7.1 Host Factors Involved in RNA Synthesis and Particle Assembly

Many host cell proteins influencing RNA synthesis and virion assembly have been identified via coimmune precipitation, yeast-two-hybrid assays, and proteomic approaches. The heat shock protein 72 (Hsp72) was shown to interact with the MeV P protein-binding motif of the N protein at its C-terminal region, resulting in an increased MeV genome transcription, replication, and virulence (Carsillo et al., 2006; Zhang et al., 2005). The host factor peroxiredoxin (Prdx1) also binds to the C-terminal region of MeV N and competes with P for binding, thereby modulating the formation of the RNP and regulating RNA synthesis. Prdx1 suppression by RNA interference reduced the level of viral mRNA and genomic RNA and repressed MeV growth (Watanabe et al., 2011). Furthermore, the MeV N protein targets the p40 subunit of eukaryotic initiation factor 3 (eIF3-p40) and inhibits the translation of cellular mRNA (Sato et al., 2007). The C protein regulates viral RNA synthesis through host factor SHC SH2 domain-binding protein 1 (SHCBP1)-mediated interaction with the MeV RNP complex (Ito et al., 2013). Other host factors that interact with MeV proteins include casein kinase II, which phosphorylates the P protein, and a series of unidentified kinases, which phosphorylate amino acid residues in N and P. N protein phosphorylation at S479 and S510 promotes viral transcription and replication, whereas P protein phosphorylation of S86 and S151 downregulates viral transcriptional activity (Hagiwara et al., 2008; Sugai et al., 2012, 2013). In RPV, downregulation of ErbB3-binding protein Ebp1 has been observed, and its overexpression leads to decreased genome transcription and translation of viral proteins, suggesting an antiviral activity (Gopinath et al., 2010).

For intracellular transport, viruses either hijack the intracellular trafficking machinery, or they interact with the cytoskeletal components. In the morbillivirus life cycle, stable actin filaments are required for intracellular trafficking of viral RNPs to the plasma membrane, whereas actin dynamics are necessary for budding at the plasma membrane (Dietzel et al., 2013). It has been shown that F-actin modulates MeV syncytium formation and assembly by controlling the interaction between the M protein and the cytoplasmic tail of the H protein (Wakimoto et al., 2013). Increased phosphorylation of the actin-modulating protein Cofilin after MeV infection promotes RNP complex formation via interaction with N and controls assembly, budding, and cell–cell fusion through actin remodeling (Koga et al., 2015). Actin filaments also play a major role during CDV replication by affecting M protein localization and by reducing viral infectivity (Klauschies et al., 2010). Transport of the MeV RNP complex in polarized epithelial cells is microtubule-dependent and mediated by recycling endosomes containing the Ras-related protein Rab11 (Nakatsu et al., 2013). Due to the structural and functional similarities among morbilliviruses, it is safe to assume that many of these interactions are conserved among all members of the genus.

7.2 Host Factors Involved in IFN Response

The interplay between innate immune activation and virus-mediated immunosuppression influences the course and outcome of infection. Innate immune responses are initially activated by the detection of pathogen-associated molecular patterns (PAMPS) via pattern recognition receptors (PRR) (Creagh and O'Neill, 2006; Kawai and Akira, 2010) including Toll-like receptors, melanoma differentiation–associated factor 5 (MDA-5) and retinoic-acid inducible gene (RIG)-I-like receptors (RLRs) (Kato et al., 2006) and nucleotide-binding oligomerization domain-like receptors (NLRs). Sensing of viral infections by PRRs then leads to IRF3, IRF7, and NFκB activation, resulting in the production of type I IFN-α/β, as well as inflammatory cytokines (Creagh and O'Neill, 2006; Ikegame et al., 2010).

Morbilliviruses have evolved diverse strategies to counteract different aspects of this viral RNA sensing. Like other Paramyxoviruses, MeV V protein interacts with RIG-I-like receptors MDA5 and LGP2, which is suggested to be a positive regulator of RIG-I and MDA5-mediated antiviral responses (Satoh et al., 2010), to inhibit IFN induction (Andrejeva et al., 2004; Rodriguez and Horvath, 2014). In addition, the virus escapes MDA5 detection by interaction of the V protein with the phosphatases PP1α and PP1γ, which prevents PP1-mediated dephosphorylation of MDA5 and thereby its activation (Davis et al., 2014). The MeV V protein also interacts with IRF3 and IRF7 to inhibit their transcriptional activity (Pfaller and Conzelmann, 2008). Its cysteine-rich C-terminal domain interacts with MDA5 and IκB kinase α (IKKα) to downregulate IRF7 activation (Pfaller and Conzelmann, 2008), and with NF-κB subunit p65 to repress IFN-β and cytokine production (Schuhmann et al., 2011). Independent of these V protein activities, the MeV P protein suppresses

TLR4 signaling via upregulation of ubiquitin-modifying enzyme A20, which also negatively regulates NF-κB activity (Li et al., 2008; Yokota et al., 2011). RPV and MeV C proteins target IRF-3 in the nucleus and repress IFN-β transcription without inhibiting the activation of IRF-3 (Boxer et al., 2009; Sparrer et al., 2012), but the interaction of other morbilliviruses with RLR or TLR members still needs to be explored in more detail.

Secreted type I IFNs bind to type I IFN receptors, which are associated with the Janus-activated kinases (Jaks) tyrosine kinase 2 (Tyk-2) and Jak-1. Activation of the Jaks results in phosphorylation of signal transducers and activators of transcription (STAT) 1 and STAT2, triggering their heterodimerization. The phosphorylated STAT1/STAT2 dimer associates with IRF9, forming interferon-stimulated gene factor 3 (ISGF3), which translocates to the nucleus and binds IFN-stimulated response elements (ISREs) in the promoter region of interferon-stimulated genes (ISGs), directing ISG expression. ISGs include double-stranded protein kinase (PKR), OAS/RNaseL, and adenosine deaminase acting on RNA (ADAR1). ADAR1 in turn inhibits the activation of PKR and IRF3, functioning as an important suppressor of MeV-mediated IFN-β production (Li et al., 2012; Pfaller et al., 2011).

Type II interferon (IFN-γ) binds to IFN-γ receptors, inducing phosphorylation of Jak-1 and Jak-2 which leads to STAT1 phosphorylation and its homodimerization to form gamma-activated factor (GAF). GAF in turn translocates to the nucleus and binds to the gamma activation sequence (GAS) to activate transcription of ISGs.

Morbilliviruses interfere with these IFN synthesis or signal transduction pathways at multiple levels (Fig. 3), and new interacting partners continue to be discovered. All morbillivirus V proteins interfere with phosphorylation of Tyk2 and prevent STAT1 and STAT2 activation to mediate an effective blockade on the type I IFN signaling pathway (Chinnakannan et al., 2013). Among the common well-characterized interactions is the interference with STAT1 nuclear translocation of the V protein N-terminal domain, and the interaction of the unique C-terminus with Jak-1, in some cases Tyk2, and STAT2, broadly inhibiting IFN-α/β signaling (Caignard et al., 2009; Nanda and Baron, 2006; Ramachandran et al., 2008; Rothlisberger et al., 2010). MeV and CDV carrying mutations that selectively abolish the interference with STAT1, STAT2, or mda5 signaling have shown to result in partial attenuation in macaques or ferrets, respectively, illustrating that each interaction is required to achieve the full extent of

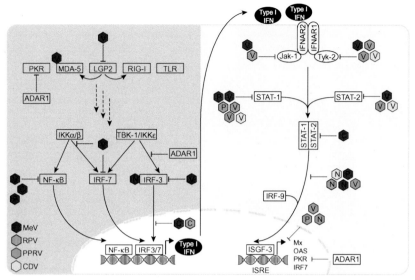

Fig. 3 Host targets of morbillivirus innate immune response interference. The signaling pathways are shown, and known interactions for each virus are indicated.

morbillivirus immune interference (Devaux et al., 2011; Svitek et al., 2014). Additional functions have been described for individual viruses: The MeV P protein STAT1 phosphorylation and nuclear translocation (Devaux et al., 2007), while MeV C protein blocks the dimerization of phosphorylated STAT1 (Yokota et al., 2011). In addition, the MeV N protein inhibits the nuclear import of activated STATs without preventing STAT and Jak activation or inducing STAT degradation (Takayama et al., 2012). Similarly, CDV and RPV N proteins interfere with the nuclear transport of STAT1 and STAT2. The RPV P protein also binds to STAT1 and blocks IFN action (Nanda and Baron, 2006), and PPRV N, P, and V proteins inhibit IFN signaling transduction via restriction of ISRE and GAS promoter expression with the V protein having the strongest effect (Ma et al., 2015). However, additional studies are needed to fully appreciate the relative importance of each activity and its relevance for innate immune interference in vivo.

8. CONCLUSIONS

This review summarizes the common aspects of morbillivirus pathogenesis and molecular virus–host interactions. Ongoing research will reveal which of these aspects are also shared with the newly discovered FeMV and other new and more phylogenetically members of the genus. Despite the existence of excellent MeV vaccines and the eradication of RPV as proof-of-principle, the eradication of MeV has yet to be achieved, highlighting the importance of a detailed understanding of virus–host interactions for the development of new prophylactic and therapeutic approaches.

REFERENCES

Abramson, O., Dagan, R., Tal, A., Sofer, S., 1995. Severe complications of measles requiring intensive care in infants and young children. Arch. Pediatr. Adolesc. Med. 149, 1237–1240.

Abu Elzein, E.M., Hassanien, M.M., Al-Afaleq, A.I., Abd Elhadi, M.A., Housawi, F.M., 1990. Isolation of peste des petits ruminants from goats in Saudi Arabia. Vet. Rec. 127, 309–310.

Ader-Ebert, N., Khosravi, M., Herren, M., Avila, M., Alves, L., Bringolf, F., Örvell, C., Langedijk, J.P., Zurbriggen, A., Plemper, R.K., Plattet, P., 2015. Sequential conformational changes in the morbillivirus attachment protein initiate the membrane fusion process. PLoS Pathog. 11, e1004880.

Amarasinghe, G.K., Bao, Y., Basler, C.F., Bavari, S., Beer, M., Bejerman, N., Blasdell, K.R., Bochnowski, A., Briese, T., Bukreyev, A., Calisher, C.H., Chandran, K., Collins, P.L., Dietzgen, R.G., Dolnik, O., Durrwald, R., Dye, J.M., Easton, A.J., Ebihara, H., Fang, Q., Formenty, P., Fouchier, R.A.M., Ghedin, E., Harding, R.M., Hewson, R., Higgins, C.M., Hong, J., Horie, M., James, A.P., Jiang, D., Kobinger, G.P., Kondo, H., Kurath, G., Lamb, R.A., Lee, B., Leroy, E.M., Li, M., Maisner, A., Muhlberger, E., Netesov, S.V., Nowotny, N., Patterson, J.L., Payne, S.L., Paweska, J.T., Pearson, M.N., Randall, R.E., Revill, P.A., Rima, B.K., Rota, P., Rubbenstroth, D., Schwemmle, M., Smither, S.J., Song, Q., Stone, D.M., Takada, A., Terregino, C., Tesh, R.B., Tomonaga, K., Tordo, N., Towner, J.S., Vasilakis, N., Volchkov, V.E., Wahl-Jensen, V., Walker, P.J., Wang, B., Wang, D., Wang, F., Wang, L.-F., Werren, J.H., Whitfield, A.E., Yan, Z., Ye, G., Kuhn, J.H., 2017. Taxonomy of the order Mononegavirales: update 2017. Arch. Virol. 162, 2493–2504.

Anderson, R.M., May, R.M., 1985. Age-related changes in the rate of disease transmission: implications for the design of vaccination programmes. J. Hyg. (Lond) 94, 365–436.

Anderson, J., McKay, J.A., 1994. The detection of antibodies against peste des petits ruminants virus in cattle, sheep and goats and the possible implications to rinderpest control programmes. Epidemiol. Infect. 112, 225–231.

Andrejeva, J., Childs, K.S., Young, D.F., Carlos, T.S., Stock, N., Goodbourn, S., Randall, R.E., 2004. The V proteins of paramyxoviruses bind the IFN-inducible RNA helicase, mda-5, and inhibit its activation of the IFN-beta promoter. Proc. Natl. Acad. Sci. U.S.A. 101, 17264–17269.

Appel, M.J., 1970. Distemper pathogenesis in dogs. J. Am. Vet. Med. Assoc. 156, 1681–1684.

Appel, M.J., Summers, B.A., 1995. Pathogenicity of morbilliviruses for terrestrial carnivores. Vet. Microbiol. 44, 187–191.

Arzt, J., White, W.R., Thomsen, B.V., Brown, C.C., 2010. Agricultural diseases on the move early in the third millennium. Vet. Pathol. 47, 15–27.

Balamurugan, V., Krishnamoorthy, P., Veeregowda, B.M., Sen, A., Rajak, K.K., Bhanuprakash, V., Gajendragad, M.R., Prabhudas, K., 2012. Seroprevalence of Peste des petits ruminants in cattle and buffaloes from Southern Peninsular India. Trop. Anim. Health Prod. 44, 301–306.

Bao, J., Wang, Z., Li, L., Wu, X., Sang, P., Wu, G., Ding, G., Suo, L., Liu, C., Wang, J., Zhao, W., Li, J., Qi, L., 2011. Detection and genetic characterization of peste des petits ruminants virus in free-living bharals (Pseudois nayaur) in Tibet, China. Res. Vet. Sci. 90, 238–240.

Baron, M.D., Diallo, A., Lancelot, R., Libeau, G., 2016. Peste des Petits Ruminants Virus. Adv. Virus Res. 95, 1–42.

Barrett, T., Visser, I.K., Mamaev, L., Goatley, L., van Bressem, M.F., Osterhaust, A.D., 1993. Dolphin and porpoise morbilliviruses are genetically distinct from phocine distemper virus. Virology 193, 1010–1012.

Beckford, A.P., Kaschula, R.O., Stephen, C., 1985. Factors associated with fatal cases of measles. A retrospective autopsy study. S. Afr. Med. J. 68, 858–863.

Black, F.L., 2013. Epidemiology of Paramyxoviridae. The Paramyxoviruses. Springer Verlag. 1 online resource.

Blixenkrone-Møller, M., Svansson, V., Have, P., Orvell, C., Appel, M., Pedersen, I.R., Dietz, H.H., Henriksen, P., 1993. Studies on manifestations of canine distemper virus infection in an urban dog population. Vet. Microbiol. 37, 163–173.

Blixenkrone-Møller, M., Bolt, G., Gottschalck, E., Kenter, M., 1994. Comparative analysis of the gene encoding the nucleocapsid protein of dolphin morbillivirus reveals its distant evolutionary relationship to measles virus and ruminant morbilliviruses. J. Gen. Virol. 75 (Pt. 10), 2829–2834.

Bodewes, R., Morick, D., van de Bildt, M.W., Osinga, N., Rubio Garcia, A., Sanchez Contreras, G.J., Smits, S.L., Reperant, L.A., Kuiken, T., Osterhaus, A.D., 2013. Prevalence of phocine distemper virus specific antibodies: bracing for the next seal epizootic in north-western Europe. Emerg. Microbes. Infect. 2, e3.

Boxer, E.L., Nanda, S.K., Baron, M.D., 2009. The rinderpest virus non-structural C protein blocks the induction of type 1 interferon. Virology 385, 134–142.

Caignard, G., Bourai, M., Jacob, Y., Tangy, F., Vidalain, P.-O., 2009. Inhibition of IFN-alpha/beta signaling by two discrete peptides within measles virus V protein that specifically bind STAT1 and STAT2. Virology 383, 112–120.

Calain, P., Roux, L., 1993. The rule of six, a basic feature for efficient replication of Sendai virus defective interfering RNA. J. Virol. 67, 4822–4830.

Carsillo, T., Traylor, Z., Choi, C., Niewiesk, S., Oglesbee, M., 2006. hsp72, a host determinant of measles virus neurovirulence. J. Virol. 80, 11031–11039.

Castaneda, S.J., Wong, T.C., 1990. Leader sequence distinguishes between translatable and encapsidated measles virus RNAs. J. Virol. 64, 222–230.

Cathomen, T., Mrkic, B., Spehner, D., Drillien, R., Naef, R., Pavlovic, J., Aguzzi, A., Billeter, M.A., Cattaneo, R., 1998. A matrix-less measles virus is infectious and elicits extensive cell fusion: consequences for propagation in the brain. EMBO J. 17, 3899–3908.

Cattaneo, R., Rebmann, G., Schmid, A., Baczko, K., ter Meulen, V., Billeter, M.A., 1987. Altered transcription of a defective measles virus genome derived from a diseased human brain. EMBO J. 6, 681–688.

Cattaneo, R., Kaelin, K., Baczko, K., Billeter, M.A., 1989. Measles virus editing provides an additional cysteine-rich protein. Cell 56, 759–764.

Cattet, M.R.L., Duignan, P.J., House, C.A., Aubin, D.J.S., 2004. Antibodies to canine distemper and phocine distemper viruses in polar bears from the Canadian arctic. J. Wildl. Dis. 40, 338–342.

Chiba, M., 2003. Measles infection in pregnancy. J. Infect. 47, 40–44.

Chinnakannan, S.K., Nanda, S.K., Baron, M.D., 2013. Morbillivirus v proteins exhibit multiple mechanisms to block type 1 and type 2 interferon signalling pathways. PLoS One 8, e57063.

Cocks, B.G., Chang, C.C., Carballido, J.M., Yssel, H., de Vries, J.E., Aversa, G., 1995. A novel receptor involved in T-cell activation. Nature 376, 260–263.

Cosby, S.L., Duprex, W.P., Hamill, L.A., Ludlow, M., McQuaid, S., 2002. Approaches in the understanding of morbillivirus neurovirulence. J. Neurovirol. 8 (Suppl. 2), 85–90.

Creagh, E.M., O'Neill, L.A.J., 2006. TLRs, NLRs and RLRs: a trinity of pathogen sensors that co-operate in innate immunity. Trends Immunol. 27, 352–357.

Daoust, P.Y., Haines, D.M., Thorsen, J., Duignan, P.J., Geraci, J.R., 1993. Phocine distemper in a harp seal (Phoca groenlandica) from the Gulf of St. Lawrence, Canada. J. Wildl. Dis. 29, 114–117.

Darold, G.M., Alfieri, A.A., Muraro, L.S., Amude, A.M., Zanatta, R., Yamauchi, K.C.I., Alfieri, A.F., Lunardi, M., 2017. First report of feline morbillivirus in South America. Arch. Virol. 162, 469–475.

Davis, M.E., Wang, M.K., Rennick, L.J., Full, F., Gableske, S., Mesman, A.W., Gringhuis, S.I., Geijtenbeek, T.B.H., Duprex, W.P., Gack, M.U., 2014. Antagonism of the phosphatase PP1 by the measles virus V protein is required for innate immune escape of MDA5. Cell Host Microbe 16, 19–30.

de Vries, R.D., McQuaid, S., van Amerongen, G., Yuksel, S., Verburgh, R.J., Osterhaus, A.D.M.E., Duprex, W.P., de Swart, R.L., 2012. Measles immune suppression: lessons from the macaque model. PLoS Pathog. 8, e1002885.

de Vries, R.D., Duprex, W.P., de Swart, R.L., 2015. Morbillivirus infections: an introduction. Virus 7, 699–706.

de Vries, R.D., Ludlow, M., de Jong, A., Rennick, L.J., Verburgh, R.J., van Amerongen, G., van Riel, D., van Run, P.R.W.A., Herfst, S., Kuiken, T., Fouchier, R.A.M., Osterhaus, A.D.M.E., de Swart, R.L., Duprex, W.P., 2017. Delineating morbillivirus entry, dissemination and airborne transmission by studying in vivo competition of multicolor canine distemper viruses in ferrets. PLoS Pathog. 13, e1006371.

Deem, S.L., Spelman, L.H., Yates, R.A., Montali, R.J., 2000. Canine distemper in terrestrial carnivores: a review. J. Zoo Wildl. Med. 31, 441–451.

Delpeut, S., Noyce, R.S., Richardson, C.D., 2014. The tumor-associated marker, PVRL4 (nectin-4), is the epithelial receptor for morbilliviruses. Virus 6, 2268–2286.

Delpeut, S., Sawatsky, B., Wong, X.-X., Frenzke, M., Cattaneo, R., von Messling, V., 2017. Nectin-4 interactions govern measles virus virulence in a new model of pathogenesis, the squirrel monkey (Saimiri sciureus). J. Virol. 91, pii: e01026-17.

Devaux, P., von Messling, V., Songsungthong, W., Springfeld, C., Cattaneo, R., 2007. Tyrosine 110 in the measles virus phosphoprotein is required to block STAT1 phosphorylation. Virology 360, 72–83.

Devaux, P., Hudacek, A.W., Hodge, G., Reyes-Del Valle, J., McChesney, M.B., Cattaneo, R., 2011. A recombinant measles virus unable to antagonize STAT1 function cannot control inflammation and is attenuated in rhesus monkeys. J. Virol. 85, 348–356.

Dietzel, E., Kolesnikova, L., Maisner, A., 2013. Actin filaments disruption and stabilization affect measles virus maturation by different mechanisms. Virol. J. 10, 249.

Domingo, M., Ferrer, L., Pumarola, M., Marco, A., Plana, J., Kennedy, S., McAliskey, M., Rima, B.K., 1990. Morbillivirus in dolphins. Nature 348, 21.

Domingo, M., Visa, J., Pumarola, M., Marco, A.J., Ferrer, L., Rabanal, R., Kennedy, S., 1992. Pathologic and immunocytochemical studies of morbillivirus infection in striped dolphins (Stenella coeruleoalba). Vet. Pathol. 29, 1–10.

Drexler, J.F., Corman, V.M., Müller, M.A., Maganga, G.D., Vallo, P., Binger, T., Gloza-Rausch, F., Cottontail, V.M., Rasche, A., Yordanov, S., Seebens, A., Knörnschild, M., Oppong, S., Adu Sarkodie, Y., Pongombo, C., Lukashev, A.N., Schmidt-Chanasit, J., Stöcker, A., Carneiro, A.J.B., Erbar, S., Maisner, A., Fronhoffs, F., Buettner, R., Kalko, E.K.V., Kruppa, T., Franke, C.R., Kallies, R., Yandoko, E.R.N., Herrler, G., Reusken, C., Hassanin, A., Krüger, D.H., Matthee, S., Ulrich, R.G., Leroy, E.M., Drosten, C., 2012. Bats host major mammalian paramyxoviruses. Nat. Commun. 3, 796.

Duignan, P.J., Geraci, J.R., Raga, J.A., Calzada, N., 1992. Pathology of morbillivirus infection in striped dolphins (Stenella coeruleoalba) from Valencia and Murcia, Spain. Can. J. Vet. Res. 56, 242–248.

Duignan, P.J., Sadove, S., Saliki, J.T., Geraci, J.R., 1993. Phocine distemper in harbor seals (Phoca vitulina) from Long Island, New York. J. Wildl. Dis. 29, 465–469.

Duignan, P.J., Saliki, J.T., St Aubin, D.J., House, J.A., Geraci, J.R., 1994. Neutralizing antibodies to phocine distemper virus in Atlantic walruses (Odobenus rosmarus rosmarus) from Arctic Canada. J. Wildl. Dis. 30, 90–94.

Durrheim, D.N., Crowcroft, N.S., Strebel, P.M., 2014. Measles—the epidemiology of elimination. Vaccine 32, 6880–6883.

El Harrak, M., Touil, N., Loutfi, C., Hammouchi, M., Parida, S., Sebbar, G., Chaffai, N., Harif, B., Messoudi, N., Batten, C., Oura, C.A.L., 2012. A reliable and reproducible experimental challenge model for peste des petits ruminants virus. J. Clin. Microbiol. 50, 3738–3740.

Enders, J.F., Peebles, T.C., 1954. Propagation in tissue cultures of cytopathogenic agents from patients with measles. Proc. Soc. Exp. Biol. Med. 86, 277–286.

Fisher, D.L., Defres, S., Solomon, T., 2015. Measles-induced encephalitis. QJM 108, 177–182.

Fox, J.P., 1983. Herd immunity and measles. Rev. Infect. Dis. 5, 463–466.

Furuse, Y., Suzuki, A., Oshitani, H., 2010. Origin of measles virus: divergence from rinderpest virus between the 11th and 12th centuries. Virol. J. 7, 52.

Gargadennec, L., Lalanne, A., 1942. La Peste des Petits Ruminants. Bull. Serv. Zoo. A. O. F. 5, 15–21.

Gibbs, E.P., Taylor, W.P., Lawman, M.J., Bryant, J., 1979. Classification of peste des petits ruminants virus as the fourth member of the genus morbillivirus. Intervirology 11, 268–274.

Gopinath, M., Raju, S., Honda, A., Shaila, M.S., 2010. Host factor Ebp1 inhibits rinderpest virus transcription in vivo. Arch. Virol. 155, 455–462.

Griffin, D.E., Ward, B.J., Esolen, L.M., 1994. Pathogenesis of measles virus infection: an hypothesis for altered immune responses. J Infect Dis 170 (Suppl. 1), S24–S31.

Groch, K.R., Colosio, A.C., Marcondes, M.C.C., Zucca, D., Diaz-Delgado, J., Niemeyer, C., Marigo, J., Brandao, P.E., Fernandez, A., Luiz Catao-Dias, J., 2014. Novel cetacean morbillivirus in Guiana dolphin, Brazil. Emerg. Infect. Dis. 20, 511–513.

Grone, A., Doherr, M.G., Zurbriggen, A., 2004. Canine distemper virus infection of canine footpad epidermis. Vet. Dermatol. 15, 159–167.

Hagiwara, K., Sato, H., Inoue, Y., Watanabe, A., Yoneda, M., Ikeda, F., Fujita, K., Fukuda, H., Takamura, C., Kozuka-Hata, H., Oyama, M., Sugano, S., Ohmi, S., Kai, C., 2008. Phosphorylation of measles virus nucleoprotein upregulates the transcriptional activity of minigenomic RNA. Proteomics 8, 1871–1879.

Harder, T.C., Osterhaus, A.D., 1997. Canine distemper virus—a morbillivirus in search of new hosts? Trends Microbiol. 5, 120–124.

Headley, S.A., Amude, A.M., Alfieri, A.F., Bracarense, A.P.F.R.L., Alfieri, A.A., Summers, B.A., 2009. Molecular detection of canine distemper virus and the immunohistochemical characterization of the neurologic lesions in naturally occurring old dog encephalitis. J. Vet. Diagn. Invest. 21, 588–597.

Hilleman, M.R., 1992. Past, present, and future of measles, mumps, and rubella virus vaccines. Pediatrics 90, 149–153.

Horikami, S.M., Moyer, S.A., 1991. Synthesis of leader RNA and editing of the P mRNA during transcription by purified measles virus. J. Virol. 65, 5342–5347.

Ikegame, S., Takeda, M., Ohno, S., Nakatsu, Y., Nakanishi, Y., Yanagi, Y., 2010. Both RIG-I and MDA5 RNA helicases contribute to the induction of alpha/beta interferon in measles virus-infected human cells. J. Virol. 84, 372–379.

Ito, M., Iwasaki, M., Takeda, M., Nakamura, T., Yanagi, Y., Ohno, S., 2013. Measles virus nonstructural C protein modulates viral RNA polymerase activity by interacting with host protein SHCBP1. J. Virol. 87, 9633–9642.

Jacob, J.M., West, K.L., Levine, G., Sanchez, S., Jensen, B.A., 2016. Initial characterization of novel beaked whale morbillivirus in Hawaiian cetaceans. Dis. Aquat. Organ. 117, 215–227.

Kato, H., Takeuchi, O., Sato, S., Yoneyama, M., Yamamoto, M., Matsui, K., Uematsu, S., Jung, A., Kawai, T., Ishii, K.J., Yamaguchi, O., Otsu, K., Tsujimura, T., Koh, C.-S., Reis e Sousa, C., Matsuura, Y., Fujita, T., Akira, S., 2006. Differential roles of MDA5 and RIG-I helicases in the recognition of RNA viruses. Nature 441, 101–105.

Kawai, T., Akira, S., 2010. The role of pattern-recognition receptors in innate immunity: update on toll-like receptors. Nat. Immunol. 11, 373–384.

Ke, G.-M., Ho, C.-H., Chiang, M.-J., Sanno-Duanda, B., Chung, C.-S., Lin, M.-Y., Shi, Y.-Y., Yang, M.-H., Tyan, Y.-C., Liao, P.-C., Chu, P.-Y., 2015. Phylodynamic analysis of the canine distemper virus hemagglutinin gene. BMC Vet. Res. 11, 164.

Kennedy, S., 1998. Morbillivirus infections in aquatic mammals. J. Comp. Pathol. 119, 201–225.

Kennedy, S., Smyth, J.A., Cush, P.F., McCullough, S.J., Allan, G.M., McQuaid, S., 1988. Viral distemper now found in porpoises. Nature 336, 21.

Kennedy, S., Smyth, J.A., Cush, P.F., Duignan, P., Platten, M., McCullough, S.J., Allan, G.M., 1989. Histopathologic and immunocytochemical studies of distemper in seals. Vet. Pathol. 26, 97–103.

Kessler, J.R., Kremer, J.R., Shulga, S.V., Tikhonova, N.T., Santibanez, S., Mankertz, A., Semeiko, G.V., Samoilovich, E.O., Tamfum, J.-J.M., Pukuta, E., Muller, C.P., 2011. Revealing new measles virus transmission routes by use of sequence analysis of phosphoprotein and hemagglutinin genes. J. Clin. Microbiol. 49, 677–683.

Khalafalla, A.I., Saeed, I.K., Ali, Y.H., Abdurrahman, M.B., Kwiatek, O., Libeau, G., Obeida, A.A., Abbas, Z., 2010. An outbreak of peste des petits ruminants (PPR) in camels in the Sudan. Acta Trop. 116, 161–165.

Kimura, A., Tosaka, K., Nakao, T., 1975. Measles rash. I. Light and electron microscopic study of skin eruptions. Arch. Virol. 47, 295–307.

Klauschies, F., Gutzkow, T., Hinkelmann, S., von Messling, V., Vaske, B., Herrler, G., Haas, L., 2010. Viral infectivity and intracellular distribution of matrix (M) protein of canine distemper virus are affected by actin filaments. Arch. Virol. 155, 1503–1508.

Koga, R., Sugita, Y., Noda, T., Yanagi, Y., Ohno, S., 2015. Actin-modulating protein Cofilin is involved in the formation of measles virus ribonucleoprotein complex at the perinuclear region. J. Virol. 89, 10524–10531.

Krakowka, S., Confer, A., Koestner, A., 1974. Evidence for transplacental transmission of canine distemper virus: two case reports. Am. J. Vet. Res. 35, 1251–1253.

Lamb, R.A., Parks, G.D., 2013. Paramyxoviridae: the viruses and their replication. In: Fields, B.N., Knipe, D.M., Howley, P.M. (Eds.), Fields Virology. Lippincott-Raven Press, Philadelphia, pp. 957–995.

Lemon, K., de Vries, R.D., Mesman, A.W., McQuaid, S., van Amerongen, G., Yuksel, S., Ludlow, M., Rennick, L.J., Kuiken, T., Rima, B.K., Geijtenbeek, T.B.H., Osterhaus, A.D.M.E., Duprex, W.P., de Swart, R.L., 2011. Early target cells of measles virus after aerosol infection of non-human primates. PLoS Pathog. 7, e1001263.

Li, L., Hailey, D.W., Soetandyo, N., Li, W., Lippincott-Schwartz, J., Shu, H.-B., Ye, Y., 2008. Localization of A20 to a lysosome-associated compartment and its role in NFkappaB signaling. Biochim. Biophys. Acta 1783, 1140–1149.

Li, Z., Okonski, K.M., Samuel, C.E., 2012. Adenosine deaminase acting on RNA 1 (ADAR1) suppresses the induction of interferon by measles virus. J. Virol. 86, 3787–3794.

Lorusso, A., Di Tommaso, M., Di Felice, E., Zaccaria, G., Luciani, A., Marcacci, M., Aste, G., Boari, A., Savini, G., 2015. First report of feline morbillivirus in Europe. Vet. Ital. 51, 235–237.

Ma, X., Yang, X., Nian, X., Zhang, Z., Dou, Y., Zhang, X., Luo, X., Su, J., Zhu, Q., Cai, X., 2015. Identification of amino-acid residues in the V protein of peste des petits ruminants essential for interference and suppression of STAT-mediated interferon signaling. Virology 483, 54–63.

Martinez-Gutierrez, M., Ruiz-Saenz, J., 2016. Diversity of susceptible hosts in canine distemper virus infection: a systematic review and data synthesis. BMC Vet. Res. 12, 78.

McCullough, S.J., McNeilly, F., Allan, G.M., Kennedy, S., Smyth, J.A., Cosby, S.L., McQuaid, S., Rima, B.K., 1991. Isolation and characterisation of a porpoise morbillivirus. Arch. Virol. 118, 247–252.

Mesman, A.W., de Vries, R.D., McQuaid, S., Duprex, W.P., de Swart, R.L., Geijtenbeek, T.B.H., 2012. A prominent role for DC-SIGN+ dendritic cells in initiation and dissemination of measles virus infection in non-human primates. PLoS One 7, e49573.

Miller, D.L., 1964. Frequency of complications of measles, 1963. Report on a national inquiry by the public health laboratory service in collaboration with the society of medical oficers of health. Br. Med. J. 2, 75–78.

Mina, M.J., Metcalf, C.J.E., de Swart, R.L., Osterhaus, A.D.M.E., Grenfell, B.T., 2015. Long-term measles-induced immunomodulation increases overall childhood infectious disease mortality. Science 348, 694–699.

Mühlebach, M.D., Mateo, M., Sinn, P.L., Prufer, S., Uhlig, K.M., Leonard, V.H.J., Navaratnarajah, C.K., Frenzke, M., Wong, X.X., Sawatsky, B., Ramachandran, S., McCray, P.B., Cichutek, K., von Messling, V., Lopez, M., Cattaneo, R., 2011. Adherens junction protein nectin-4 is the epithelial receptor for measles virus. Nature 480, 530–533.

Munir, M., 2014. Role of wild small ruminants in the epidemiology of peste des petits ruminants. Transbound. Emerg. Dis. 61, 411–424.

Nakatsu, Y., Ma, X., Seki, F., Suzuki, T., Iwasaki, M., Yanagi, Y., Komase, K., Takeda, M., 2013. Intracellular transport of the measles virus ribonucleoprotein complex is mediated by Rab11A-positive recycling endosomes and drives virus release from the apical membrane of polarized epithelial cells. J. Virol. 87, 4683–4693.

Nanda, S.K., Baron, M.D., 2006. Rinderpest virus blocks type I and type II interferon action: role of structural and nonstructural proteins. J. Virol. 80, 7555–7568.

Navaratnarajah, C.K., Leonard, V.H.J., Cattaneo, R., 2009. Measles virus glycoprotein complex assembly, receptor attachment, and cell entry. Curr. Top. Microbiol. Immunol. 329, 59–76.

Nawathe, D.R., Taylor, W.P., 1979. Experimental infection of domestic pigs with the virus of peste des petits ruminants. Tropl. Anim. Health Prod. 11, 120–122.

Njeumi, F., Taylor, W., Diallo, A., Miyagishima, K., Pastoret, P.-P., Vallat, B., Traore, M., 2012. The long journey: a brief review of the eradication of rinderpest. Rev. Sci. Tech. 31, 729–746.

Nourjah, P., Frerichs, R.R., 1995. Minimum attack rate for measuring measles vaccine efficacy. Int. J. Epidemiol. 24, 834–841.

Noyce, R.S., Bondre, D.G., Ha, M.N., Lin, L.-T., Sisson, G., Tsao, M.-S., Richardson, C.D., 2011. Tumor cell marker PVRL4 (nectin 4) is an epithelial cell receptor for measles virus. PLoS Pathog. 7, e1002240.

Okada, H., Kobune, F., Sato, T.A., Kohama, T., Takeuchi, Y., Abe, T., Takayama, N., Tsuchiya, T., Tashiro, M., 2000. Extensive lymphopenia due to apoptosis of uninfected lymphocytes in acute measles patients. Arch. Virol. 145, 905–920.

Osterhaus, A.D., Vedder, E.J., 1988. Identification of virus causing recent seal deaths. Nature 335, 20.

Park, E.-S., Suzuki, M., Kimura, M., Mizutani, H., Saito, R., Kubota, N., Hasuike, Y., Okajima, J., Kasai, H., Sato, Y., Nakajima, N., Maruyama, K., Imaoka, K., Morikawa, S., 2016. Epidemiological and pathological study of feline morbillivirus infection in domestic cats in Japan. BMC Vet. Res. 12, 228.

Pfaller, C.K., Conzelmann, K.-K., 2008. Measles virus V protein is a decoy substrate for IkappaB kinase alpha and prevents toll-like receptor 7/9-mediated interferon induction. J. Virol. 82, 12365–12373.

Pfaller, C.K., Li, Z., George, C.X., Samuel, C.E., 2011. Protein kinase PKR and RNA adenosine deaminase ADAR1: new roles for old players as modulators of the interferon response. Curr. Opin. Immunol. 23, 573–582.

Pillet, S., von Messling, V., 2009. Canine distemper virus selectively inhibits apoptosis progression in infected immune cells. J. Virol. 83, 6279–6287.

Plattet, P., Alves, L., Herren, M., Aguilar, H.C., 2016. Measles virus fusion protein: structure, function and inhibition. Virus 8, 112.

Plowright, W., 1962. Rinderpest virus. Ann. N. Y. Acad. Sci. 101, 548–563.

Plumet, S., Duprex, W.P., Gerlier, D., 2005. Dynamics of viral RNA synthesis during measles virus infection. J. Virol. 79, 6900–6908.

Pope, R.A., Parida, S., Bailey, D., Brownlie, J., Barrett, T., Banyard, A.C., 2013. Early events following experimental infection with Peste-des-Petits ruminants virus suggest immune cell targeting. PLoS One 8, e55830.

Ramachandran, A., Parisien, J.-P., Horvath, C.M., 2008. STAT2 is a primary target for measles virus V protein-mediated alpha/beta interferon signaling inhibition. J. Virol. 82, 8330–8338.

Ramazzini, B., 1712. De Contagiosa Epidemia Quae in Patavino Agro et tota fere Veneta Ditione in Boves Irrepsit Dissertatio. Conzattus.

Richetta, C., Grégoire, I.P., Verlhac, P., Azocar, O., Baguet, J., Flacher, M., Tangy, F., Rabourdin-Combe, C., Faure, M., 2013. Sustained autophagy contributes to measles virus infectivity. PLoS Pathog. 9, e1003599.

Rima, B.K., Wishaupt, R.G., Welsh, M.J., Earle, J.A., 1995. The evolution of morbilliviruses: a comparison of nucleocapsid gene sequences including a porpoise morbillivirus. Vet. Microbiol. 44, 127–134.

Rodriguez, K.R., Horvath, C.M., 2014. Paramyxovirus V protein interaction with the antiviral sensor LGP2 disrupts MDA5 signaling enhancement but is not relevant to LGP2-mediated RLR signaling inhibition. J. Virol. 88, 8180–8188.

Rothlisberger, A., Wiener, D., Schweizer, M., Peterhans, E., Zurbriggen, A., Plattet, P., 2010. Two domains of the V protein of virulent canine distemper virus selectively inhibit STAT1 and STAT2 nuclear import. J. Virol. 84, 6328–6343.

Rudd, P.A., Cattaneo, R., von Messling, V., 2006. Canine distemper virus uses both the anterograde and the hematogenous pathway for neuroinvasion. J. Virol. 80, 9361–9370.

Ryon, J.J., Moss, W.J., Monze, M., Griffin, D.E., 2002. Functional and phenotypic changes in circulating lymphocytes from hospitalized zambian children with measles. Clin. Diagn. Lab. Immunol. 9, 994–1003.

Sakaguchi, S., Nakagawa, S., Yoshikawa, R., Kuwahara, C., Hagiwara, H., Asai, K.-i., Kawakami, K., Yamamoto, Y., Ogawa, M., Miyazawa, T., 2014. Genetic diversity of feline morbilliviruses isolated in Japan. J. Gen. Virol. 95, 1464–1468.

Sato, H., Masuda, M., Kanai, M., Tsukiyama-Kohara, K., Yoneda, M., Kai, C., 2007. Measles virus N protein inhibits host translation by binding to eIF3-p40. J. Virol. 81, 11569–11576.

Satoh, T., Kato, H., Kumagai, Y., Yoneyama, M., Sato, S., Matsushita, K., Tsujimura, T., Fujita, T., Akira, S., Takeuchi, O., 2010. LGP2 is a positive regulator of RIG-I- and MDA5-mediated antiviral responses. Proc. Natl. Acad. Sci. U. S. A. 107, 1512–1517.

Schuhmann, K.M., Pfaller, C.K., Conzelmann, K.-K., 2011. The measles virus V protein binds to p65 (RelA) to suppress NF-kappaB activity. J. Virol. 85, 3162–3171.

Shanks, G.D., Waller, M., Briem, H., Gottfredsson, M., 2015. Age-specific measles mortality during the late 19th-early 20th centuries. Epidemiol. Infect. 143, 3434–3441.

Sharp, C.R., Nambulli, S., Acciardo, A.S., Rennick, L.J., Drexler, J.F., Rima, B.K., Williams, T., Duprex, W.P., 2016. Chronic infection of domestic cats with feline morbillivirus, United States. Emerg. Infect. Dis. 22, 760–762.

Sidhu, M.S., Chan, J., Kaelin, K., Spielhofer, P., Radecke, F., Schneider, H., Masurekar, M., Dowling, P.C., Billeter, M.A., Udem, S.A., 1995. Rescue of synthetic measles virus minireplicons: measles genomic termini direct efficient expression and propagation of a reporter gene. Virology 208, 800–807.

Siebert, U., Gulland, F., Harder, T., Jauniaux, T., Seibel, H., Wohlsein, P., Baumgärtner, W., 2010. Epizootics in harbour seals (Phoca vitulina): clinical aspects. NAMMCOSP 8, 265.

Slifka, M.K., Homann, D., Tishon, A., Pagarigan, R., Oldstone, M.B.A., 2003. Measles virus infection results in suppression of both innate and adaptive immune responses to secondary bacterial infection. J. Clin. Invest. 111, 805–810.

Sourimant, J., Plemper, R.K., 2016. Organization, function, and therapeutic targeting of the morbillivirus RNA-dependent RNA polymerase complex. Virus 8.

Sparrer, K.M.J., Pfaller, C.K., Conzelmann, K.-K., 2012. Measles virus C protein interferes with Beta interferon transcription in the nucleus. J. Virol. 86, 796–805.

Stephens, N., Duignan, P.J., Wang, J., Bingham, J., Finn, H., Bejder, L., Patterson, A.P., Holyoake, C., 2014. Cetacean morbillivirus in coastal Indo-Pacific bottlenose dolphins, Western Australia. Emerg. Infect. Dis. 20, 666–670.

Sugai, A., Sato, H., Yoneda, M., Kai, C., 2012. Phosphorylation of measles virus phosphoprotein at S86 and/or S151 downregulates viral transcriptional activity. FEBS Lett. 586, 3900–3907.

Sugai, A., Sato, H., Yoneda, M., Kai, C., 2013. Phosphorylation of measles virus nucleoprotein affects viral growth by changing gene expression and genomic RNA stability. J. Virol. 87, 11684–11692.

Summers, B.A., Appel, M.J., 1994. Aspects of canine distemper virus and measles virus encephalomyelitis. Neuropathol. Appl. Neurobiol. 20, 525–534.

Summers, B.A., Greisen, H.A., Appel, M.J., 1979. Early events in canine distemper demyelinating encephalomyelitis. Acta Neuropathol. 46, 1–10.

Suringa, D.W., Bank, L.J., Ackerman, A.B., 1970. Role of measles virus in skin lesions and Koplik's spots. N. Engl. J. Med. 283, 1139–1142.

Svitek, N., von Messling, V., 2007. Early cytokine mRNA expression profiles predict morbillivirus disease outcome in ferrets. Virology 362, 404–410.

Svitek, N., Gerhauser, I., Goncalves, C., Grabski, E., Doring, M., Kalinke, U., Anderson, D.E., Cattaneo, R., von Messling, V., 2014. Morbillivirus control of the interferon response: relevance of STAT2 and mda5 but not STAT1 for canine distemper virus virulence in ferrets. J. Virol. 88, 2941–2950.

Tahara, M., Takeda, M., Yanagi, Y., 2007. Altered interaction of the matrix protein with the cytoplasmic tail of hemagglutinin modulates measles virus growth by affecting virus assembly and cell-cell fusion. J. Virol. 81, 6827–6836.

Tahara, M., Ito, Y., Brindley, M.A., Ma, X., He, J., Xu, S., Fukuhara, H., Sakai, K., Komase, K., Rota, P.A., Plemper, R.K., Maenaka, K., Takeda, M., 2013. Functional and structural characterization of neutralizing epitopes of measles virus hemagglutinin protein. J. Virol. 87, 666–675.

Tahara, M., Bürckert, J.-P., Kanou, K., Maenaka, K., Muller, C.P., Takeda, M., 2016. Measles virus hemagglutinin protein epitopes: the basis of antigenic stability. Virus 8.

Takayama, I., Sato, H., Watanabe, A., Omi-Furutani, M., Sugai, A., Kanki, K., Yoneda, M., Kai, C., 2012. The nucleocapsid protein of measles virus blocks host interferon response. Virology 424, 45–55.

Tatsuo, H., Ono, N., Tanaka, K., Yanagi, Y., 2000. SLAM (CDw150) is a cellular receptor for measles virus. Nature 406, 893–897.

Tatsuo, H., Ono, N., Yanagi, Y., 2001. Morbilliviruses use signaling lymphocyte activation molecules (CD150) as cellular receptors. J. Virol. 75, 5842–5850.

Taubenberger, J.K., Tsai, M.M., Atkin, T.J., Fanning, T.G., Krafft, A.E., Moeller, R.B., Kodsi, S.E., Mense, M.G., Lipscomb, T.P., 2000. Molecular genetic evidence of a novel morbillivirus in a long-finned pilot whale (Globicephalus melas). Emerg. Infect. Dis. 6, 42–45.

Taylor, W., 2016. The global eradication of peste des petits ruminants (PPR) within 15 years—is this a pipe dream? Tropl. Anim. Health Prod. 48, 559–567.

Truong, T., Boshra, H., Embury-Hyatt, C., Nfon, C., Gerdts, V., Tikoo, S., Babiuk, L.A., Kara, P., Chetty, T., Mather, A., Wallace, D.B., Babiuk, S., 2014. Peste des petits ruminants virus tissue tropism and pathogenesis in sheep and goats following experimental infection. PLoS One 9, e87145.

van Bressem, M.-F., Duignan, P.J., Banyard, A., Barbieri, M., Colegrove, K.M., de Guise, S., Di Guardo, G., Dobson, A., Domingo, M., Fauquier, D., Fernandez, A., Goldstein, T., Grenfell, B., Groch, K.R., Gulland, F., Jensen, B.A., Jepson, P.D., Hall, A., Kuiken, T., Mazzariol, S., Morris, S.E., Nielsen, O., Raga, J.A., Rowles, T.K., Saliki, J., Sierra, E., Stephens, N., Stone, B., Tomo, I., Wang, J., Waltzek, T., Wellehan, J.F.X., 2014. Cetacean morbillivirus: current knowledge and future directions. Virus 6, 5145–5181.

van de Bildt, M.W., Martina, B.E., Vedder, E.J., Androukaki, E., Kotomatas, S., Komnenou, A., Sidi, B.A., Jiddou, A.B., Barham, M.E., Niesters, H.G., Osterhaus, A.D., 2000. Identification of morbilliviruses of probable cetacean origin in carcases of Mediterranean monk seals (Monachus monachus). Vet. Rec. 146, 691–694.

Visser, I.K., van Bressem, M.F., Swart, R.L.d., van de Bildt, M.W., Vos, H.W., van der Heijden, R.W., Saliki, J.T., Orvell, C., Kitching, P., Kuiken, T., 1993. Characterization of morbilliviruses isolated from dolphins and porpoises in Europe. J. Gen. Virol. 74 (Pt 4), 631–641.

von Messling, V., Springfeld, C., Devaux, P., Cattaneo, R., 2003. A ferret model of canine distemper virus virulence and immunosuppression. J. Virol. 77, 12579–12591.

von Messling, V., Milosevic, D., Cattaneo, R., 2004. Tropism illuminated: lymphocyte-based pathways blazed by lethal morbillivirus through the host immune system. Proc. Natl. Acad. Sci. U.S.A. 101, 14216–14221.

Wakimoto, H., Shimodo, M., Satoh, Y., Kitagawa, Y., Takeuchi, K., Gotoh, B., Itoh, M., 2013. F-actin modulates measles virus cell-cell fusion and assembly by altering the interaction between the matrix protein and the cytoplasmic tail of hemagglutinin. J. Virol. 87, 1974–1984.

Wang, Z., Bao, J., Wu, X., Liu, Y., Li, L., Liu, C., Suo, L., Xie, Z., Zhao, W., Zhang, W., Yang, N., Li, J., Wang, S., Wang, J., 2009. Peste des petits ruminants virus in Tibet, China. Emerg. Infect. Dis. 15, 299–301.

Wang, L.-F., Collins, P.L., Fouchier, R.A.M., Kurath, G., Lamb, R.A., Randall, R.E., Rima, B.K. (Eds.), 2011. Virus Taxonomy: Classification and Nomenclature of Viruses: Ninth Report of the International Committee on Taxonomy of Viruses: Family Paramyxoviridae, 9th ed. Academic Press, London.

Watanabe, M., Hirano, A., Stenglein, S., Nelson, J., Thomas, G., Wong, T.C., 1995. Engineered serine protease inhibitor prevents furin-catalyzed activation of the fusion glycoprotein and production of infectious measles virus. J. Virol. 69, 3206–3210.

Watanabe, A., Yoneda, M., Ikeda, F., Sugai, A., Sato, H., Kai, C., 2011. Peroxiredoxin 1 is required for efficient transcription and replication of measles virus. J. Virol. 85, 2247–2253.

Welsh, M.J., Lyons, C., Trudgett, A., Rima, B.K., McCullough, S.J., Orvell, C., 1992. Characteristics of a cetacean morbillivirus isolated from a porpoise (Phocoena phocoena). Arch. Virol. 125, 305–311.

West, K.L., Levine, G., Jacob, J., Jensen, B., Sanchez, S., Colegrove, K., Rotstein, D., 2015. Coinfection and vertical transmission of Brucella and morbillivirus in a neonatal sperm whale (Physeter macrocephalus) in Hawaii, USA. J. Wildl. Dis. 51, 227–232.

Woo, P.C.Y., Lau, S.K.P., Wong, B.H.L., Fan, R.Y.Y., Wong, A.Y.P., Zhang, A.J.X., Wu, Y., Choi, G.K.Y., Li, K.S.M., Hui, J., Wang, M., Zheng, B.-J., Chan, K.H., Yuen, K.-Y., 2012. Feline morbillivirus, a previously undescribed paramyxovirus associated with tubulointerstitial nephritis in domestic cats. Proc. Natl. Acad. Sci. U.S.A. 109, 5435–5440.

Yokota, S.-I., Okabayashi, T., Fujii, N., 2011. Measles virus C protein suppresses gamma-activated factor formation and virus-induced cell growth arrest. Virology 414, 74–82.

Zhang, X., Bourhis, J.-M., Longhi, S., Carsillo, T., Buccellato, M., Morin, B., Canard, B., Oglesbee, M., 2005. Hsp72 recognizes a P binding motif in the measles virus N protein C-terminus. Virology 337, 162–174.

FURTHER READING

Casalone, C., Mazzariol, S., Pautasso, A., Di Guardo, G., Di Nocera, F., Lucifora, G., Ligios, C., Franco, A., Fichi, G., Cocumelli, C., Cersini, A., Guercio, A., Puleio, R., Goria, M., Podesta, M., Marsili, L., Pavan, G., Pintore, A., de Carlo, E., Eleni, C., Caracappa, S., 2014. Cetacean strandings in Italy: an unusual mortality event along the Tyrrhenian Sea coast in 2013. Dis. Aquat. Organ. 109, 81–86.

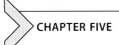

CHAPTER FIVE

Viruses of Plant-Interacting Fungi

Bradley I. Hillman*,[1], Aulia Annisa[†], Nobuhiro Suzuki[†,1]

*Plant Biology and Pathology, Rutgers University, New Brunswick, NJ, United States
[†]Institute of Plant Science and Resources (IPSR), Okayama University, Kurashiki, Japan
[1]Corresponding authors: e-mail address: hillman@aesop.rutgers.edu; nsuzuki@okayama-u.ac.jp

Contents

Abstract

Plant-associated fungi are infected by viruses at the incidence rates from a few % to over 90%. Multiple viruses often coinfect fungal hosts, and occasionally alter their phenotypes, but most of the infections are asymptomatic. Phenotypic alterations are grouped into two types: harmful or beneficial to the host fungi. Harmful interactions between viruses and hosts include hypovirulence and/or debilitation that are documented in a number of phytopathogenic fungi, exemplified by the chestnut blight, white root rot, and rapeseed rot fungi. Beneficial interactions are observed in a limited number of plant endophytic and pathogenic fungi where heat tolerance and virulence are enhanced, respectively. Coinfections of fungi provided a platform for discoveries of interesting virus/virus interactions that include synergistic, as in the case for those in plants, and unique antagonistic and mutualistic interactions between unrelated RNA viruses. Also discussed here are coinfection-induced genome rearrangements and frequently observed coinfections by the simplest positive-strand RNA virus, the mitoviruses.

Advances in Virus Research, Volume 100
ISSN 0065-3527
https://doi.org/10.1016/bs.aivir.2017.10.003

1. INTRODUCTION

According to the latest list of fungal viruses approved by the International Committee on Taxonomy of Viruses (ICTV) (ICTV Master Species List 2016 v1.3), fungal viruses or mycoviruses span at least 12 families. Some show similarity to plant and/or animal viruses, while others constitute their own families. Their numbers will soon be considerably increased given the pace of discoveries of new viruses that is particularly accelerated by metagenomics/next-generation sequencing approaches (Marzano and Domier, 2016; Nerva et al., 2016). Such studies along with conventional fungal virus hunting have greatly enhanced our understanding of virus diversity and evolution. Double-stranded (ds) and positive-sense (+) RNA viruses were known to prevail in fungi and no viruses with other genome types had been reported until recently. In the past decade, however, (−) RNA viruses with phylogenetic affinity to mononegaviruses or segmented (−)RNA viruses have been reported from ascomycetes (e.g., Kondo et al., 2013a; Liu et al., 2014). In addition, gemini-like single-stranded DNA viruses first identified in fungi (Yu et al., 2010) now are classified in the family *Genomoviridae* together with those reported from various environmental samples (Krupovic et al., 2016). Among fungal viruses are peculiar ones that challenge "virus rules," as exemplified by capsidless viruses (Dawe and Nuss, 2013; Hillman and Cai, 2013; Zhang et al., 2016) and infectious viruses as naked dsRNA (Kanhayuwa et al., 2015).

Fungal viruses are generally transmitted vertically via spores and horizontally via anastomosis, with no extracellular phase of the infection cycle. One exception to this is the genomovirus, Sclerotinia gemycircularvirus 1 (SGCV1) that enters host fungal cells on media, and infects a mycophagous insect, which transmits the virus between fungal host colonies in fields (Liu et al., 2016). The transmission of fungal viruses by vector organisms has been implicated for a long time (Hillman et al., 2004; Petrzik et al., 2016; Yaegashi et al., 2013), and there are likely other organisms that serve as vectors of fungal viruses in nature. Interhyphal transmission is readily achieved during anastomosis when the two hyphae are vegetatively compatible (Choi et al., 2012; Zhang et al., 2014), and transmission across species boundaries has been inferred from field samples and demonstrated in the laboratory (Liu et al., 2003). Fungal vegetative incompatibility, a self/nonself-recognition system, is governed genetically by multiple loci called VIC loci (Glass and Dementhon, 2006; Zhang et al., 2014). Cell-to-cell movement though septal pores should be possible given that cellular organelles including nuclei can move through them.

The principles of intracellular replication of fungal viruses are assumed to be similar to plant or animal viruses with the same genome type. The yeast *Saccharomyces cerevisiae*, host to a number of its own viruses, has been used effectively as an experimental host for several plant and animal viruses to probe essential replication-associated host genes (Janda and Ahlquist, 1993; Nagy, 2016, for review). Wickner and colleagues reported on a number of viral and host factors whose mutations affect different steps of the replication of a dsRNA virus, Saccharomyces cerevisiae virus L-A (Wickner et al., 2013). However, little is known about the genome replication of mycoviruses in filamentous fungi at the molecular level. Only a few host factors were shown to be essential for the efficient replication/maintenance of (+) RNA viruses (Son et al., 2013; Sun et al., 2008). As in the case of other eukaryotes, fungi operate cellular level antiviral defense, i.e., RNA silencing that affects virus replication. Recent progress on fungal RNA silencing as an antiviral defense and an apparently proviral mechanism is notable (Andika et al., 2017; Chiba and Suzuki, 2015; Eusebio-Cope and Suzuki, 2015; Segers et al., 2007; Sun et al., 2009).

In this review article, we focus on intriguing interplays between coinfecting viruses, between viruses and hosts, and among three associated players, viruses/fungi/plants. Readers are also referred to other excellent recent reviews (Ghabrial, 2013; Ghabrial et al., 2015; Xie and Jiang, 2014).

2. TYPES OF VIRUS/HOST INTERACTIONS

Effects of virus infections on host fungi are diverse, involving alterations in the host transcriptome, small RNAome, proteome, metabolome, lipidome, and epigenome. Fungal viruses may cause beneficial, neutral (little or no), or harmful effects on the development, vegetative growth, and other physiological properties of host fungi, as in the case for other hosts. Importantly, due to technical advances in artificial introduction and curing of viruses (Kondo et al., 2013b), viral etiology has been established for these phenotypic alterations in a number of virus/host fungal systems. Most fungal virus infections are asymptomatic, but even apparently asymptomatic infections may affect host physiology and phenotype under stress conditions. In addition, Vainio and colleagues reported that interactions of even single partitiviruses or related viruses are complex, at some times beneficial and at other times harmful, depending on host strain (genotype) and environ-mental conditions (Vainio and Hantula, 2016).

2.1 Beneficial Interactions With Host Fungi

There are a few examples in which virus infection exerts beneficial effects on its fungal host. One of the most fascinating examples is the tripartite mutu-alism among a panic grass, an endophytic fungus, and a mycovirus. Curvularia thermal tolerance virus, a bisegmented genome virus belonging to a cluster of unassigned dsRNA viruses, infects a fungus (*Curvularia protuberia*) endophytic to plants and confers heat tolerance not only to the fungal host but also to plant hosts of the fungus (Marquez et al., 2007). The virus/fungus was originally discovered in a grass (*Dichanthelium lanuginosum*) in Yellowstone National Park. Interestingly virus-infected fungi can render experimental dicots including tomato heat tolerant (Marquez et al., 2007), but how the virus confers heat tolerance remains elusive.

There are several examples of combinations of viruses enhancing phyto-pathogenic fungi on plant hosts. Ahn and Lee (2001) reported a hyp-ervirulence phenomenon where a virus with a 6-kbp dsRNA genome confers enhanced virulence to the host fungus, *Nectria radicicola* that causes root rot in ginseng. It is of interest to note that the virus-encoded RdRp shows sequence similarity to those of partitiviruses, despite the fact that its genome appears to be nonsegmented and much larger than those of partitiviruses. Hypervirulence-associated traits of increased levels of con-idiation and pigmentation may be related to the alteration of two signaling pathways: cAMP-dependent and Ca^{2+}-dependent pathways. The upregulation of cAMP-dependent protein kinase and downregulation of Ca^{2+}-dependent protein kinase are commonly observed in the 6-kbp dsRNA-induced hypervirulence in *N. radicicola* (Ahn and Lee, 2001) and Cryphonectria hypovirus 1 (CHV1)-mediated hypovirulence in *Cryphonectria parasitica* (Nuss, 1996). Another example of increased viru-lence was described for a virus infecting *Alternaria alternata,* which produces host-specific toxins and causes black spot in Japanese pear (Fuke et al., 2011) (H. Moriyama, personal communication). The virus increases the virulence of the host fungus by enhancing host-specific toxin production while caus-ing irregular vegetative growth and pigmentation. It will be an intriguing challenge to explore which step of the pathway for host-specific toxin syn-thesis is perturbed. Note that the "beneficial effects" in these and examples below may not always confer higher ecological fitness to their hosts.

Recently discovered examples of animal/fungus/virus systems similar to the plant/fungus/virus examples include the mild hypervirulence conferred by a four-segmented dsRNA virus of the human pathogen *Aspergillus fumigatus*, Aspergillus fumigatus tetramycovirus-1 (AfuTmV1) (Kanhayuwa et al., 2015), and by a multisegmented virus complex of the entomopathogenic fungus *Beauveria bassiana* (Kotta-Loizou and Coutts, 2017). Another similar system involves a gammapartitivirus, *Pseudogymnoascus destructans* partitivirus-pa that may enhance pigmentation and conidiation of its host fungus that causes fatal white-nose syndrome in bats in North America (Thapa et al., 2016).

2.2 Harmful Interactions With Host Fungi

Technical advances in artificial introduction and curing of viruses have led to determination of viral etiology for a number of virus/host fungal systems (Kondo et al., 2013b; Suzuki, 2017). Harmful interactions are well exemplified by reduced fungal virulence, or "hypovirulence" induced by several viruses (Ghabrial et al., 2015). Thus, fungal viruses also could be potential virocontrol agents if they infect plant pathogenic fungi (Yu et al., 2013), as in the case for hypoviruses that are used to help manage chestnut blight in Europe (Rigling and Prospero, 2017). Hypovirulence is usually associated with other phenotypic alterations like reduced pigmentation, reduced sporulation, and growth defects. The best-studied example is CHV1/ *C. parasitica*, a long-established system that has provided particularly good tools for studying virus–fungus interactions (Dawe and Nuss, 2013). Using reverse genetics available for a mild and a severe CHV1 strain, a domain responsible for hypovirulence was shown to reside on the 3′-portion of the ORFB-coding domain. Other hypovirulence-inducing *C. parasitica*-infecting examples include CHV2, CHV3, mycoreovirus 1 (MyRV1), and MyRV2 (Hillman and Suzuki, 2004). Rosellinia necatrix megabirnavirus 1 (RnMBV1) and MyRV3 were shown to reduce virulence of the white root rot fungus (Chiba et al., 2009; Kanematsu et al., 2010). RnMBV1 is stably maintained in the host, thus being regarded as a potential virocontrol agent, while MyRV3 is unstable and occasionally lost in the host. *Sclerotinia sclerotiorum* is an important plant pathogenic fungus in which the most hypovirulence-conferring viruses were identified (Xie and Jiang, 2014). Of particular note is the first description of a gemini-like ssDNA virus (Yu et al., 2010), SsHADV1 and a mononegavirus, Sclerotinia sclerotiorum negative-stranded RNA virus 1 (SsNSRV-1) (Liu et al., 2014) associated with hypovirulence. Two other viruses,

Sclerotinia sclerotiorum hypovirus 2 (SsHV2) (Marzano et al., 2015) and Sclerotinia sclerotiorum partitivirus 1 (SsPV1) (Xiao et al., 2014), also cause hypovirulence in *S. sclerotiorum*, the latter noteworthy in that most partitiviruses show asymptomatic infections, whether their hosts are plants or fungi. There are many other examples of hypovirulence-causing viruses spanning diverse virus families. Host fungi shown to be displaying hypovirulent phenotypes are largely restricted to ascomycetes, and relatively little is known about viral or host factors responsible for the phenotypic changes caused by these viruses.

3. TYPES OF VIRUS/VIRUS INTERACTIONS

Coinfections of single fungal host strains by multiple viruses are common, but constraints on the accumulation of multiple viruses in a single host remain unclear. Fungal viruses were recently shown to be horizontally transferred in a natural setting, possibly by small animals (Yaegashi et al., 2013), and to suppress vegetative incompatibility responses and facilitate horizontal transmission via anastomosis (Wu et al., 2017). These may enhance mixed infections of single fungal strains. Below are several recognizable virus/virus interactions in fungi (see Table 1 for their typing).

3.1 Synergistic Interactions Between Viruses

Synergistic interactions are well established in plant/virus systems (Pruss et al., 1997; Tatineni et al., 2010) and are classically defined as increased virus titer and symptom severity in coinfections relative to single infections. For example, coinfection of tobacco by a potexvirus, potato virus X, and a potyvirus, potato virus Y, enhances symptoms and allows for more PVX accumulation than respective single infections (Vance, 1991). One-way synergism was found in coinfections of *C. parasitica* by CHV1 and MyRV1, where CHV1 enhances MyRV1 accumulation, but not vice versa. The alteration in symptoms and MyRV1 accumulation is partially mediated by transgenic expression of an RNA silencing suppressor encoded by CHV1, p29 (Sun et al., 2006). Another example was found in *Rosellinia necatrix* doubly infected by a megabirnavirus, RnMBV2 and a partitivirus, RnPV1 (Sasaki et al., 2016). This example is distinct from the earlier cases in that neither RnMBV2 nor RnPV1 causes phenotypic alteration; only coinfection leads to hypovirulence and reduced colony growth regardless of host fungal strains. Furthermore, RnMBV2 enhances the accumulation of RnPV1 by approximately twofold. The domain responsible for this effect may be on dsRNA2 of RnMBV2, given the observation that

Table 1 Types of Virus/Virus Interactions in Coinfections

Type	Definition and Remarks	Example (Host Fungus)	Reference
Synergistic interactions	One virus enhances replication and symptom induction of the other virus unilaterally or mutually	MyRV1/CHV1 (*Cryphonectria parasitica*)	Sun et al. (2006)
		RnPV1/RnMBV2 (*Rosellinia necatrix*)	Sasaki et al. (2016)
Mutualistic interactions	One virus confers the viability to the other in their natural lifecycles unilaterally or mutually	YnV1/YkV1 (*R. necatrix*)	Zhang et al. (2016)
		PaTV1/PaFIV1[a] (*Penicillium aurantiogriseum*)	Nerva et al. (2016)
		FpVV1/FpMV2[a] (*Fusarium poae*)	Osaki et al. (2016)
		AfV-S1/AfV-S2[a] (*Aspergillus foetidus*)	Kozlakidis et al. (2013)
Antagonistic interactions	One virus impairs an infection step(s) of the other virus unilaterally or mutually	RnVV1/MyRV1 (*C. parasitica*)	Chiba and Suzuki (2015)
		RnVV1/CHV1-Δp69[b] (*C. parasitica*)	Chiba and Suzuki (2015)
		RnVV1/RnPV3 (*C. parasitica*)	Chiba et al. (unpublished data)
Induced genome rearrangements	One virus generates genome recombination of the other virus. This phenomenon is associated with suppression of RNA silencing. Only one example described in the next column has been reported thus far.	MyRV1 (reovirus) genome rearrangements induced by CHV1 (hypovirus) in *C. parasitica*.	Sun and Suzuki. (2008), Tanaka et al. (2011), and Eusebio-Cope and Suzuki (2015)

[a] For these virus/virus combinations, a mutualistic interaction similar to the YnV1/YkV1 is predicted, but should be substantiated.
[b] CHV1-Δp69 is a mutant lacking ORFA encoding p29 (RNA silencing suppressor) and p40 (replication enhancer).

replication-competent RnMBV2 dsRNA1 cannot increase RnPV1 accumulation, which awaits further experimental validation.

3.2 Mutualistic Interactions Between Viruses

Mutualistic interactions in this subdivision deal with dependent relations rather than two-way synergistic interactions that involve two independent viruses. However, mutualistic interactions between viruses are distinct from satellite/helper viruses or defective/helper viruses, which are not relationships between bona fide viruses but between viruses and subviral molecules (satellites and defective nucleic acids). Subviral molecules do not encode a replicase essential for autonomous replication, which is the hallmark gene for viruses. Mutualistic interactions recently discovered in *R. necatrix* represent a different virus lifestyle. A capsidless (+)RNA virus termed yado-kari virus 1 (YkV1) is hosted by a dsRNA virus designated as yado–nushi virus 1 (YnV1). According to the model proposed by Zhang et al. (2016), YnV1 is an independent virus able to complete its replication cycle like other dsRNA viruses, while YkV1 diverts YnV1 CP at the replication sites where *trans*-encapsidated YkV1 RdRp synthesize its own RNA as if it was a dsRNA virus. This replication strategy with virion-associated replicase is generally employed by a dsRNA virus. "Yado" in Japanese literally means home or house, while "kari" and "nushi" refer to "borrower" and "owner," respectively. This model needs to be validated by site-directed mutagenesis of available infectious YkV1 cDNA and biochemical analysis with purified heterocapsids. There may be similar mutualistic interactions in other fungi such as *Aspergillus foetidus* (Kozlakidis et al., 2013; Nerva et al., 2016; Osaki et al., 2016). More thorough discussion will be featured elsewhere (Fig. 1) (Hisano et al., 2018).

3.3 Antagonistic Interactions Between Viruses

RNA silencing operates as antiviral defense at the cellular level in fungi as in other eukaryotic organisms. Two key genes in *C. parasitica*, Dicer-like 2 (*dcl2*) and Argonaute-like 2 (*agl2*), play important roles in antiviral defense. Like plant viruses, some fungal viruses are known to counteract RNA silencing using silencing suppressors as exemplified by CHV1 p29. CHV1 has an undivided (+) RNA genome, belonging to the expanded picorna-like supergroup, that possesses two ORFs, A and B. ORFA encodes a multifunctional protein p29 and a basic protein p40 that are released by the self-cleavage activity (papain-like cysteine protease) of p29. p29 is also

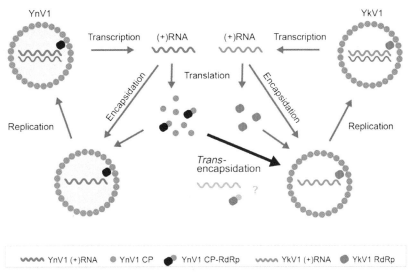

Fig. 1 A proposed model for the interplay between YnV1 and YkV1. YnV1 as an independent dsRNA virus can complete its replication cycle. YkV1 diverts the YnV1 capsid protein to *trans*-encapsidate its genomic, plus-sense RNA, and RNA-dependent RNA polymerase. In the model, heterocapsids serve as the replication sites for the synthesis of YkV1 minus-sense RNA (replication) and plus-sense RNA (transcription). YkV1, thus, is replicated as if it were a dsRNA despite the fact YkV1 has a (+) RNA virus genome.

involved in virus viability, symptom expression, and RNA silencing suppression in addition to polyprotein processing, while p40 enhances the replication and vertical transmission of CHV1 (Hillman and Suzuki, 2004). In this subdivision, two other RNA viruses are included: MyRV1 (a reovirus) with an 11-segmented dsRNA genome and Rosellinia necatrix victorivirus 1 (RnVV1, a totivirus) with an undivided dsRNA genome.

Antagonistic interactions between coinfecting viruses were found in *C. parasitica* in which one virus, a CHV1 mutant lacking p29 and p40 (CHV1-Δp69), interferes with the replication and horizontal transmission of another virus, RnVV1. An indistinguishable antagonism was observed between MyRV1 and RnVV1 in *C. parasitica*. This phenomenon appears to be phenotypically similar but mechanistically dissimilar to virus interference (crossprotection) that is well known in plants, or vaccination in vertebrates, both of which involve two closely related viruses. In *C. parasitica*, RnVV1 was impaired by coinfection with MyRV1 or CHV1-Δp69 (Chiba and Suzuki, 2015). Even preexisting RnVV1 is eliminated by a challenge with either of these viruses. Antiviral RNA silencing is involved in this phenomenon. MyRV1 and CHV1-Δp69 markedly activate antiviral RNA silencing via transcriptional upregulation of *dcl2* and *agl2* (Chiba and Suzuki, 2015). The *dcl2* and *agl2* upregulation and its suppression by CHV1 p29 were first noted by Nuss and colleagues (Sun et al., 2009; Zhang et al., 2012). RnVV1 is demonstrably more susceptible to activated RNA silencing than MyRV1 and CHV1-Δp69. Andika et al. (2017) showed the SAGA (Spt–Ada–Gcn5 acetyltransferase) complex, a general coactivator conserved across eukaryotes, to mediate the transcriptional induction of *dcl2* and *agl2*. The histone acetyltransferase (HAT) activity of SAGA is the major regulator of the *dcl2* upregulation, while SAGA's HAT and deubiquitinase activities control *agl2* induction. Interestingly, DCL2 and AGL2 are important as positive feedback players in this antiviral RNA silencing activation; DCL2 is essential for the induction of both genes by either virus, while AGL2 is required only for their full-scale induction by CHV1 but not for that by MyRV1 (Andika et al., 2017).

3.4 Genome Rearrangements During Coinfection

Induced genome rearrangements of fungal viruses were first observed in *C. parasitica* coinfected by MyRV1 and CHV1 (Sun and Suzuki, 2008). The coinfection leads to the frequent appearance of rearranged MyRV1 segment S10. These rearrangements are associated with compromised RNA silencing by the CHV1 p29 RNA silencing suppressor. Transgenic expression of CHV1 p29 or disruption of key genes in the RNA silencing pathway results in generation of MyRV1 genome rearrangements to segments S1–S4, S6, and S10 (Eusebio-Cope and Suzuki, 2015; Sun and Suzuki, 2008; Tanaka et al., 2011, 2012). Rearrangements include large extensions and deletions. Extended sizes range from almost double-sizes for S1–S3 and S6, to 1.5-fold for S2 and S3, while deletions include minor to ~90% deletions of the S4 and S10 coding regions (S4ss and S10ss). Among these rearranged MyRV1 segments, S4ss and S10ss also appear infrequently in the wild-type fungal strain under laboratory conditions (Eusebio-Cope et al., 2010). The RNA silencing suppression-mediated rearrangement mechanism remains largely unknown.

RNA silencing appears to have yin and yang effects on virus genome stability, depending on the individual viruses. In the earlier examples RNA silencing contributes to MyRV1 genome stability, whereas RNA silencing is associated with instability of CHV1 RNAs. Defective CHV1 RNAs are generated in RNA silencing-competent host strains and are lost upon lateral transfer of the virus to mutant host strains that are defective in RNA silencing (Sun et al., 2009). This phenomenon is related to the observed genetic instability of CHV1-based vector constructs in RNA silencing-competent wild-type strains. CHV1-defective RNAs were hypothesized to be unable to move laterally to or replicate in RNA silencing-deficient strains. Given the relatively stable maintenance of defective RNAs of the CHV1 mutant Δp69 in the dicer-deficient fungal mutant Δ*dcl2* (Chiba and Suzuki, 2015), defective RNAs appear not to be transferred during hyphal fusion. These hypovirus behaviors in RNA silencing-deficient mutants warrant further exploration. Genome rearrangements have also been reported in nature and in laboratories in partitiviruses (Chiba et al., 2013, 2016) and megabirnaviruses (Kanematsu et al., 2014) after virion transfection. Association of these examples with compromised RNA silencing has yet to be examined.

3.5 Implication of Coinfections by Multiple Mito- and Mito-Like Viruses

Mitoviruses were identified as the first autonomous RNA elements that appeared to complete their life cycles within mitochondria (Polashock and Hillman, 1994; reviewed in Hillman and Cai, 2013). Although many of their properties remain to be elucidated, we now know much more about these important members of the mycovirus community. More than 100 such elements have been identified based on nucleotide sequence, and several such elements have been examined in some biological detail. One of the key distinguishing features of mitoviruses compared to all other viruses is their use of UGA to encode Trp rather than translation termination: their coding sequences are usually predicted to be nontranslatable in the cytoplasm.

The difficulty in teasing apart mitovirus–host interactions involves their essential nature as mitochondrial elements. It is, in effect, an interaction of a virus in a host within a host. Coinfections of a single fungal thallus with a mitovirus and a cytoplasmic virus (e.g., Ran et al., 2016) or with multiple mitoviruses appear to be a common occurrence (e.g., Hong et al., 1999; Khalifa and Pearson, 2013; Wu et al., 2016; Xie and Ghabrial, 2012). Indeed, the first mitovirus system characterized at the biological level was the complex *Ophiostoma novo-ulmi* (Dutch elm disease) fungus–virus system, which contained many such elements that appeared to contribute to the fungal phenotype in varying ways (e.g., Hong et al., 1999; Rogers et al., 1986, 1987). Unambiguously clarifying the effects of specific mitovirus elements on fungal phenotype requires their characterization and infection of isogenic fungal strains with individual elements. Doing research such as this highlights the difficulty of performing reverse genetics with elements that replicate in mitochondria, where the lack of straightforward transfection systems that are available for cytoplasmic elements and complexities of mitochondrial biology lead to difficulties in interpreting virus transmission results (Polashock et al., 1997). The confounding factor of mitochondrial disease in fungi that is not associated with virus infection (e.g., Baidyaroy et al., 2011) underscores the importance of isolating only the effects of individual mitoviruses on fungal phenotype, which turns out to be quite challenging.

The number of mitovirus sequences and corresponding fungal host mitochondrial sequences deposited in GenBank has accumulated to a high enough level that a systematic study comparing relative codon usage could be accomplished. In doing so, Nibert (2017) recently found a positive correlation between the two: thus, mitoviral RNAs that contain abundant UGA codons tend to infect fungal hosts whose use of Trp-encoding UGA codons is also high, and low UGA(Trp) codon use in the host in turn corresponds to low presence in associated viruses. This important insight not only greatly advances our understanding of mitoviruses but also our understanding of the fungal host, as this variability in fungal mitochondrial codon usage had not been documented previously. Of course, this has profound implications not only for mitovirus–fungus coevolution but also for host range predictions and expectations of coinfections of a host by different mitoviruses.

Mitoviruses may also provide key insights to understanding fundamental biology of virus–host interactions. Although mitoviruses have been identified only in filamentous fungi, mitovirus-related sequences have been identified in many plants as well, integrated as DNA copies in both nuclear and mitochondrial genomes (Hong et al., 1998; Marienfeld et al., 1997; Xu et al., 2015). Interestingly, integrated mitoviral sequences form a monophyletic group and are found even in the most ancient vascular plants, suggesting that integration into plants, and specifically to plant mitochondrial DNA, was itself an ancient event that likely happened only once (Bruenn et al., 2015). The timing of such horizontal transfer—possibly by infection with ancestral mitoviruses (bacterial leviviruses) not long after the ancestors of mitochondria (alphaproteobacteria) became plant endosymbionts—is a matter of speculation. Expression of the mitochondrial but not the nuclear copy of an integrated mitovirus-related sequence in *Arabidopsis* also raises interesting questions of function, including the possible function as part of an RNA-mediated defense system (Bruenn et al., 2015).

4. CONCLUSIONS AND PROSPECTS

Our understanding of the phylogenetic breadth and the biological properties of fungal viruses have advanced markedly over the last few years, resulting in discoveries that will lead scientists down new paths. Some of these advances result from advancing technologies, especially the widespread use of environmental sampling and new sequencing technologies that allow for discovery of many new viruses without fungal culture. Many significant advances also have come from new laboratories worldwide whose focus has been on fungal virus discovery and application. The many exceptional research accomplishments on the *C. parasitica*/virus system over the last 40 + years showed the broader research community what could be accomplished on such a system given good tools, a tractable and biologically interesting system, and highly capable scientists with sufficient resources to do focused, long-term research. Now, other fungal virus systems have emerged with equal or greater potential. Among these, particular progress has been made with Sclerotinia, Rosellinia, and Fusarium viruses.

Research on horizontal transmission of mycoviruses has progressed in several systems. The ability of invertebrate vectors to transmit viruses of filamentous fungi, which was only an occasional speculation a few years ago, has now been demonstrated convincingly in at least one insect system (Liu et al., 2016) and suggested for mites (Bouneb et al., 2016). This opens up new lines of research examining the movement of fungal viruses in the environment by methods other than hyphal anastomosis, and the possible role of invertebrate vectors in expanding the host ranges of fungal viruses. Moreover, the demonstrated replication of a fungal virus in its insect vector (Liu et al., 2016) further broadens this research area.

Passive, nonvectored mycovirus particle transmission simply by bringing purified virus particles into contact with mycelium is another transmission mechanism whose ecological importance is unknown (Yu et al., 2013). Is this simply an oddity that is peculiar to a single experimental system, or is it a more generalizable mechanism that has not yet been adequately explored? And finally, the recently demonstrated virus-mediated suppression of fungal vegetative incompatibility genes in *S. sclerotiorum*, with attendant increased transmission of heterologous coinfecting viruses (Wu et al., 2017), offers another mechanism for expanding mycovirus host range and transmission in natural settings. Although the vegetative incompatibility system of *C. parasitica* is less complex than that of *S. sclerotiorum*, the recent characterization and systematic disruption of VIC genes in

C. parasitica (Zhang and Nuss, 2016) will likely inform other systems including *S. sclerotiorum*.

In the relatively recent past, it was dogma that almost all mycoviruses contained dsRNA genomes, a few ssRNA. The characterization of many viruses with negative-sense RNA genomes and some with DNA genomes, and an increasing diversity of viruses identified through environmental sampling suggest that we have much to learn about fungal virus diversity. The challenge still is to dissect newly discovered fungal virus interactions systematically, including the many virus–virus interactions in these systems. Such work requires a high level of competence and resources, and the exceptional work that is now being carried out on several systems is very encouraging for the future of the science.

ACKNOWLEDGMENTS

This study was supported in part by Yomogi Inc. and Grants-in-Aid for Scientific Research (A) and on Innovative Areas from the Japanese Ministry of Education, Culture, Sports, Science, and Technology (KAKENHI 25252011 and 16H06436, 16H06429, and 16K21723 to N.S.). Funding to B.I.H was from the New Jersey Agricultural Experiment Station and the USDA-NIFA. We also wish to thank Hideki Kondo, Hiromitsu Moriyama and Atsuko Sasaki for their fruitful discussion and sharing unpublished data with us.

REFERENCES

Ahn, I.P., Lee, Y.H., 2001. A viral double-stranded RNA up regulates the fungal virulence of *Nectria radicicola*. Mol. Plant Microbe Interact. 14, 496–507.

Andika, I.B., Jamal, A., Kondo, H., Suzuki, N., 2017. SAGA complex mediates the transcriptional up-regulation of antiviral RNA silencing. Proc. Natl. Acad. Sci. U.S.A. 114 (17), E3499–E3506.

Baidyaroy, D., Hausner, G., Hafez, M., Michel, F., Fulbright, D.W., Bertrand, H., 2011. A 971-bp insertion in the rns gene is associated with mitochondrial hypovirulence in a strain of *Cryphonectria parasitica* isolated from nature. Fungal Genet. Biol. 48, 775–783.

Bouneb, M., Turchetti, T., Nannelli, R., Roversi, P.F., Paoli, F., Danti, R., Simoni, S., 2016. Occurrence and transmission of mycovirus Cryphonectria hypovirus 1 from dejecta of *Thyreophagus corticalis* (Acari, Acaridae). Fungal Biol. 120, 351–357.

Bruenn, J.A., Warner, B.E., Yerramsetty, P., 2015. Widespread narnavirus sequences in plant genomes. Peer J. 3, e876.

Chiba, S., Suzuki, N., 2015. Highly activated RNA silencing via strong induction of dicer by one virus can interfere with the replication of an unrelated virus. Proc. Natl. Acad. Sci. U.S.A. 112 (35), E4911–E4918.

Chiba, S., Salaipeth, L., Lin, Y.H., Sasaki, A., Kanematsu, S., Suzuki, N., 2009. A novel bipartite double-stranded RNA mycovirus from the white root rot fungus *Rosellinia necatrix*: molecular and biological characterization, taxonomic considerations, and potential for biological control. J. Virol. 83, 12801–12812.

Chiba, S., Lin, Y.H., Kondo, H., Kanematsu, S., Suzuki, N., 2013. Effects of defective-interfering RNA on symptom induction by, and replication of, a novel partitivirus from a phytopathogenic fungus *Rosellinia necatrix*. J. Virol. 87, 2330–2341.

Chiba, S., Lin, Y.H., Kondo, H., Kanematsu, S., Suzuki, N., 2016. A novel betapartitivirus RnPV6 from *Rosellinia necatrix* tolerates host RNA silencing but is interfered by its defective RNAs. Virus Res. 219, 62–72.

Choi, G.H., Dawe, A.L., Churbanov, A., Smith, M.L., Milgroom, M.G., Nuss, D.L., 2012. Molecular characterization of vegetative incompatibility genes that restrict hypovirus transmission in the chestnut blight fungus *Cryphonectria parasitica*. Genetics 190, 113–127.

Dawe, A.L., Nuss, D.L., 2013. Hypovirus molecular biology: from Koch's postulates to host self-recognition genes that restrict virus transmission. Adv. Virus Res. 86, 109–147.

Eusebio-Cope, A., Suzuki, N., 2015. Mycoreovirus genome rearrangements associated with RNA silencing deficiency. Nucleic Acids Res. 43 (7), 3802–3813.

Eusebio-Cope, A., Sun, L., Hillman, B.I., Suzuki, N., 2010. Mycoreovirus 1 S4-coded protein is dispensable for viral replication but necessary for efficient vertical transmission and normal symptom induction. Virology 397, 399–408.

Fuke, K., Takeshita, K., Aoki, N., Fukuhara, T., Egusa, M., Kodama, M., Moriyama, H., 2011. The presence of double-stranded RNAs in Alternaria alternata Japanese pear pathotype is associated with morphological changes. J. Gen. Plant Pathol. 77 (4), 248–252.

Ghabrial, S.A., 2013. Mycoviruses. Adv. Virus Res. 86, 376.

Ghabrial, S.A., Caston, J.R., Jiang, D., Nibert, M.L., Suzuki, N., 2015. 50-plus years of fungal viruses. Virology 479–480, 356–368.

Glass, N.L., Dementhon, K., 2006. Non-self recognition and programmed cell death in filamentous fungi. Curr. Opin. Microbiol. 9, 553–558.

Hillman, B.I., Cai, G., 2013. The family *Narnaviridae*: simplest of RNA viruses. Adv. Virus Res. 86, 149–176.

Hillman, B.I., Suzuki, N., 2004. Viruses of the chestnut blight fungus, *Cryphonectria parasitica*. Adv. Virus Res. 63, 423–472.

Hillman, B.I., Supyani, S., Kondo, H., Suzuki, N., 2004. A reovirus of the fungus *Cryphonectria parasitica* that is infectious as particles and related to the *Coltivirus* genus of animal pathogens. J. Virol. 78 (2), 892–898.

Hisano, S., Zhang, R., Faruk, M.I., Kondo, H., Suzuki, N., 2018. A neo-virus lifestyle exhibited by a (+)ssRNA virus hosted in an unrelated dsRNA virus: taxonomic and evolutionary considerations. Virus Res. 244, 75–83.

Hong, Y.G., Cole, T.E., Brasier, C.M., Buck, K.W., 1998. Evolutionary relationships among putative RNA-dependent RNA polymerases encoded by a mitochondrial virus-like RNA in the Dutch elm disease fungus, *Ophiostoma novo-ulmi*, by other viruses and virus-like RNAs and by the *Arabidopsis* mitochondrial genome. Virology 246, 158–169.

Hong, Y.G., Dover, S.L., Cole, T.E., Brasier, C.M., Buck, K.W., 1999. Multiple mitochondrial viruses in an isolate of the Dutch elm disease fungus Ophiostoma novo-ulmi. Virology 258 (1), 118–127.

Janda, M., Ahlquist, P., 1993. RNA-dependent replication, transcription, and persistence of brome mosaic virus RNA replicons in *S. cerevisiae*. Cell 72, 961–970.

Kanematsu, S., Sasaki, A., Onoue, M., Oikawa, Y., Ito, T., 2010. Extending the fungal host range of a partitivirus and a mycoreovirus from *Rosellinia necatrix* by inoculation of protoplasts with virus particles. Phytopathology 100, 922–930.

Kanematsu, S., Shimizu, T., Salaipeth, L., Yaegashi, H., Sasaki, A., Ito, T., Suzuki, N., 2014. Genome rearrangement of a mycovirus Rosellinia necatrix megabirnavirus 1 affecting its ability to attenuate virulence to the host fungus. Virology 450–451, 308–315.

Kanhayuwa, L., Kotta-Loizou, I., Ozkan, S., Gunning, A.P., Coutts, R.H., 2015. A novel mycovirus from *Aspergillus fumigatus* contains four unique dsRNAs as its genome and is infectious as dsRNA. Proc. Natl. Acad. Sci. U.S.A. 112 (29), 9100–9105.

Khalifa, M.E., Pearson, M.N., 2013. Molecular characterization of three mitoviruses co-infecting a hypovirulent isolate of *Sclerotinia sclerotiorum* fungus. Virology 441, 22–30.

Kondo, H., Chiba, S., Sasaki, A., Kanematsu, S., Suzuki, N., 2013a. Evidence for negative-strand RNA virus infection in fungi. Virology 435, 201–209.

Kondo, H., Kanematsu, S., Suzuki, N., 2013b. Viruses of the white root rot fungus, *Rosellinia necatrix*. Adv. Virus Res. 86, 177–214.

Kotta-Loizou, I., Coutts, R.H.A., 2017. Studies on the Virome of the Entomopathogenic fungus Beauveria bassiana reveal novel dsRNA elements and mild hypervirulence. PLoS Pathog. 13 (1), e1006183. https://doi.org/10.1371/journal.ppat.1006183.

Kozlakidis, Z., Herrero, N., Ozkan, S., Bhatti, M.F., Coutts, R.H., 2013. A novel dsRNA element isolated from the *Aspergillus foetidus* mycovirus complex. Arch. Virol. 158 (12), 2625–2628.

Krupovic, M., Ghabrial, S.A., Jiang, D., Varsani, A., 2016. *Genomoviridae*: a new family of widespread single-stranded DNA viruses. Arch. Virol. 161 (9), 2633–2643.

Liu, Y.C., Linder-Basso, D., Hillman, B.I., Kaneko, S., Milgroom, M.G., 2003. Evidence for interspecies transmission of viruses in natural populations of filamentous fungi in the genus *Cryphonectria*. Mol. Ecol. 12, 1619–1628.

Liu, L., Xie, J., Cheng, J., Fu, Y., Li, G., Yi, X., Jiang, D., 2014. Fungal negative-stranded RNA virus that is related to bornaviruses and nyaviruses. Proc. Natl. Acad. Sci. U.S.A. 111 (33), 12205–12210.

Liu, S., Xie, J.T., Cheng, J.S., Li, B., Chen, T., Fu, Y.P., Li, G.Q., Wang, M.Q., Jin, H.A., Wan, H., Jiang, D.H., 2016. Fungal DNA virus infects a mycophagous insect and utilizes it as a transmission vector. Proc. Natl. Acad. Sci. U.S.A. 113 (45), 12803–12808.

Marienfeld, J.R., Unseld, M., Brandt, P., Brennicke, A., 1997. Viral nucleic acid sequence transfer between fungi and plants. Trends Genet. 13, 260–261.

Marquez, L.M., Redman, R.S., Rodriguez, R.J., Roossinck, M.J., 2007. A virus in a fungus in a plant: three-way symbiosis required for thermal tolerance. Science 315 (5811), 513–515.

Marzano, S.Y.L., Domier, L.L., 2016. Novel mycoviruses discovered from metatranscriptomics survey of soybean phyllosphere phytobiomes. Virus Res. 213, 332–342.

Marzano, S.Y.L., Hobbs, H.A., Nelson, B.D., Hartman, G.L., Eastburn, D.M., McCoppin, N.K., Domier, L.L., 2015. Transfection of Sclerotinia sclerotiorum with in vitro transcripts of a naturally occurring interspecific recombinant of Sclerotinia sclerotiorum hypovirus 2 significantly reduces virulence of the fungus. J. Virol. 89 (9), 5060–5071.

Nagy, P.D., 2016. Tombusvirus-Host Interactions: co-opted evolutionarily conserved host factors take center court. Annu. Rev. Virol. 3, 491–515.

Nerva, L., Ciuffo, M., Vallino, M., Margaria, P., Varese, G.C., Gnavi, G., Turina, M., 2016. Multiple approaches for the detection and characterization of viral and plasmid symbionts from a collection of marine fungi. Virus Res. 219, 22–38.

Nibert, M.L., 2017. Mitovirus UGA(Trp) codon usage parallels that of host mitochondria. Virology 507, 96–100.

Nuss, D.L., 1996. Using hypoviruses to probe and perturb signal transduction processes underlying fungal pathogenesis. Plant Cell 8 (10), 1845–1853.

Osaki, H., Sasaki, A., Nomiyama, K., Tomioka, K., 2016. Multiple virus infection in a single strain of *Fusarium poae* shown by deep sequencing. Virus Genes 52 (6), 835–847.

Petrzik, K., Sarkisova, T., Stary, J., Koloniuk, I., Hrabakova, L., Kubesova, O., 2016. Molecular characterization of a new monopartite dsRNA mycovirus from mycorrhizal *Thelephora terrestris* (Ehrh.) and its detection in soil oribatid mites (Acari: Oribatida). Virology 489, 12–19.

Polashock, J.J., Hillman, B.I., 1994. A small mitochondrial double-stranded (ds) RNA element associated with a hypovirulent strain of the chestnut blight fungus and ancestrally related to yeast cytoplasmic T and W dsRNAs. Proc. Natl. Acad. Sci. U.S.A. 91 (18), 8680–8684.

Polashock, J.J., Bedker, P.J., Hillman, B.I., 1997. Movement of a small mitochondrial double-stranded RNA element of *Cryphonectria parasitica*: ascospore inheritance and implications for mitochondrial recombination. Mol. Gen. Genet. 256 (5), 566–571.

Pruss, G., Ge, X., Shi, X.M., Carrington, J.C., Bowman Vance, V., 1997. Plant viral synergism: the potyviral genome encodes a broad-range pathogenicity enhancer that transactivates replication of heterologous viruses. Plant Cell 9 (6), 859–868.

Ran, H., Liu, L., Li, B., Cheng, J., Fu, Y., Jiang, D., Xie, J., 2016. Co-infection of a hypovirulent isolate of *Sclerotinia sclerotiorum* with a new botybirnavirus and a strain of a mitovirus. Virol. J. 13, 92–101.

Rigling, D., Prospero, S., 2017. *Cryphonectria parasitica*, the causal agent of chestnut blight: invasion history, population biology and disease control. Mol. Plant Pathol. https://doi.org/10.1111/mpp.12542.

Rogers, H.J., Buck, K.W., Brasier, C.M., 1986. Transmission of double-stranded RNA and a disease factor in *Ophiostoma ulmi*. Plant Pathol. 35, 277–287.

Rogers, H.J., Buck, K.W., Brasier, C.M., 1987. A mitochondrial target for double-stranded-RNA in diseased Isolates of the fungus that causes Dutch elm disease. Nature 329, 558–560.

Sasaki, A., Nakamura, H., Suzuki, N., Kanematsu, S., 2016. Characterization of a new megabirnavirus that confers hypovirulence with the aid of a co-infecting partitivirus to the host fungus, *Rosellinia necatrix*. Virus Res. 219, 73–82.

Segers, G.C., Zhang, X., Deng, F., Sun, Q., Nuss, D.L., 2007. Evidence that RNA silencing functions as an antiviral defense mechanism in fungi. Proc. Natl. Acad. Sci. U.S.A. 104, 12902–12906.

Son, M., Lee, K.M., Yu, J., Kang, M., Park, J.M., Kwon, S.J., Kim, K.H., 2013. The HEX1 gene of *Fusarium graminearum* is required for fungal asexual reproduction and pathogenesis and for efficient viral RNA accumulation of fusarium graminearum virus 1. J. Virol. 87 (18), 10356–10367.

Sun, L., Suzuki, N., 2008. Intragenic rearrangements of a mycoreovirus induced by the multifunctional protein p29 encoded by the prototypic hypovirus CHV1-EP713. RNA 14, 2557–2571.

Sun, L., Nuss, D.L., Suzuki, N., 2006. Synergism between a mycoreovirus and a hypovirus mediated by the papain-like protease p29 of the prototypic hypovirus CHV1-EP713. J. Gen. Virol. 87, 3703–3714.

Sun, Q., Choi, G.H., Nuss, D.L., 2008. Hypovirus-responsive transcription factor gene pro1 of the chestnut blight fungus Cryphonectria parasitica is required for female fertility, asexual spore development and stable maintenance of hypovirus infection. Eukaryot. Cell 8, 262–270.

Sun, Q., Choi, G.H., Nuss, D.L., 2009. A single Argonaute gene is required for induction of RNA silencing antiviral defense and promotes viral RNA recombination. Proc. Natl. Acad. Sci. U.S.A. 106 (42), 17927–17932.

Suzuki, N., 2017. Frontiers in fungal virology. J. Gen. Plant. Pathol. 83, 419–423.

Tanaka, T., Sun, L., Tsutani, K., Suzuki, N., 2011. Rearrangements of mycoreovirus 1 S1, S2 and S3 induced by the multifunctional protein p29 encoded by the prototypic hypovirus Cryphonectria hypovirus 1 strain EP713. J. Gen. Virol. 92, 1949–1959.

Tanaka, T., Eusebio-Cope, A., Sun, L., Suzuki, N., 2012. Mycoreovirus genome alterations: similarities to and differences from rearrangements reported for other reoviruses. Front. Microbiol. 3, 186.

Tatineni, S., Graybosch, R.A., Hein, G.L., Wegulo, S.N., French, R., 2010. Wheat cultivar-specific disease synergism and alteration of virus accumulation during co-infection with Wheat streak mosaic virus and Triticum mosaic virus. Phytopathology 100 (3), 230–238.

Thapa, V., Turner, G.G., Hafenstein, S., Overton, B.E., Vanderwolf, K.J., Roossinck, M.J., 2016. Using a novel partitivirus in Pseudogymnoascus destructans to understand the epidemiology of white-nose syndrome. PLoS Pathog. 12 (12), e1006076. https://doi.org/10.1371/journal.ppat.1006076.

Vainio, E.J., Hantula, J., 2016. Taxonomy, biogeography and importance of *Heterobasidion* viruses. Virus Res. 219, 2–10.

Vance, V.B., 1991. Replication of potato virus X RNA is altered in coinfections with potato virus Y. Virology 182 (2), 486–494.

Wickner, R.B., Fujimura, T., Esteban, R., 2013. Viruses and prions of *Saccharomyces cerevisiae*. Adv. Virus Res. 86, 1–36.

Wu, M., Deng, Y., Zhou, Z., He, G., Chen, W., Li, G., 2016. Characterization of three mycoviruses co-infecting the plant pathogenic fungus Sclerotinia nivalis. Virus Res. 223, 28–38.

Wu, S., Cheng, J., Fu, Y., Chen, T., Jiang, D., Ghabrial, S.A., Xie, J., 2017. Virus-mediated suppression of host non-self recognition facilitates horizontal transmission of heterologous viruses. PLoS Pathog. 13 (3), e1006234.

Xiao, X., Cheng, J., Tang, J., Fu, Y., Jiang, D., Baker, T.S., Ghabrial, S.A., Xie, J., 2014. A novel partitivirus that confers hypovirulence on plant pathogenic fungi. J. Virol. 88 (17), 10120–10133.

Xie, J., Ghabrial, S.A., 2012. Molecular characterization of two mitoviruses co-infecting a hypovirulent isolate of the plant pathogenic fungus *Sclerotinia sclerotiorum* [corrected]. Virology 428, 77–85.

Xie, J., Jiang, D., 2014. New insights into mycoviruses and exploration for the biological control of crop fungal diseases. Annu. Rev. Phytopathol. 52, 45–68.

Xu, Z., Wu, S., Liu, L., Cheng, J., Fu, Y., Jiang, D., Xie, J., 2015. A mitovirus related to plant mitochondrial gene confers hypovirulence on the phytopathogenic fungus *Sclerotinia sclerotiorum*. Virus Res. 197, 127–136.

Yaegashi, H., Nakamura, H., Sawahata, T., Sasaki, A., Iwanami, Y., Ito, T., Kanematsu, S., 2013. Appearance of mycovirus-like double-stranded RNAs in the white root rot fungus, *Rosellinia necatrix*, in an apple orchard. FEMS Microbiol. Ecol. 83, 49–62.

Yu, X., Li, B., Fu, Y., Jiang, D., Ghabrial, S.A., Li, G., Peng, Y., Xie, J., Cheng, J., Huang, J., Yi, X., 2010. A geminivirus-related DNA mycovirus that confers hypovirulence to a plant pathogenic fungus. Proc. Natl. Acad. Sci. U.S.A. 107, 8387–8392.

Yu, X., Li, B., Fu, Y., Xie, J., Cheng, J., Ghabrial, S.A., Li, G., Yi, X., Jiang, D., 2013. Extracellular transmission of a DNA mycovirus and its use as a natural fungicide. Proc. Natl. Acad. Sci. U.S.A. 110 (4), 1452–1457.

Zhang, D.X., Nuss, D.L., 2016. Engineering super mycovirus donor strains of chestnut blight fungus by systematic disruption of multilocus vic genes. Proc. Natl. Acad. Sci. U.S.A. 113, 2062–2067.

Zhang, X., Shi, D., Nuss, D.L., 2012. Variations in hypovirus interactions with the fungal-host RNA-silencing antiviral-defense response. J. Virol. 86 (23), 12933–12939.

Zhang, D.X., Spiering, M.J., Dawe, A.L., Nuss, D.L., 2014. Vegetative incompatibility loci with dedicated roles in allorecognition restrict mycovirus transmission in chestnut blight fungus. Genetics 197 (2), 701–714.

Zhang, R., Hisano, S., Tani, A., Kondo, H., Kanematsu, S., Suzuki, N., 2016. A capsidless ssRNA virus hosted by an unrelated dsRNA virus. Nat. Microbiol. 1. https://doi.org/10.1038/NMICROBIOL.2015.1031.

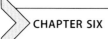

CHAPTER SIX

Protein Localization and Interaction Studies in Plants: Toward Defining Complete Proteomes by Visualization

Michael M. Goodin[1]
University of Kentucky, Lexington, KY, United States
[1]Corresponding author: e-mail address: mgoodin@uky.edu

Contents

Abstract

Protein interaction and localization studies in plants are a fundamental component of achieving mechanistic understanding of virus:plant interactions at the systems level. Many such studies are conducted using transient expression assays in leaves of *Nicotiana benthamiana*, the most widely used experimental plant host in virology, examined by laser-scanning confocal microscopy. This chapter provides a workflow for protein interaction and localization experiments, with particular attention to the many control and supporting assays that may also need to be performed. Basic principles of microscopy are introduced to aid researchers in the early stages of adding imaging techniques to their experimental repertoire. Three major types of imaging-based experiments are

Advances in Virus Research, Volume 100
ISSN 0065-3527
https://doi.org/10.1016/bs.aivir.2017.10.004

117

discussed in detail: (i) protein localization using autofluorescent proteins, (ii) colocalization studies, and (iii) bimolecular fluorescence complementation, with emphasis on judicious interpretation of the data obtained from these approaches. In addition to establishing a general framework for protein localization experiments in plants, the need for proteome-scale localization projects is discussed, with emphasis on nuclear-localized proteins.

1. INTRODUCTION

The reason that "cells" are so-called derives from plants and Robert Hooke, who examined thin slices of cork using a compound microscope of his own invention c.1665. In "Observation XVIII" of the *Micrographia*, Hooke provided drawings of the "pores or cells," observed under his microscope. Since that time, every iteration of technical advancement yields microscopes that can peer into cells at increasing resolution (Schubert, 2017) or provide quantitative data pertaining to the localization, interaction, concentration, physiological condition such as pH, of components of the cellular milieu (Germond et al., 2016; Kerppola, 2008; Rodriguez et al., 2017). Presently, it is possible to track the movement of single virus particles in living cells (Kelich et al., 2015; Yu, 2016), observe processes such as membrane fusion (Oum et al., 2016), or determine the site(s) of accumulation of every protein encoded by a particular genome (Uhlen et al., 2015). As such, modern microscopy literally brings to light phenomena that cannot be revealed by other molecular, genetics, biochemical, or computational approaches.

Regardless of the sophistication of the instrumentation, communication of microscopy data requires both technical accuracy and attention to the fundamental principles of photography. In his classic book, "The Negative," Ansel Adams ruminated on the lack of recognition of the "Zone System" for determination of the optimal exposure in photography by the scientific community. He wrote, "The reason appears to be that scientists are not concerned with the kind of photography that relates to intangible qualities of imagination, as distinct from the laboratory standards of exact physical values" (Adams and Baker, 1981). Therefore, the aim of this chapter is to introduce basic concepts that need to be considered prior to embarking on protein localization and interaction studies in plant cells. The imaging experiments considered are most likely to be conducted on laser-scanning confocal microscopes (hereafter called confocals), although other types of instrumentation such as total internal reflection fluorescence (TIRF) and spinning disk microscopes should be considered (Ettinger and Wittmann, 2014; Martin-Fernandez et al., 2013). Whatever the instrument used, the fundamental operating principles derive from standard epifluorescence microscopy, which the reader is encouraged to assimilate. Many of the control experiments described later can be performed on any modern epifluorescence microscope, with greater speed and lower cost, prior to conducting experiments on confocals. Far more detailed information than can be provided here is available via comprehensive texts on confocal microscopy (Pawley, 2006; Price and Jerome, 2011; Ruzin, 1999), and on the information-rich tutorials provided online by all manufacturers of confocals. However, such reference materials can be daunting in the hands of researchers at the early stages of enhancing their research efforts via microscopy techniques.

Accurate determination of the site of subcellular localization is an essential part of determining the biological function(s) of a protein of interest (Babajani and Kermode, 2014; Cho et al., 2012; Gong et al., 2015; Lutz et al., 2015; Martin et al., 2009; Min et al., 2010; Mohannath et al., 2014; Schoelz et al., 2016; Smolarkiewicz et al., 2014; Tian et al., 2004; Tripathi et al., 2015; Tzfira et al., 2005; Uchiyama et al., 2014; Wu et al., 2013; Xie et al., 2017). As such, in order to communicate image-based data effectively researchers require competency in the molecular techniques required to express and detect proteins in plant cells, the physics of fluorescence in biological systems, and photography in its artistic and scientific contexts. The amount of effort that goes into producing high-quality micrographs is often greatly underestimated relative to assumptions made about molecular techniques. Thus, the following sections provide a decision-making framework for designing protein interaction and localization studies in plants, with the hopes of developing a comprehensive definition of the plant proteome via visual data (Fig. 1).

2. THE PERFECT IMAGE

Confocals are point-scan/point-detection instruments that assemble the final image from an array of user-specified pixels. The larger the number of pixels the longer the time required to acquire the image. Further, the scan-rate, i.e., the time that the lasers/detector are positioned at a pixel, typically 2–10 ms/pixel, can significantly impact the quality of the final image, with longer dwell times naturally leading to longer times to acquire

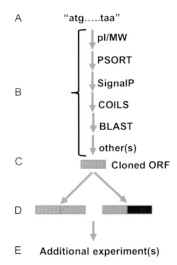

Fig. 1 Generalized workflow for conducing protein localization. (A) Generate sequence of coding sequence (genomic and/or cDNA) for protein of interest. (B) Generate as much information as reasonable using online sequence analysis tools. At minimum, determine the molecular weight and predicted isoelectric point, search for signal peptides and putative subcellular targeting sequences, as well as homology searches. These analyses can be coded into automated sequence analysis pipelines or can be performed ad hoc. (C) The coding ORF or genomic clone needs to be cloned into appropriate construction vector, and sequence verified. (D) Proteins should be expressed as both amino- and carboxy-terminal fusions. (E) Depending on the type of characterization required, localization data can be integrated into a plethora of molecular, biochemical, and genetics experiments.

the complete image. Both the power output of the lasers and the sensitivity of the detectors are user-controlled in most confocal instruments. All of these settings will have to be adjusted relative to the expression level and brightness of the protein of interest being detected. As such, the perfect image is an integration of all the technical requirements of image acquisition, as well as the aesthetic qualities of the micrograph that will be used to communicate scientific data (Fig. 2).

The question of what constitutes a perfect image is one that beginning users should think about prior to engaging in localization experiments. In fact, Ansel Adams' advice that photographers, and by extension microscopists, should "see" the final composition image before they take the picture remains a sound recommendation (Adams and Baker, 1980). That is, to think about how the data should be represented pictorially before one goes to the microscope. This is not a strategy to bias the data. To the contrary,

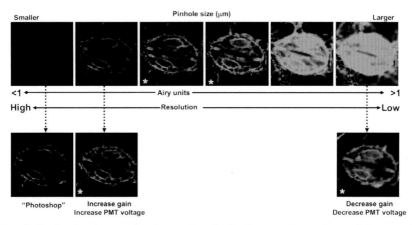

Fig. 2 Confocal micrograph of guard cells in the abaxial surface of transgenic *N. benthamiana* expressing GFP targeted to the ER. The "correct" image is a compromise of the control settings for laser output, pinhole size, detector sensitivity, and/or digital enhancement. Users should be well versed in the basic operations of microscopes prior to attempting advanced imaging techniques. By manipulating various exposure control setting, at least three or four of these images may be suitable for publication (see *asterisk**).

this is a consideration of how best to communicate the data knowing that one or a few images will represent the entire range of variation observed in different cells.

How will the final images be used? If the plan is to display the data in multipanel figures composed of one to dozens of images of 1-in. square micrographs, then images collected at a resolution of 512 × 512 pixels are probably sufficient. Will a single image showing great detail in small regions of interest in a large field be needed? Then perhaps a resolution of 1024 × 1024 or greater is required. Mobile structures in living cells may have to be imaged at lower resolution than the same structures in fixed cells. However, it may be technically easier and more time efficient to use live-cell imaging, particularly if a large number of samples have to be processed.

It is important to note that the appropriate resolution of an image is not an arbitrary selection. Ideally, the resolution selected should fulfill the Nyquist theorem of sampling (Hibbs, 2004; Ruzin, 1999). Briefly, a pixel resolution that is one-half of the optical resolution should be selected. In turn, optical resolution for confocal imaging is both a function of the wavelength (shorter wavelength = higher resolution) and the numerical aperture (NA) of the objective being used (higher NA = greater resolution). For practical purposes, lower wavelengths of light (e.g., 405 nm to excite cyan fluorescent protein, CFP) permit thinner optical slices to be taken than when longer wavelengths are used (e.g., 561 for red fluorescent protein, RFP). Consideration of this issue becomes critical when trying to assess colocalization, particularly in three-dimensional reconstructions (Hibbs, 2004; Pawley, 2006; Ruzin, 1999).

As will become evident in the sections later, the final published image is "perfect" only within the context of communicating scientific advances. Every micrograph is unique and cannot be replicated with pixel-for-pixel identity in independent studies by other researchers using different microscopes in the way that polymerase chain reaction, Western immunoblotting, or other molecular procedures can. Researchers therefore must take great care in the acquisition and selection of publication-quality micrographs. Quality microscopy done correctly requires a significant investment of time.

3. GETTING STARTED: WHAT IS THE QUESTION THAT NEEDS TO BE ADDRESSED?

A simplified workflow for conducting protein interaction and localization experiments in plant cells is provided in Fig. 1. These experiments should commence correctly with an analysis of the amino acid-coding sequence using any of a variety of algorithms available online (Liu et al., 2013; Nakai and Kanehisa, 1991, 1992) (Fig. 1). This approach will help to identify functional domains in proteins such as nuclear localization signals, signal peptides, and others. While this is often a useful first step, the results can be misleading or erroneous. Regardless of what in silico methods are used, validation in vivo will have to be performed, as localization prediction algorithms still cannot determine suborganellar sites (e.g., nuclear envelope or pore vs nucleus per se).

The most versatile vector systems for protein expression in plant cells permit expression of either carboxyl- or amino-terminal fusions to autofluorescent proteins (Chakrabarty et al., 2007; Goodin et al., 2002; Hecker et al., 2015; Martin et al., 2009). Researchers are encouraged to express proteins of interest (POI) in both orientations. More elaborate cloning strategies insert autofluorescent protein-coding sequences into exons predicted as the best to accept fluorescent tags with minimal impact on protein function (Tian et al., 2004). In the end, however, the orientation that yields biologically relevant localization patterns can only be determined empirically. Researchers should move away from conventional wisdom that contends that proteins with amino-terminal signal peptides be expressed with AFPs fused to their carboxy-terminus. While this is often the case, there are exceptions! To date, glycoproteins of all plant-adapted rhabdoviruses tested are correctly localized only when expressed as amino-terminal fusions to AFPs (Bandyopadhyay et al., 2010; Dietzgen et al., 2012; Goodin et al., 2007b; Martin et al., 2012; Ramalho et al., 2014). Lack of expression, or mislocalization, of G-protein–AFP fusions is likely due to interference with their carboxy-terminal transmembrane/oligomerization domains. In rarer cases, some POI are sensitive to the particular AFP to which they are fused, such as the nucleocapsid protein of *Sonchus yellow net virus*, which is mislocalized when fused to DRONPA, but not other AFPs (Martin et al., 2009). While the majority of protein localization studies employ green and red fluorescent proteins (GFP; RFP), a wide variety of AFPs of different colors are available (Rodriguez et al., 2017). A good general starting point is to express POI as GFP:POI and POI:RFP fusions. If necessary, the reciprocal RFP:POI and POI:GFP fusions can be tested. The advantage of this strategy is twofold: (i) it informs about the physical properties of a protein of interest with respect to its tolerance of having its termini manipulated, and (ii) it provides a rapid route to defining functional GFP/RFP fusions that can be used in downstream coexpression/colocalization studies. In all localization experiments, protein fusions should be expressed in cells that have at least one subcellular locus marked. For example, transgenic *Nicotiana benthamiana* lines expressing fluorescent marker proteins targeted to the ER or nuclei provide ideal references for protein localization (Martin et al., 2009) (Fig. 3).

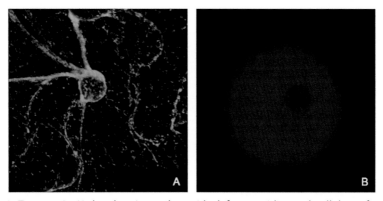

Fig. 3 Transgenic *N. benthamiana* plants ideal for providing subcellular reference markers for protein localization assays. (A) The "16c" line expresses GFP-HDEL targeted to the endoplasmic reticulum. Whole-cell view. (B) Line "103" expressing mRFP-Histone 2B, which serves as a nuclear marker.

4. A STARTLING ARRAY OF IMAGING TECHNOLOGIES AND INSTRUMENTATION

Researchers using microscopy are faced with an increasingly complex array of instrumentation and methods with such catchy terms as, superresolution (Shelden et al., 2016), light sheet, multiphoton, FRET, FRAP, FLIM, photoactivation, and TIRF, to name a few (Follain et al., 2017; Goodin et al., 2007a; Lummer et al., 2013). More recently, instrumentation that pushes beyond the limits of resolution first defined by Ernst Abbe over a century ago is gaining rapid acceptance (Cremer et al., 2017). The practical limit on imaging EGFP using the highest numerical aperture objectives is approximately 200 nm (x–y) in the lateral dimension and 500 nm in the axial (z). Incredibly, STORM, STED, PALM, and a host of other acronyms define techniques that increase resolution by 10-fold or more (Cremer et al., 2017; Follain et al., 2017).

Despite the ever-increasing sophistication of imaging technologies, the fundamentals of imaging should be assimilated prior to progressing to increasingly complex experiments, such as knowing the excitation and emission maxima for the fluors that one is using. While enthusiasm to utilize the most advanced technologies should be appreciated and encouraged, it behooves the user to learn that there is no such thing as a "GFP laser" and, more importantly, that many controls must be included in every imaging experiment. Directors of biological imaging facilities are happy to discuss the technical requirements for imaging experiments prior to attempting them.

A very brief guide for some of the common fluorescent dyes and proteins are provided in Fig. 4.

Key points to note are that the wavelength of light used to excite fluorescent molecules is always shorter (higher energy) than the resulting fluorescence detected. Importantly, the wavelengths used to excite fluors will be a function of what laser lines are available on the particular confocal microscope being used. As such, the wavelength of the laser may not necessarily correspond to the excitation maxima of the fluor. More than one laser line can be used to excite the same fluor. For example, the 543 line of a He–Ne laser or the 561 nm line of the newer solid-state lasers can be used to excite Tag-RFP. CFP can be excited with either 405 nm or 440 nm laser lines. Regardless of the excitation wavelength used, the emission spectrum of a fluor does not change. Therefore, the collected light will always be within a narrow band around the emission maximum of each fluor used in an

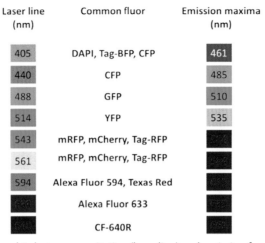

Laser line (nm)	Common fluor	Emission maxima (nm)
405	DAPI, Tag-BFP, CFP	461
440	CFP	485
488	GFP	510
514	YFP	535
543	mRFP, mCherry, Tag-RFP	
561	mRFP, mCherry, Tag-RFP	
594	Alexa Fluor 594, Texas Red	
	Alexa Fluor 633	
	CF-640R	

Fig. 4 The relationship between excitation (laser line) and emission from a select few of the hundreds of available fluors. Note that laser lines that span from UV to infrared are available. The laser lines selected for confocal microscopy experiments are those required to excite the fluors being used. The emission from the excited fluor will always be at a longer wavelength (lower energy) than that used for excitation. Additionally, multiple laser lines may be suitable for excitation of a particular fluor.

experiment. Thoughtful selection of the dazzling array of fluorescent proteins and dyes must be considered prior to initiation of localization studies. Users are most often constrained not by the availability of autofluorescent proteins per se but by the availability of these proteins in particular expression vectors. Purchasing of AFPs is an expensive proposition, and validating published AFPs is a time-consuming exercise. Many AFPs are initially characterized in bacterial or human cell lines. Utility in these cell lines, or in vitro, may or may not translate to their usefulness in plant systems. The incorporation of next-generation AFPs into plant expression vectors lags far behind their initial reporting (Lummer et al., 2013; Martin et al., 2009). When testing novel AFPs it is important to evaluate them relative to the present standards such as EGFP, EYFP, mRFP, and mCherry, as some AFPs do not perform well in plant imaging applications (Martin et al., 2009).

5. VALIDATING EXPRESSION

Detection of fluorescent protein fusions is extremely sensitive, and therefore proper targeting of the fusion to a particular subcellular locus is the best indicator of expression. However, the researcher may wish to validate their initial observations by second method analyses such as immunoblotting. Antibodies to the most commonly used AFPs are commercially available. Alternatively, an epitope tag (Myc, HA, FLAG) or other can be incorporated into the protein sequence by PCR, or such tags may be part of the AFP reading frame in the expression vector.

If detection of the AFP fusion by fluorescence or immunoblotting is difficult, an RNA silencing suppressor (such as potyvirus HC-Pro, Cucumber mosaic virus 2b, or others) may be coexpressed with the protein fusions (Wu et al., 2010). Coexpression will often result in a several-fold increase in the steady-state accumulation. It is common that interaction with a partner protein results in stabilization of certain proteins. Alternatively, such interactions may result in a change in localization patterns relative to the proteins being expressed separately (Goodin et al., 2001, 2007b; Min et al., 2010; Ramalho et al., 2014).

6. POINTS OF REFERENCE

Publication standards today will likely and correctly result in the rejection of protein localization data that lack a subcellular localization marker. The easiest means to obtain images with subcellular markers is to employ one of the several transgenic lines expressing autofluorescent protein fusions targeted to a variety of loci (Chakrabarty et al., 2007; Martin et al., 2009; Nelson et al., 2007; Wu et al., 2013). Alternatively, marker proteins can be coexpressed along with the POI:AFP fusion. Finally, in lieu of marker proteins, a wide variety of loci-selective dyes are available that can be infiltrated into leaf tissues shortly before imaging. Dyes such as DAPI, *FM 4-64*, and CellTrace BODIPY TR Methyl Ester are commonly used for counterstaining nuclei and endomembranes (Levy et al., 2015; Uchiyama et al., 2014; Wang et al., 2015). The advantage of using stable transgenics is consistency in the intensity of the marked loci (Martin et al., 2009; Wu et al., 2013). Additionally, there can be a significant saving in time and money if localization is conducted in transgenics, which in turn increases throughput. The two most commonly used marker plants employed in our laboratory are *N. benthamiana* plants expressing RFP:Histone 2B, RFP-HDEL, for marking nuclei and membranes, respectively. These plants are ideal for localizing GFP fusions. Alternatively, transgenic plants expressing CFP:Histone2B are ideal for bimolecular fluorescence complementation (BiFC) experiments that employ YFP protein fusions.

7. AVOIDING CROSS TALK

It is common that coexpression experiments are included in detailed characterization of proteins. Such investigations require that a variety of AFPs be expressed in the same cells. Common coexpression partners are CFP/YFP, GFP/RFP, and TagBFP/GFP/RFP. It is essential that each protein fusion be tested individually before conducting colocalization studies. It is not uncommon for investigators to produce "colocalization" micrographs that have pixel-for-pixel match for each fluor, only to later determine that detection of one of the AFPs was simply an artifact of (i) bleed-through fluorescence from one of the AFPs into a second channel and (ii) failure of one of the AFP fusions to express (Fig. 5).

It is commonly, and erroneously, assumed that colocalization and protein–protein interaction are one in the same phenomenon. However, it is quite possible that two proteins accumulate in the same subcellular

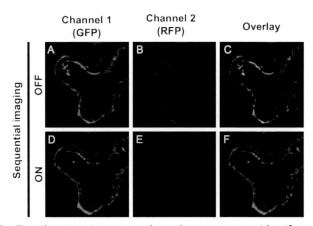

Fig. 5 While all modern imaging systems have the means to avoid artifactual data, failure to implement the proper controls can lead to egregious outcomes. One of the most common errors is the capture of fluorescence from the lower emission wavelength fluor in another channel. Shown here are confocal micrographs of a transgenic *N. benthamiana* leaf epidermal cell expressing GFP targeted to the ER (A and D). In the *top panel* fluorescence is collected simultaneously in both channels 1 and 2, resulting in what appears to be "RFP" signal in Channel 2 (B). The resulting "overlay" provides a pixel-for-pixel "colocalized" match (C). In the *bottom panel*, fluorescence is collected sequentially, resulting in lack of fluorescence detection in Channel 2 (E), and only GFP in the overlay (F). When conducting multichannel experiments all constructs should be tested independently prior to coexpression, and bleed-through fluorescence needs to be controlled for.

locus without interacting. If it is the interaction of two proteins that is relevant to a research question, then further experiments will have to be performed after their colocalization is determined (see BiFC in Section 13, later).

8. COLOCALIZATION: WHAT IT IS, AND WHAT IT IS NOT

Many excellent guides to colocalization have been published (Costes et al., 2004; Dunn et al., 2011; Hecker et al., 2015; Pawley, 2006). Despite the available scholarly material, manuscripts still arrive for review with figures that claim to show colocalization but which actually do not. One of the more common mistakes is to claim colocalization of a protein present in punctate loci against another protein whose localization occupies the entire area of the micrograph (Fig. 6).

Colocalization has two major components: (i) the spatial overlap of two fluors, which can be evaluated subjectively and (ii) correlation, wherein two fluors not only overlap but are distributed proportionally in multiple loci. Neither of these conditions can be taken as evidence for detecting molecular interactions. It is simply not possible to identify the interaction of proteins via a comparison of their patterns of distribution in micrographs.

Colocalization data are often presented colorimetrically such that "merged" micrographs are presented with a color change where positions of fluors overlap. For example, when GFP and RFP fusions are expressed together, regions of colocalization will be represented by yellow (Fig. 6).

Alternatively, such data can be presented graphically as scatterplots where the intensity of one fluor is plotted vs that of a second fluor. The slope of a least squares line through these data will indicate the ratio of fluorescence of the two fluors. Fluors of equal intensity that accumulate exclusively in the same loci (e.g., peroxisomes and mitochondria) will yield a graph showing a near 1:1 correspondence for flours of equivalent brightness. While these images and plots are good first steps, confidence that the two fluors are indeed colocalized will be increased by quantifying the colocalization using the Pearson's correlation coefficient statistic (Costes et al., 2004; Dunn et al., 2011).

Colocalization studies are most appropriately interpreted in the context of associating proteins to the same subcellular locus (e.g., nuclei, microtubules, or Golgi). Such interpretation is limited by resolution. Typically, lower magnification analyses are insufficient to determine colocalization

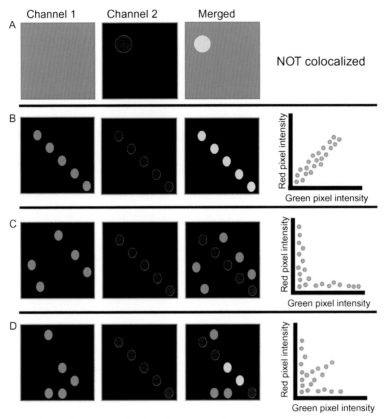

Fig. 6 Idealized depictions of colocalization analyses commonly presented in manuscripts submitted for publication. Operating software on all present-day confocal instrumentation allows merged images of fluorescence captured in multiple channels to be generated. Where, for example, *green* (GFP) fluorescence overlaps that of *red* (RFP), *yellow* is depicted in the merged image. (A) If Channel 1 fluorescence occupies all, or most of, the region of interest depicted in the micrograph, then no argument for "colocalization" of Channel 2 signal can be made. While seemingly trivial, this is a very common mistake. (B) True colocalization will result in both a total, or nearly total overlap of signals in Channels 1 and 2, and a graph of *red* vs *green* pixel intensity with a slope near to 1. In this scenario, an important control is to make sure that the Channel 2 signal is not bleed through from Channel 1 (see Section 7). (C) In the absence of colocalization, there is neither significant overlap of channel signals nor correlation of pixel intensities. (D) Partial colocalization results in merged images and graphs intermediate to those shown in (C) and (D). The biological relevance of partial colocalization will require substantial supporting data beyond micrographs in manuscripts claiming it to be significant.

accurately. At some point, all cellular loci coalesce and so colocalization should be performed at the magnification and resolution appropriate for the size of the subcellular locus in which the POI are expected to be colocalized.

9. DOES THE LOCALIZATION PATTERN MAKE BIOLOGICAL SENSE?

Localization experiments should be conducted with the biology of the particular protein(s) in mind. It is inappropriate to simply accept whatever appears under the microscope. It is very easy to produce artifactual data, particularly if image manipulation software is employed. Physiological state, infection by pathogens (e.g., viruses), and developmental stage can all influence the localization pattern of a protein. Depending on the research question, it may be necessary to conduct localization experiments under a specific set of conditions, such as virus–infected cells, for example (Goodin et al., 2007b). If the protein of interest is small (<30 kDa), it may still be below cutoff for diffusion into plant nuclei when expressed as an AFP fusion. In such cases, it may be difficult to differentiate localization of the AFP fusion from the AFP itself, in which case immunoblotting to determine that the correct–sized fusion was expressed is required.

If computational analyses have been conducted, then the researcher should consider localization patterns relevant to (i) signal peptides, (ii) nuclear import/export signals, (iii) other subcellular targeting motifs (e.-g., transmembrane domains), and (iv) similarity to proteins that have been characterized in greater detail.

Vectors with duplicated promotors (e.g., Double 35S) may result in much higher levels of expression than single promoter vectors. This could lead to mislocalization of the POI:AFP fusion. If this is a concern, the researcher can compare expression from both single and double promoter vectors. Transient expression, particularly by Agroinfiltration, may result in higher steady-state accumulation of protein fusions than might occur in a transgenic plant. However, the speed and efficiency of transient assays often far outweigh the time and expense of making transgenic plants.

10. WHAT SUPPORTING DATA ARE NEEDED?

Diverse data are often required as part of a comprehensive investigation into protein function. As such, rarely will localization data provide a stand-alone study. As noted earlier, protein interaction data may be required to determine the relationship between colocalization and interaction. A commonly employed procedure is to conduct BiFC assays, which has the advantage of providing both interaction and localization data. The basis of BiFC is to reconstitute a functional (fluorescent) YFP (or other AFP) by coexpressing it as two fragments (an amino-terminal, "nYFP" and carboxy-terminal, "cYFP") fused separately to two proteins. Interaction of the proteins brings the YFP fragments into close proximity resulting in detectable fluorescence at the site of interaction (Kerppola, 2008; Martin et al., 2009; Pusch et al., 2011). While simple in principle, BiFC experiments must be well controlled in order to yield meaningful results (Fig. 7). There are six permutations by which two different proteins can be coexpressed, as the nYFP and cYFP fusions should be made for each protein. Additionally, each of these fusions must be tested against a nonbinding control protein. Therefore, up to 12 coexpressed fusions need to be tested for every protein pair, assuming two different proteins are being used. A means to justify the testing of fewer combinations is to express each of the proteins for the BiFC experiments first as AFP:POI and POI:AFP fusions. If one orientation is not biologically meaningful, then the same orientation can be avoided in the BiFC experiments. It is typical that BiFC reports only the most stable complex of the two proteins. Therefore, coexpression experiments using two different AFPs may not yield the same localization pattern(s) to those observed with BiFC.

The vector platform selected for BiFC experiments should be evaluated for the level of background produced by the empty vectors prior to conducting interaction studies. Ideally, coexpression of the amino- and carboxy-terminal YFP fragments should not result in detectable fluorescence. The original pSAT-based BiFC system was susceptible to such background. However, conversion of these vectors to their pSITEII derivatives, which employed Gateway™ cloning technology, resulted in BiFC vectors that do not produce detectable YFP signal when the nYFP and cYFP fragments were coexpressed (Martin et al., 2009). While this result increases the confidence in scoring positive interactions, it is not the only control that needs to be performed. Each protein fusion, nYFP:POI-1, cYFP:POI-1, POI:nYFP-2, and POI:cYFP-2, must be tested for interaction against a nonbinding control protein. In my laboratory we routinely use glutathione-S-transferase (GST) as the nonbinding control given the long-established history of using GST for protein purification and biochemistry (Hakes and Dixon, 1992). It is important to keep in mind that

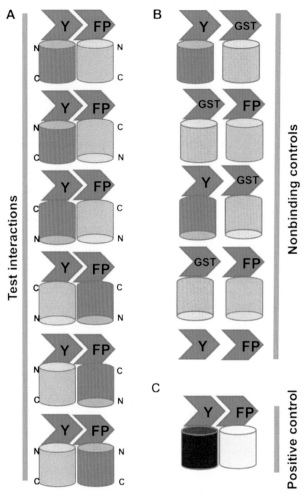

Fig. 7 Experimental plan for BiFC experiments. (A) Up to six combinations of coexpressed fusions may have to be tested for each pair of proteins (*yellow* and *blue* cylinders). (B) Each split YFP construct (two N-fragment and two C-fragment) need to be tested against a "nonbinding" control protein such as GST (*gray cylinders*). An "empty vector" to express just the YFP fragments should be included as well. (C) A positive control using proteins (*red* and *light green cylinders*) that are known to interact using two independent interaction assays must be included to set initial exposure settings for the experiment.

the linker sequences at the amino- and carboxy-termini of proteins introduced after the Gateway™ recombination-based cloning are quite basic. The amino-terminal attB1 SLYKKAG and carboxy-terminal attB2 PAFLYKV sequences have isoelectric points of 9.7 and 9.0, respectively.

Depending on the cloning orientation and strategy, one of these sequences can be excluded from the expressed fusion. However, the convenience of making only one entry vector means cloning ORFs lacking stop codons, which results in fusions at both termini. In rare cases, we have found that some proteins interact with the basic linker sequences. As such, alternate vectors/cloning strategies must be used. Once all such controls have been evaluated, users can proceed with BiFC assays to test POI between proteins.

Confidence in BiFC data is increased if the assays are conducted using confocal microscope settings within the range commensurate with standard imaging of AFP fusions. Neither increasing detector sensitivity, gain, and offset beyond reasonable settings to detect interactions nor decreasing them to avoid finding interactions is appropriate. The idea with BiFC is not to identify the interactions that one wants to see but to have an unbiased assay for bona fide interactions. As such, every BiFC assay must include both positive and negative controls. As mentioned earlier, GST vs GST is a convenient negative control, while a rhabdoviral nucleocapsid protein vs phosphoprotein interaction that has been validated via GST pulldowns and yeast two-hybrid assays (i.e., validated in two independent protein . interaction assays) serves as a positive control in my laboratory assays (Deng et al., 2007; Goodin et al., 2001).

Use the negative control to establish background levels and then set voltage, gain, and offset according to the positive control. The remaining interactions should, at least in the initial assay, be tested at the settings used for the positive control. It has been estimated that the detection limit of GFP is 1 µM in Vero cells, with lower levels of detection if fusions are targeted to subcellular loci (Niswender et al., 1995). Detection levels in plants are likely to be higher given higher levels of autofluorescence. However, the vastly increased sensitivity of present day microscopes and their much improved spectral selection capabilities probably put the detection level of GFP in plant cells well below micromolar concentrations. With the use of duplicated 35S promoters and suppressors of RNA silencing to increase AFP fusion expression in plant cells, false positives are likely to be of greater concern than false negatives in BiFC assays, particularly if immunodetectable levels are produced.

The more critical the determination of protein:protein interaction is to the research question, the greater the supporting data need to be. Many journals will insist on two independent protein assays before accepting protein interaction data for publication.

In addition to interaction per se, a lack of interaction may be equally informative. In such cases as mapping nuclear localization signals, BiFC between a protein and nuclear import receptor (e.g., Importin-α) is often performed. In this case, the mutant protein, lacking the putative NLS, should test negative in a BiFC experiment if nuclear accumulation of the mutant protein (lacking an NLS) is also lost (Anderson et al., 2012). In such experiments, it is critical to provide data to show that both the wild-type and mutant proteins are expressed at detectable levels at steady state (Anderson et al., 2012).

11. THE PUBLISHED MICROGRAPH IS THE LOCALIZATION PATTERN

When considering micrographs for publication it is best to review the exact requirements for a particular journal to which your manuscript will be submitted. All journals have specifications for digital media in their instructions for authors. Generally acceptable manipulations include linear adjustments to brightness, contrast, and color. These manipulations must apply to the entire image and not just specific areas within the micrograph. Additionally, the elements highlighted in the final image must have been present in the original data. Removal, deletion, copying and pasting, repositioning, and/or selective enhancement are forbidden as this is unethical in scientific data presentation.

It may seem obvious but it is far easier, and less prone to the faults described above, if a quality image is taken initially, rather than trying to "correct" subpar images. A good starting point is to take at least 3–6 quality images of every localized protein. In many cases low magnification (whole-cell) and high magnification (subcellular locus) views need to be captured. Moreover, ensure that the information presented in each channel (e.g., GFP and RFP) is in focus. Finally, all protein fusions should be tested in at least two to three independent plants.

Depending on the concentration of the *Agrobacterium* suspensions used, age of plants, and time allowed for protein expression (2 vs 4 days), protein localization patterns may vary from experiment to experiment. The published micrograph should reflect the predominant (and biologically relevant) localization pattern, which may require viewing up to several hundred independent cells to determine. Collectively then, it may take several hours of imaging and dozens of micrographs to obtain the one, or few, images that confidently represent the localization pattern for a particular protein. Once published, a particular micrograph will represent the localization pattern for a particular protein. Great care should therefore be taken to honestly represent the imaging data.

12. THE CASE FOR A PROTEIN ATLAS FOR PLANT PROTEINS

Upon mastery of the techniques and experimental plans earlier, researchers may wish to consider grander localization projects that would broadly impact virology and plant biology in general. Despite exceptional attempts to establish this, the plant biology community has never sustained efforts to determine the subcellular localization of entire plant proteomes, even with the advent of large-scale interactome projects (Braun et al., 2011; Martinez et al., 2016; Rodrigo et al., 2016).

A fundamental requirement in understanding protein function to a high degree of competency is identification of its subcellular localization under differing physiological states, including viral infection. For this reason, global protein localization maps have been generated for a variety of organisms (Lindskog, 2015; Mazumder et al., 2013; Uhlen et al., 2015). Of these maps, the most comprehensive databases for protein localization are for yeast and humans, the latter which localized some 90% of the proteome ($>16,000$ proteins) in all major ($n = 44$) tissue and organ types, and cancerous derivatives, with RNA profiling analysis for 32 tissue types (Uhlen et al., 2015). The result is an impressive protein atlas, the official web portal for which (http://www.proteinatlas.org/) provides unprecedented insight into protein function, regardless of experimental system.

While there are increasingly sophisticated proteome analyses for plants (Braun et al., 2011; Martinez et al., 2016) and plant–virus interactions (Martinez et al., 2016), the proteome-scale supporting protein localization data lag far behind that in any of the major experimental systems (Lindskog, 2015; Mazumder et al., 2013; Uhlen et al., 2015). Additionally, emerging evidence suggests that microexons that are differentially spliced in altered physiological conditions primarily affect protein interaction sites (Irimia et al., 2014; Scheckel and Darnell, 2015). Thus, mapped protein interactomes most likely will differ under a variety of physiological conditions, which in turn may explain in part, global changes in polyadenylation and dramatic relocation of proteins in response to stress (Graber et al., 2013; Mazumder et al., 2013), including biotic stress during viral infection.

Another very important consideration is that current algorithms for protein localization prediction are reasonably accurate in identifying localization at the suborganelle level. More importantly, they are entirely incapable of predicting subcellular targeting or changes in localization in altered physiological states. For these reasons, we have initiated mapping of the plant nuclear-associated proteins using *N. benthamiana* as a model system. Choice of this model plant is valid given that it can serve as an experimental host to the broadest range of viruses of any experimental plant model (Goodin et al., 2008). Additionally, transient expression of proteins in this plant is more easily achieved than in other plants systems. While the unique features of *N. benthamiana* related to RNA silencing differentiate it from other plant systems, clearly it possesses all factors required for viral replication and systemic movement (Goodin et al., 2008; Wylie et al., 2015).

13. THE NUCLEUS IN VIRUS–HOST INTERACTIONS

The role of the nucleus and nuclear-associated factors, as well as the need for a database of plant nuclear proteins, to understand the replication cycles of viruses that replicate in this organelle is intuitive (Goodin et al., 2005; Jackson and Li, 2016; Ramalho et al., 2014). Less so is the role of the nucleus in the replication of cytoplasmic viruses. The emerging view however is that conversion of the host cell into a "virus factory" results in targeting diverse subcellular loci, independent of where viral replication complexes are established (Laliberte and Zheng, 2014; Nagy, 2016; Wang, 2015). In the case of picornaviruses, the viral proteinase 3CD^{pro} has been shown to enter the nucleus where it degrades the TATA box-binding protein-associated factor RNA polymerase I subunit C, which results in inhibition of RNA polymerase I transcription. Pol II transcription is inhibited in enterovirus-infected cells by cleavage of TATA-box-binding-protein1, cyclic AMP-responsive element-binding protein 1, and POU domain, class 2, transcription factor 1 (Oct-1) by 3CD^{pro} (Yarbrough et al., 2014).

The nuclear pore complex (NPC) itself is modified by some viruses. For example, three variants of the matrix protein of *Vesicular stomatitis virus* (VSV), typically considered a structural protein, have additional functions including that of targeting Nup98 of NPCs, resulting in a shutdown of mRNA export (Petersen et al., 2000; Redondo et al., 2015). Additionally, the normally nuclear resident heterogeneous ribonucleoproteins, hnRNPA1, hnRNPK, and hnRNPC1/C2, but not hnRNPB1 or lamin A/C, are relocalized to the cytoplasm during VSV infection

(Pettit Kneller et al., 2009). Similarly, plant viruses have been shown to require nuclear factors for their life cycle. The Triple gene block protein 1 (TGBP1) of *Potato mop-top virus* facilitates virus systemic movement in an importin alpha-dependent manner (Lukhovitskaya et al., 2015). Also, nuclear proteins can function as antivirals, as in the case of WW-domain proteins that are antagonists of the *Tomato bushy stunt virus* (Barajas et al., 2015).

Taken together, these examples illustrate two points: (i) that nuclear factors play a significant role in the ability of viruses to reprogram host cellular functions and (ii) that viruses can serve as intrinsic probes to determine functions of subnuclear loci. Further advancing our current understanding of nuclear architecture and function in plants (Herud et al., 2016; Meier and Somers, 2011; Wang et al., 2014; Xu and Meier, 2008; Zhao and Meier, 2011), our present efforts will shed new light on the nucleus. Fig. 8 provides examples of the types of data that this project is generating. With the abundance of markers for subnuclear loci we will be better able to address: (i) proteins capable of receptor-mediated entry into the nucleus that may be observed in the cytoplasm at steady state, (ii) nuclear-associated proteins that may be localized to nonnuclear subcellular loci, such as microtubules (Min et al., 2010), (iii) nuclear-associated proteins that may localize to undefined loci within nuclei, and (iv) extensive alteration of nuclear architecture by viruses. Little is known about the effects of this alteration of the nucleome per se.

Visualization of nuclear-associated proteins in plants will support a broad range of virology and plant biology research. Contributions to plant protein localization databases to come will require well-trained microscopists.

Imaging instrumentation and methods are rapidly expanding what can be achieved beyond what was unimaginable even a few years ago. However, sophisticated our ability to manipulate light in biological imaging systems becomes, the base principles for image acquisition remain the same, as is the need to accept intangible qualities of imagination, when communicating science via micrographs.

14. BRIEF PROTOCOL FOR EXPRESSION OF PROTEINS IN PLANT CELLS USING AGROINFILTRATION

Transform a tractable *Agrobacterium* strain (e.g., LBA4404, C58C1) with an expression vector of choice (e.g., pGD, pSITE). Inoculate transformants onto LB agar amended with the appropriate antibiotics and incubate at 28°C. Transformed colonies should be streaked onto said LB plates

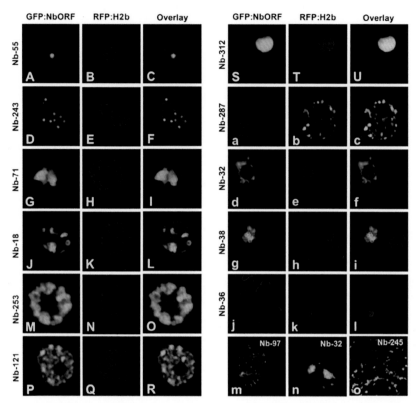

Fig. 8 Nuclear-localized *N. benthamiana* proteins selected from a screen to characterize the plant nucleome. (A–U) Nuclear localized GFP fusions expressed in leaf epidermal cells of transgenic *N. benthamiana* expressing Histone 2B fused to GFP. Identity codes of cDNAs expressed as GFP fusions are presented on the *left hand side* as "Nb-#." Fluorescence from GFP fusions is presented as GFP:NbORF. Location of the RFP-tagged nucleus is shown in panels labeled RFP:H2b, with the merged images in the column marked "overlay." The proteins designated in lower case, (a–o), are nonnuclear localized proteins, except for Nb-287 (a–c), which uses RFP targeted to endomembranes as a subcellular reference. (d–f) Perinuclear ER. (g–i) Cytoplasmic accumulation that could be confused for nucleus, but for the subcellular marker. (J–l) Cell periphery. Proteins localized without subcellular reference (m–o) demonstrate the importance of having a subcellular marker for accurate determination of localization.

and incubated overnight (up to several days) at 28°C. Harvest cells with an inoculation loop and resuspend in agroinfiltration buffer (10 mM MES, 10 mM MgCl₂, 150 μM acetosyringone, pH 5.9), to an optical density of 0.3–1.0. Suspensions can be infiltrated into leaves immediately or incubated at room temperature (18–22°C) at least 2–3 h prior to use. Leaves of *N. benthamiana* plants can be infiltrated with a 1-mL (tuberculin) syringe barrel by pressing the tip to the abaxial surface of the leaf. Infiltrated plants are incubated with illumination at 18–28°C for 48–96 h. Increased levels of protein expression and/or extending the length of time tissue is suitable for experiments that can be achieved if a suppressor of RNA silencing is coinfiltrated with the constructs of interest. If there is a need to coexpress two or more proteins by agroinfiltration, simply mix equal parts of suspensions of cells transformed with different constructs. If transgenic marker lines are not available, the nucleus can be stained by infiltrating leaves 30 min prior to microscopy using MES buffer containing 0.5 mM diamidino-2-phenylindole (DAPI). Other cell-permeant dyes can be introduced in this manner as needed. Wet-mounted leaf pieces ($\sim$1 cm^2) are adequate for confocal or epifluorescence microscopy (Goodin et al., 2002).

ACKNOWLEDGMENTS

This publication recognizes support from the Kentucky Science & Engineering Foundation (KSEF-3490-RDE-019). Students and colleagues who provided constructive feedback were vital to the preparation of the manuscript, particularly Steven Ruzin. Apologies to collaborators and colleagues whose work, for want of space, is not cited here.

REFERENCES

Adams, A., Baker, R., 1980. The Camera. New York Graphic Society, Boston.

Adams, A., Baker, R., 1981. The Negative. New York Graphic Society, Boston.

Anderson, G., Wang, R., Bandyopadhyay, A., Goodin, M., 2012. The nucleocapsid protein of potato yellow dwarf virus:protein interactions and nuclear import mediated by a non-canonical nuclear localization signal. Front. Plant Sci. 3, 14.

Babajani, G., Kermode, A.R., 2014. Alteration of the proteostasis network of plant cells promotes the post-endoplasmic reticulum trafficking of recombinant mutant (L444P) human beta-glucocerebrosidase. Plant Signal. Behav. 9. e28714.

Bandyopadhyay, A., Kopperud, K., Anderson, G., Martin, K., Goodin, M., 2010. An integrated protein localization and interaction map for potato yellow dwarf virus, type species of the genus Nucleorhabdovirus. Virology 402, 61–71.

Barajas, D., Kovalev, N., Qin, J., Nagy, P.D., 2015. Novel mechanism of regulation of tomato bushy stunt virus replication by cellular WW-domain proteins. J. Virol. 89, 2064–2079.

Braun, P., Carvunis, A.R., Charloteaux, B., Dreze, M., Ecker, J.R., Hill, D.E., Roth, F.P., Vidal, M., Galli, M., Balumuri, P., Bautista, V., Chesnut, J.D., Kim, R.C., de los Reyes, C., Gilles, P., Kim, C.J., Matrubutham, U., Mirchandani, J., Olivares, E., Patnaik, S., Quan, R., Ramaswamy, G., Shinn, P., Swamilingiah, G.M., Wu, S., Ecker, J.R., Dreze, M., Byrdsong, D., Dricot, A., Duarte, M., Gebreab, F., Gutierrez, B.J., Macwilliams, A., Monachello, D., Mukhtar, M.S., Poulin, M.M., Reichert, P., Romero, V., Tam, S., Waaijers, S., Weiner, E.M., Vidal, M., Hill, D.E., Braun, P., Galli, M., Carvunis, A.R., Cusick, M.E., Dreze, M., Romero, V., Roth, F.P., Tasan, M., Yazaki, J., Braun, P., Ecker, J.R., Carvunis, A.R., Ahn, Y.Y., Barabasi, A.L., Charloteaux, B., Chen, H.M., Cusick, M.E., Dangl, J.L., Dreze, M., Ecker, J.R., Fan, C.Y., Gai, L.T., Galli, M., Ghoshal, G., Hao, T., Hill, D.E., Lurin, C., Milenkovic, T., Moore, J., Mukhtar, M.S., Pevzner, S.J., Przulj, N.,

Rabello, S., Rietman, E.A., Rolland, T., Roth, F.P., Santhanam, B., Schmitz, R.J., Spooner, W., Stein, J., Tasan, M., Vandenhaute, J., Ware, D., Braun, P., Vidal, M., Braun, P., Carvunis, A.R., Charloteaux, B., Dreze, M., Galli, M., Vidal, M., Arabidopsis Interactome Mapping Consortium, 2011. Evidence for network evolution in an Arabidopsis Interactome map. Science 333, 601–607.

Chakrabarty, R., Banerjee, R., Chung, S.M., Farman, M., Citovsky, V., Hogenhout, S.A., Tzfira, T., Goodin, M., 2007. PSITE vectors for stable integration or transient expression of autofluorescent protein fusions in plants: probing Nicotiana benthamiana-virus interactions. Mol. Plant Microbe Interact. 20, 740–750.

Cho, S.Y., Cho, W.K., Choi, H.S., Kim, K.H., 2012. Cis-acting element (SL1) of potato virus X controls viral movement by interacting with the NbMPB2Cb and viral proteins. Virology 427, 166–176.

Costes, S.V., Daelemans, D., Cho, E.H., Dobbin, Z., Pavlakis, G., Lockett, S., 2004. Automatic and quantitative measurement of protein-protein colocalization in live cells. Biophys. J. 86, 3993–4003.

Cremer, C., Szczurek, A., Schock, F., Gourram, A., Birk, U., 2017. Super-resolution microscopy approaches to nuclear nanostructure imaging. Methods 123, 11–32.

Deng, M., Bragg, J.N., Ruzin, S., Schichnes, D., King, D., Goodin, M.M., Jackson, A.O., 2007. Role of the sonchus yellow net virus N protein in formation of nuclear viroplasms. J. Virol. 81, 5362–5374.

Dietzgen, R.G., Martin, K.M., Anderson, G., Goodin, M.M., 2012. In planta localization and interactions of impatiens necrotic spot tospovirus proteins. J. Gen. Virol. 93, 2490–2495.

Dunn, K.W., Kamocka, M.M., McDonald, J.H., 2011. A practical guide to evaluating colocalization in biological microscopy. Am. J. Physiol. Cell Physiol. 300, C723–42.

Ettinger, A., Wittmann, T., 2014. Fluorescence live cell imaging. Methods Cell Biol. 123, 77–94.

Follain, G., Mercier, L., Osmani, N., Harlepp, S., Goetz, J.G., 2017. Seeing is believing—multi-scale spatio-temporal imaging towards in vivo cell biology. J. Cell Sci. 130, 23–38.

Germond, A., Fujita, H., Ichimura, T., Watanabe, T.M., 2016. Design and development of genetically encoded fluorescent sensors to monitor intracellular chemical and physical parameters. Biophys. Rev. 8, 121–138.

Gong, X., Hurtado, O., Wang, B., Wu, C., Yi, M., Giraldo, M., Valent, B., Goodin, M., Farman, M., 2015. pFPL vectors for high-throughput protein localization in fungi: detecting cytoplasmic accumulation of putative effector proteins. Mol. Plant Microbe Interact. 28, 107–121.

Goodin, M.M., Austin, J., Tobias, R., Fujita, M., Morales, C., Jackson, A.O., 2001. Interactions and nuclear import of the N and P proteins of sonchus yellow net virus, a plant nucleorhabdovirus. J. Virol. 75, 9393–9406.

Goodin, M.M., Dietzgen, R.G., Schichnes, D., Ruzin, S., Jackson, A.O., 2002. pGD vectors: versatile tools for the expression of green and red fluorescent protein fusions in agroinfiltrated plant leaves. Plant J. 31, 375–383.

Goodin, M., Yelton, S., Ghosh, D., Mathews, S., Lesnaw, J., 2005. Live-cell imaging of rhabdovirus-induced morphological changes in plant nuclear membranes. Mol. Plant Microbe Interact. 18, 703–709.

Goodin, M.M., Chakrabarty, R., Banerjee, R., Yelton, S., Debolt, S., 2007a. New gateways to discovery. Plant Physiol. 145, 1100–1109.

Goodin, M.M., Chakrabarty, R., Yelton, S., Martin, K., Clark, A., Brooks, R., 2007b. Membrane and protein dynamics in live plant nuclei infected with Sonchus yellow net virus, a plant-adapted rhabdovirus. J. Gen. Virol. 88, 1810–1820.

Goodin, M.M., Zaitlin, D., Naidu, R.A., Lommel, S.A., 2008. Nicotiana benthamiana: its history and future as a model for plant-pathogen interactions. Mol. Plant Microbe Interact. 21, 1015–1026.

Graber, J.H., Nazeer, F.I., Yeh, P.C., Kuehner, J.N., Borikar, S., Hoskinson, D., Moore, C.L., 2013. DNA damage induces targeted, genome-wide variation of poly(A) sites in budding yeast. Genome Res. 23, 1690–1703.

Hakes, D.J., Dixon, J.E., 1992. New vectors for high level expression of recombinant proteins in bacteria. Anal. Biochem. 202, 293–298.

Hecker, A., Wallmeroth, N., Peter, S., Blatt, M.R., Harter, K., Grefen, C., 2015. Binary 2in1 vectors improve in planta (co)localization and dynamic protein interaction studies. Plant Physiol. 168, 776–787.

Herud, O., Weijers, D., Lau, S., Jurgens, G., 2016. Auxin responsiveness of the MONOPTEROS-BODENLOS module in primary root initiation critically depends on the nuclear import kinetics of the Aux/IAA inhibitor BODENLOS. Plant J. 85, 269–277.

Hibbs, A.R., 2004. Confocal Microscopy for Biologists. Kluwer Academic/Plenum Publishers, New York.

Irimia, M., Weatheritt, R.J., Ellis, J.D., Parikshak, N.N., Gonatopoulos-Pournatzis, T., Babor, M., Quesnel-Vallieres, M., Tapial, J., Raj, B., O'hanlon, D., Barrios-Rodiles, M., Sternberg, M.J.E., Cordes, S.P., Roth, F.P., Wrana, J.L., Geschwind, D.H., Blencowe, B.J., 2014. A highly conserved program of neuronal microexons is misregulated in autistic brains. Cell 159, 1511–1523.

Jackson, A.O., Li, Z., 2016. Developments in plant negative-strand RNA virus reverse genetics. Annu. Rev. Phytopathol. 54, 469–498.

Kelich, J.M., Ma, J., Dong, B., Wang, Q., Chin, M., Magura, C.M., Xiao, W., Yang, W., 2015. Super-resolution imaging of nuclear import of adeno-associated virus in live cells. Mol. Ther. Methods Clin. Dev. 2. 15047.

Kerppola, T.K., 2008. Bimolecular fluorescence complementation (BiFC) analysis as a probe of protein interactions in living cells. Annu. Rev. Biophys. 37, 465–487.

Laliberte, J.F., Zheng, H., 2014. Viral manipulation of plant host membranes. Annu. Rev. Virol. 1, 237–259.

Levy, A., Zheng, J.Y., Lazarowitz, S.G., 2015. Synaptotagmin SYTA forms ER-plasma membrane junctions that are recruited to plasmodesmata for plant virus movement. Curr. Biol. 25, 2018–2025.

Lindskog, C., 2015. The potential clinical impact of the tissue-based map of the human proteome. Expert Rev. Proteomics 12, 213–215.

Liu, L., Zhang, Z., Mei, Q., Chen, M., 2013. PSI: a comprehensive and integrative approach for accurate plant subcellular localization prediction. PLoS One 8. e75826.

Lukhovitskaya, N.I., Cowan, G.H., Vetukuri, R.R., Tilsner, J., Torrance, L., Savenkov, E.I., 2015. Importin-alpha-mediated nucleolar localization of potato mop-top virus TRIPLE GENE BLOCK1 (TGB1) protein facilitates virus systemic movement, whereas TGB1 self-interaction is required for cell-to-cell movement in Nicotiana benthamiana. Plant Physiol. 167, 738–752.

Lummer, M., Humpert, F., Wiedenlubbert, M., Sauer, M., Schuttpelz, M., Staiger, D., 2013. A new set of reversibly photoswitchable fluorescent proteins for use in transgenic plants. Mol. Plant 6, 1518–1530.

Lutz, L., Okenka, G., Schoelz, J., Leisner, S., 2015. Mutations within A 35 amino acid region of P6 influence self-association, inclusion body formation, and Caulimovirus infectivity. Virology 476, 26–36.

Martin, K., Kopperud, K., Chakrabarty, R., Banerjee, R., Brooks, R., Goodin, M.M., 2009. Transient expression in Nicotiana benthamiana fluorescent marker lines provides enhanced definition of protein localization, movement and interactions in planta. Plant J. 59, 150–162.

Martin, K.M., Dietzgen, R.G., Wang, R., Goodin, M.M., 2012. Lettuce necrotic yellows cytorhabdovirus protein localization and interaction map, and comparison with nucleorhabdoviruses. J. Gen. Virol. 93, 906–914.

Martinez, F., Rodrigo, G., Aragones, V., Ruiz, M., Lodewijk, I., Fernandez, U., Elena, S.F., Daros, J.A., 2016. Interaction network of tobacco etch potyvirus NIa protein with the host proteome during infection. BMC Genomics 17, 87.

Martin-Fernandez, M.L., Tynan, C.J., Webb, S.E., 2013. A 'pocket guide' to total internal reflection fluorescence. J. Microsc. 252, 16–22.

Mazumder, A., Pesudo, L.Q., Mcree, S., Bathe, M., Samson, L.D., 2013. Genome-wide single-cell-level screen for protein abundance and localization changes in response to DNA damage in S. cerevisiae. Nucleic Acids Res. 41, 9310–9324.

Meier, I., Somers, D.E., 2011. Regulation of nucleocytoplasmic trafficking in plants. Curr. Opin. Plant Biol. 14, 538–546.

Min, B.E., Martin, K., Wang, R., Tafelmeyer, P., Bridges, M., Goodin, M., 2010. A host-factor interaction and localization map for a plant-adapted rhabdovirus implicates cytoplasm-tethered transcription activators in cell-to-cell movement. Mol. Plant Microbe Interact. 23, 1420–1432.

Mohannath, G., Jackel, J.N., Lee, Y.H., Buchmann, R.C., Wang, H., Patil, V., Adams, A.K., Bisaro, D.M., 2014. A complex containing SNF1-related kinase (SnRK1) and adenosine kinase in Arabidopsis. PLoS One 9. e87592.

Nagy, P.D., 2016. Tombusvirus-host interactions: co-opted evolutionarily conserved host factors take center court. Annu. Rev. Virol. 3, 491–515.

Nakai, K., Kanehisa, M., 1991. Expert system for predicting protein localization sites in gram-negative bacteria. Proteins 11, 95–110.

Nakai, K., Kanehisa, M., 1992. A knowledge base for predicting protein localization sites in eukaryotic cells. Genomics 14, 897–911.

Nelson, B.K., Cai, X., Nebenfuhr, A., 2007. A multicolored set of in vivo organelle markers for co-localization studies in Arabidopsis and other plants. Plant J. 51, 1126–1136.

Niswender, K.D., Blackman, S.M., Rohde, L., Magnuson, M.A., Piston, D.W., 1995. Quantitative imaging of green fluorescent protein in cultured cells: comparison of microscopic techniques, use in fusion proteins and detection limits. J. Microsc. 180, 109–116.

Oum, Y.H., Desai, T.M., Marin, M., Melikyan, G.B., 2016. Click labeling of unnatural sugars metabolically incorporated into viral envelope glycoproteins enables visualization of single particle fusion. J. Virol. Methods 233, 62–71.

Pawley, J.B., 2006. Handbook of Biological Confocal Microscopy. Springer, New York, NY.

Petersen, J.M., Her, L.S., Varvel, V., Lund, E., Dahlberg, J.E., 2000. The matrix protein of vesicular stomatitis virus inhibits nucleocytoplasmic transport when it is in the nucleus and associated with nuclear pore complexes. Mol. Cell. Biol. 20, 8590–8601.

Pettit Kneller, E.L., Connor, J.H., Lyles, D.S., 2009. hnRNPs relocalize to the cytoplasm following infection with vesicular stomatitis virus. J. Virol. 83, 770–780.

Price, R.L., Jerome, W.G., 2011. Basic Confocal Microscopy. Springer, New York.

Pusch, S., Dissmeyer, N., Schnittger, A., 2011. Bimolecular-fluorescence complementation assay to monitor kinase-substrate interactions in vivo. Methods Mol. Biol. 779, 245–257.

Ramalho, T.O., Figueira, A.R., Sotero, A.J., Wang, R., Geraldino Duarte, P.S., Farman, M., Goodin, M.M., 2014. Characterization of coffee ringspot virus-Lavras: a model for an emerging threat to coffee production and quality. Virology 464-465C, 385–396.

Redondo, N., Madan, V., Alvarez, E., Carrasco, L., 2015. Impact of vesicular stomatitis virus M proteins on different cellular functions. PLoS One 10. e0131137.

Rodrigo, G., Daros, J.A., Elena, S.F., 2016. Virus-host interactome: putting the accent on how it changes. J. Proteomics 156, 1–4.

Rodriguez, E.A., Campbell, R.E., Lin, J.Y., Lin, M.Z., Miyawaki, A., Palmer, A.E., Shu, X., Zhang, J., Tsien, R.Y., 2017. The growing and glowing toolbox of fluorescent and photoactive proteins. Trends Biochem. Sci. 42, 111–129.

Ruzin, S.E., 1999. Plant Microtechnique and Microscopy. Oxford University Press, New York.

Scheckel, C., Darnell, R.B., 2015. Microexons-tiny but mighty. EMBO J. 34, 273–274.

Schoelz, J.E., Angel, C.A., Nelson, R.S., Leisner, S.M., 2016. A model for intracellular movement of cauliflower mosaic virus: the concept of the mobile virion factory. J. Exp. Bot. 67, 2039–2048.

Schubert, V., 2017. Super-resolution microscopy—applications in plant cell research. Front. Plant Sci. 8, 531.

Shelden, E.A., Colburn, Z.T., Jones, J.C., 2016. Focusing super resolution on the cytoskeleton. F1000Res 5.

Smolarkiewicz, M., Skrzypczak, T., Michalak, M., Lesniewicz, K., Walker, J.R., Ingram, G., Wojtaszek, P., 2014. Gamma-secretase subunits associate in intracellular membrane compartments in Arabidopsis thaliana. J. Exp. Bot. 65, 3015–3027.

Tian, G.W., Mohanty, A., Chary, S.N., Li, S., Paap, B., Drakakaki, G., Kopec, C.D., Li, J., Ehrhardt, D., Jackson, D., Rhee, S.Y., Raikhel, N.V., Citovsky, V., 2004. High-throughput fluorescent tagging of full-length Arabidopsis gene products in planta. Plant Physiol. 135, 25–38.

Tripathi, D., Raikhy, G., Goodin, M.M., Dietzgen, R.G., Pappu, H.R., 2015. In vivo localization of iris yellow spot tospovirus (Bunyaviridae)-encoded proteins and identification of interacting regions of nucleocapsid and movement proteins. PLoS One 10. e0118973.

Tzfira, T., Tian, G.W., Lacroix, B., Vyas, S., Li, J., Leitner-Dagan, Y., Krichevsky, A., Taylor, T., Vainstein, A., Citovsky, V., 2005. pSAT vectors: a modular series of plasmids for autofluorescent protein tagging and expression of multiple genes in plants. Plant Mol. Biol. 57, 503–516.

Uchiyama, A., Shimada-Beltran, H., Levy, A., Zheng, J.Y., Javia, P.A., Lazarowitz, S.G., 2014. The Arabidopsis synaptotagmin SYTA regulates the cell-to-cell movement of diverse plant viruses. Front. Plant Sci. 5, 584.

Uhlen, M., Fagerberg, L., Hallstrom, B.M., Lindskog, C., Oksvold, P., Mardinoglu, A., Sivertsson, A., Kampf, C., Sjostedt, E., Asplund, A., Olsson, I., Edlund, K., Lundberg, E., Navani, S., Szigyarto, C.A., Odeberg, J., Djureinovic, D., Takanen, J.O., Hober, S., Alm, T., Edqvist, P.H., Berling, H., Tegel, H., Mulder, J., Rockberg, J., Nilsson, P., Schwenk, J.M., Hamsten, M., Von Feilitzen, K., Forsberg, M., Persson, L., Johansson, F., Zwahlen, M., Von Heijne, G., Nielsen, J., Ponten, F., 2015. Proteomics. Tissue-based map of the human proteome. Science 347. 1260419.

Wang, A., 2015. Dissecting the molecular network of virus-plant interactions: the complex roles of host factors. Annu. Rev. Phytopathol. 53, 45–66.

Wang, Y., Wang, W., Cai, J., Zhang, Y., Qin, G., Tian, S., 2014. Tomato nuclear proteome reveals the involvement of specific E2 ubiquitin-conjugating enzymes in fruit ripening. Genome Biol. 15, 548.

Wang, H., Han, S., Siao, W., Song, C., Xiang, Y., Wu, X., Cheng, P., Li, H., Jasik, J., Micieta, K., Turna, J., Voigt, B., Baluska, F., Liu, J., Wang, Y., Zhao, H., 2015. Arabidopsis Synaptotagmin 2 participates in pollen germination and tube growth and is delivered to plasma membrane via conventional secretion. Mol. Plant 8, 1737–1750.

Wu, Q., Wang, X., Ding, S.W., 2010. Viral suppressors of RNA-based viral immunity: host targets. Cell Host Microbe 8, 12–15.

Wu, Q., Luo, A., Zadrozny, T., Sylvester, A., Jackson, D., 2013. Fluorescent protein marker lines in maize: generation and applications. Int. J. Dev. Biol. 57, 535–543.

Wylie, S.J., Zhang, C., Long, V., Roossinck, M.J., Koh, S.H., Jones, M.G., Iqbal, S., Li, H., 2015. Differential responses to virus challenge of laboratory and wild accessions of australian species of nicotiana, and comparative analysis of RDR1 gene sequences. PLoS One 10. e0121787.

Xie, W., Nielsen, M.E., Pedersen, C., Thordal-Christensen, H., 2017. A split-GFP gateway cloning system for topology analyses of membrane proteins in plants. PLoS One 12. e0170118.

Xu, X.M., Meier, I., 2008. The nuclear pore comes to the fore. Trends Plant Sci. 13, 20–27.

Yarbrough, M.L., Mata, M.A., Sakthivel, R., Fontoura, B.M., 2014. Viral subversion of nucleocytoplasmic trafficking. Traffic 15, 127–140.

Yu, J., 2016. Single-molecule studies in live cells. Annu. Rev. Phys. Chem. 67, 565–585.

Zhao, Q., Meier, I., 2011. Identification and characterization of the Arabidopsis FG-repeat nucleoporin Nup62. Plant Signal. Behav. 6, 330–334.

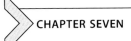

CHAPTER SEVEN

So What Have Plant Viruses Ever Done for Virology and Molecular Biology?

George P. Lomonossoff[1]

John Innes Centre, Norwich, United Kingdom
[1]Corresponding author: e-mail address: george.lomonossoff@jic.ac.uk

Contents

Abstract

The discovery of a new class of pathogen, viruses, in the late 19th century, ushered in a period of study of the biochemical and structural properties of these entities in which plant viruses played a prominent role. This was, in large part, due to the relative ease with which sufficient quantities of material could be produced for such analyses. As analytical techniques became increasingly sensitive, similar studies could be performed on the viruses from other organisms. However, plant viruses continued to play an important role in the development of molecular biology, including the demonstration that RNA can be infectious, the determination of the genetic code, the mechanism by which viral RNAs are translated, and some of the early studies on gene silencing. Thus, the study of plant viruses should not be considered a "niche" subject but rather part of the mainstream of virology and molecular biology.

Advances in Virus Research, Volume 100
ISSN 0065-3527
https://doi.org/10.1016/bs.aivir.2017.12.001

145

1. INTRODUCTION

As I am sure most readers of this chapter will be aware, the field of what is now termed "Virology" has its origins in the study of plant viruses in the late 19th century. In a series of seminal papers, Mayer (1886), Iwanovski (1892), and Beijerinck (1898) reported that a disease of tobacco was not caused by any known bacterium that the pathogenic entity could pass through filters which retained bacteria and could multiply when introduced into new hosts. In his 1898 paper, Beijerinck described this new type of pathogen (now known as tobacco mosaic virus, TMV) as a "contagium vivum fluidum" in the title of his paper and subsequently used the term "virus" within the body of the manuscript. The word is simply Latin for "poison" or "slime," but the name stuck for the new class of pathogen and the rest, as they say, is history (for those interested in reading the original papers referred to here, I recommend the translations that appear in "Phytopathological classics, No. 7" published by the American Phytopathological Society). In the same year as the publication of Beijerinck's classic paper, 1898, Loeffler and Frosch (1898) characterized an animal pathogen that was also filterable and which was subsequently termed foot-and-mouth-disease virus (FMDV). In both cases the newly discovered class of pathogen was able to multiply in previously uninfected hosts, ruling out the possibility that it was a toxic substance. Thus, both plant and animal virology can be said to have been born in the same year. After this, many other diseases of both plants and animal were shown to be caused by viruses and, a few years later, viruses infecting bacteria (bacteriophage) were also discovered (Twort, 1915).

The purpose of this review is to evaluate the contribution that plant viruses have played in the development of modern virology and molecular biology. To do this I have attempted to put the discoveries made with plant viruses in the context of discoveries made with other systems (Fig. 1). I should stress that my motive for doing this is not a complaint about an unfair lack of recognition of the subject, but rather an attempt to understand how different areas of science can interact to provide a greater understanding of the natural world. That said, I can still recall the days when the introduction of speaker who was going to talk about a plant virus could empty an auditorium as quickly as if they had shouted "fire"!

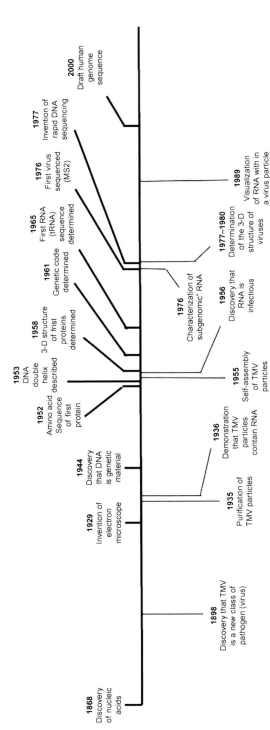

Fig. 1 Timeline of major discoveries in molecular biology and virology. The events described *above the line* relate to well-known discoveries to "bench-mark" the timeline. Those *below the line* relate to discoveries made with plant viruses. The timeline is not to scale and the choice of those discoveries to highlight is essentially a personal one.

2. BIOCHEMICAL CHARACTERIZATION

After the initial discovery of viruses as a novel form of pathogen, detailed analysis of their nature was greatly hampered in the early 20th century by the fact that they could not be grown in culture, could not be purified using standard biochemical techniques, and could not even be seen using the light microscopes available at the time. Essentially all that was known was that they were far smaller than bacteria (hence the ability to pass through filters), but their precise dimensions remained unknown. Beijerinck (1898) attempted to obtain some idea of the size of the infectious agent by examining its rate of diffusion though agar and concluded that the pathogen should be "regarded as liquid or soluble and not as corpuscular." Loeffler and Frosch (1898), however, concluded that their filterable agent was a tiny particle rather than a liquid. The distinction between the two descriptions is essentially sematic, since virus preparations are actually colloids, which lie at the boundary of solutions and suspensions.

The detailed characterization of the nature of viruses had to await developments of technologies such as protein fractionation, ultracentrifugation, and electron microscopy. In the pre-World War II era, plant viruses had a distinct advantage over other viruses for such studies as large amounts of infected material could be readily produced and, as it transpired, many plant viral particles are very stable. Thus, much of our understanding of the biochemical nature of viruses was obtained using plant viruses, particularly TMV. A major milestone in the biochemical characterization of TMV was the purification by Stanley (1935) of "a crystalline protein possessing the properties of TMV." The idea that one could actually purify and crystallize a pathogen was quite revolutionary for the time; it also started a debate, still ongoing to this day, as to whether viruses are actually "alive" or simply complex macromolecules. To get some idea of Stanley's task and the sensitivity of the techniques available to him, it is worth noting his comment that "little more than 10 GRAMS of active crystalline protein have been obtained"! From his studies he concluded that TMV (and, by implication, other viruses) was an autocatalytic protein that could multiply in a susceptible host. After the discovery that the genetic material is nucleic acid rather than protein, such a conclusion may seem somewhat quaint. However, more recently, apparently infectious proteins (prions) have been identified as causing a number of severe animal diseases (Prusiner, 2013).

Around the same time as Stanley's work in the United States, Bawden and Pirie, working in the United Kingdom, produced a preparation of TMV that they showed contained 0.5% phosphorus and 2.5% carbohydrate, which they showed were due to the presence of "nucleic acid of the ribose type" (in other words, RNA). In collaboration with Bernal and Fankuchen, they showed that the material they had purified had a regular substructure, the foundation of the idea that viruses have a regular structure (Bawden et al., 1936). In his commentary on the nature of TMV, Harrison (1999) discussed the correspondence between the US and UK groups that eventually led to the accepted conclusion that TMV is ribonucleoprotein rather than a protein. He also hypothesizes that had Bawden and Pirie been able to demonstrate the infectivity of their RNA preparations, the role of nucleic acids as the genetic carrier would have been demonstrated about 10 years earlier than was the case (Avery et al., 1944). As it was, the demonstration that the RNA within TMV was alone able to cause an infection had to wait another 20 years (Gierer and Schramm, 1956), by which time Hershey and Chase (1952) had performed their classic experiments with bacteriophage, showing that nucleic acid (in this case DNA) alone can cause a virus infection.

3. STRUCTURAL STUDIES

As a follow-up to their collaboration with Bawden and Pirie, Bernal and Fankuchen conducted a detailed analysis of the structure of a number of plant viruses using X-ray diffraction (Bernal and Fankuchen, 1937, 1941). These studies not only confirmed the repeating nature of the TMV structure but also revealed that virus such as potato virus X and tomato bushy stunt virus (TBSV) were likely to have a different overall architecture. However, with the techniques then available, it was impossible to get an overall view of what the particles actually looked like. Imaging of particles awaited the development of electron microscopy by Ernst Ruska in the 1930s though the technology was not initially applied to biological specimens (Kruger et al., 2000). It was left to Ernst Ruska's brother, Helmut, to produce the first images of a virus particle, once again TMV (Kausche et al., 1939). To demonstrate the authenticity of their images, Kausche et al. analyzed their data in the light of previous information on the structure of TMV particles obtained from the biochemical and X-ray studies described earlier. The apparent consistency of the data obtained from the different methods was instrumental in convincing the biological community of the usefulness of the electron microscope. Indeed, to this day, particles of viruses such as TMV are used as standards for calibrating electron microscopes.

The knowledge of the architecture of viral particles obtained by electron microscopy and X-ray diffraction was subsequently supplemented by the carboxypeptidase digestion studies of Harris and Knight (1952). These experiments revealed that digestion of intact TMV virions rapidly released 3400 threonine residues per mole of virus, with no other amino acid being released. This implied the presence of multiple subunits each with the same C-terminus. Though it is now known that each particle of TMV contains only 2130, rather than 3400, subunits, this experiment paved the way for our current understanding that viruses are built up from multiple copies of repeated subunits, though, as was shown later, there may be more than one type of these. Increasing resolution of both microscopy and diffraction techniques led to a generalized understanding that simple viruses, from whatever source, were symmetrical and had commonalities in structure (Crick and Watson, 1956; Finch and Klug, 1959; Watson, 1954). Although these studies concentrated on the arrangement of the protein components of virus particles, Franklin (1956) used a comparison of the fiber diffraction patterns obtained with authentic TMV and repolymerized coat protein to deduce the location of the RNA within the virus particles, the first characterization of the structure of a nucleic within an infectious entity. This was seen as such an important step in the understanding of virus structure that a model designed by Rosalind Franklin was exhibited at the World's Fair in Brussels in 1958 (Fig. 2). Caspar and Klug (1962) eventually combined these observations in the classic paper describing the underlying principles for the construction of regular viruses, be they from plants, animals, or bacteria, though most of the data used had been obtained from either plant viruses or bacteriophage. Basing their ideas, in part, upon the architectural principles of Buckminster Fuller, Caspar and Klug introduced the world to such concepts as "quasi-equivalence" and "triangulation numbers" which continue to inform our understanding of virus structures to this day. Inevitably, with our increased understanding of the structure and dynamics of protein molecules, some exceptions to the principles outlined in 1962 have emerged, such as the all-pentamer structure of polyomavirus (Rayment et al., 1982). Nonetheless, the principles outlined 55 years ago have stood the test of time remarkably well.

With the underlying principles of virus architecture established, attention turned to a detailed understanding of the structures of the components

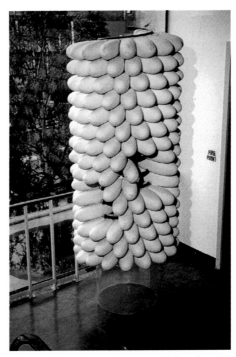

Fig. 2 Rosalind's Franklin's model of TMV that was exhibited at the Brussels World's Fair in 1958. *The photograph was taken on a landing in the Laboratory of Molecular Biology in Cambridge where the model was subsequently exhibited for many years, including the period when the author was studying for his PhD there. © MRC Laboratory of Molecular Biology.*

that make up the particles. For many years, this detailed analysis relied on diffraction methods, either fiber or crystal, but recent advances in cryo-electron microscopy (EM) have made this the method of choice for virus structure determination. Plant viruses played the leading role in the detailed determination of virus structures by X-ray methods, primarily because of the larger amounts of material that could be produced. Thus, the first helical virus for which a detailed atomic or near-atomic resolution structure was determined was TMV (Bloomer et al., 1978; Stubbs et al., 1977), while the first two icosahedral viruses resolved at this level of detail were TBSV (Harrison et al., 1978) and southern bean mosaic virus (Abad-Zapatero et al., 1980). As a result of these studies, a number of critical techniques for solving virus structures were developed and applied to animal and bacterial viruses. These structures showed that many viral coat proteins, from whatever source, adopted common folds, such as the 8-stranded antiparallel β-barrel (or jelly-roll) motif commonly found in icosahedral viruses or an α-helical bundle adopted by the coat proteins of helical viruses. These comparative studies revealed how structural commonalities between proteins can be observed even when no direct amino acid sequence identity can be detected (Rossmann and Johnson, 1989).

Though huge advances were made in the determination of the structures of the protein components of viruses throughout the 1980s, the structure(s) adopted by the nucleic acids within icosahedral particles remained elusive. This was partly a reflection of crystallographic techniques used to solve the structure of the particles, which averaged the structure of the RNA within them; resolution of the RNA structure would require that segments of the sequence adopted a precise and repetitive structure related to the arrangement of the subunits. This, in fact, was seen in the case of the particles of bean pod mottle virus, a bipartite RNA plant virus, that contain the smaller of the RNA components, RNA-2 (Chen et al., 1989). In this case, seven ordered ribonucleotides could be seen in every asymmetric unit. The advent of high-resolution cryo-EM has greatly facilitated the observation of RNA within virus particles, including those of several plant viruses. However, the current prize for the most detailed structure of an RNA molecule within a virus particle must be awarded to the bacteriophage MS2 (Dai et al., 2017).

4. LIFE CREATED IN A TEST-TUBE

A major landmark in molecular biology was the demonstration by Frankel-Conrat and Williams (1955) that infectious particles of a virus (once again, TMV) could be formed in vitro through the mixing of, what at the time were believed to be, noninfectious components (the purified protein and RNA). So dramatic was this demonstration that it led to headlines to the effect that scientists had created life in the test-tube. Of course, as mentioned earlier, it soon transpired that the RNA component alone was infectious if suitable precautions were taken to prevent its degradation. Nonetheless, the experiments demonstrated that a specific interaction takes place between the protein and nucleic acid to ensure the efficient assembly of particles. The experiments also led to the discovery that virus assembly proceeded most quickly if the coat protein was supplied in the form of two-layer disks rather than in the form of smaller aggregates (Butler and Klug, 1971). This idea that "subassemblies" of components can play a vital role in virus assembly was subsequently demonstrated for other viral systems.

Further studies with TMV revealed the specificity of assembly for the natural viral RNA over other sequences. This was shown to arise from the presence of an origin-of-assembly sequence (OAS) within the viral RNA that can adopt a hairpin structure (Zimmern, 1977; Zimmern and Butler, 1977). An unexpected twist to the story came with the discovery that the OAS was not, as anticipated, located at one end of the genomic RNA but was located approximately 5/6 of the distance from the 5′ end (Zimmern and Wilson, 1976). This unexpected location of OAS led to the development of an "inside-out" model for viral assembly, with encapsidation of the RNA proceeding bidirectionally with the major 3′ to 5′ direction ultilizing a "traveling loop" mechanism (Butler et al., 1977; Lebeurier et al., 1977). Subsequently, this proposed mechanism, obtained entirely from in vitro studies, was validated in vivo (Wu and Shaw, 1996). The concepts developed through these studies on TMV, coupled with research on RNA bacteriophage (Beckett and Uhlenbeck, 1988; Bernardi and Spahr, 1972) led to the concept that viral nucleic acids contain "packaging signals" that are responsible for the recognition of a viral nucleic acid by its cognate coat protein. This has proved relevant for many other viruses (Patel et al., 2015; Stockley et al., 2013).

5. MOLECULAR GENETICS

When one thinks of the classic pieces of research that led to the unraveling of the genetic code, one immediately thinks of the classic experiments conducted in bacterial systems (for example, those of Nirenberg and Matthaei, 1961). What is rather less well recognized nowadays is the important role that the analysis of TMV mutants played in the early stages of understanding the nature of the genetic code. As Crick et al. (1961) acknowledged in their seminal paper on the universality of the genetic code, the painstaking characterization of changes to the amino acid sequence of the coat protein of nitrous acid-induced mutants of TMV (summarized in Wittmann and Wittmann-Liebold, 1963) effectively ruled out the possibility that the code was overlapping. Furthermore, it was possible to correlate the chemical changes induced by nitrous acid (converting cytosine to uracil) with the amino acid substitutions found in the mutant coat proteins, supporting the idea that the code was degenerate and universal (Wittmann and Wittmann-Liebold, 1966). If the idea of analyzing changes in nucleotide sequences by looking for changes in amino acids seems strange in the modern era, it is important to note that protein sequencing developed before nucleic acid sequencing; the report of the first protein to be completely sequenced (insulin) occurred more than 10 years before that of the first RNA molecule (yeast tRNA$_{Ala}$). (For a review of the history of protein and nucleic acid sequencing, see Sanger, 1988.)

The study of RNA plant viruses also played a vital role in unraveling the basis of how the various open reading frames on the genomic RNA of a virus are translated. Early in vitro translation studies on TMV RNA showed that it could act as an mRNA—the first time that this had been shown for a viral RNA (Tsugita et al., 1962); however, unexpectedly, the coat protein was not among the products of translation (Aach et al., 1964). A clue as to what was happening was provided by studies on brome mosaic virus (BMV) that showed that the sequence of one of the four RNA components (RNA-4) isolated from particles, which is not required for infectivity, was also present in the next larger RNA, RNA-3 (Shih et al., 1972). Though RNA-4 could act as an efficient mRNA for the synthesis of the viral coat protein, translation of RNA-3 mainly gave rise to a larger product (now known as 3a) and very little coat protein (Shih and Kaesberg, 1973). Though the term was not used at the time, the BMV data pointed to the fact that RNA-4 was a subgenomic RNA. That the occurrence of subgenomic RNAs is not limited to multipartite viruses, such as BMV, was shown by the classic experiments on the expression of TMV coat protein by Hunter et al. (1976). These showed that, during infection, TMV produces a subgenomic RNA which encodes the coat protein but which, in the case of the common or U1 strain, is not encapsidated. It was subsequently found that the mechanism of translation of multiple open reading frames on a single viral genomic RNA via the synthesis of subgenomic RNAs is actually a common strategy for many eukaryotic RNA viruses.

6. GENOMIC SEQUENCES

Because of the small size of their genomes, viruses were the first organisms to be targeted for complete nucleotide sequence analysis. The honor of being the first organism to be sequenced belongs to the bacteriophage MS2 (Fiers et al., 1976). This was done the "hard way"—direct sequencing of radiolabeled RNA fragments. Using similar approaches, some progress had been made on the determination of the nucleotide sequence of portions of the genomes of a number of RNA plant viruses, including the 5' and 3' ends of TMV RNA (Guilley et al., 1975; Richards et al., 1977). However, around that time, rapid DNA sequencing methods were developed that revolutionized the determination of genomic sequencing. These methods were initially also applied to viruses resulting in the determination of the complete nucleotide sequence of the ssDNA bacteriophage phi x174 (Sanger et al., 1977), rapidly followed by that of the mammalian DNA virus, Simian virus 40 (Fiers et al., 1978), and the DNA plant virus cauliflower mosaic virus (Franck et al., 1980). With the development of efficient methods for the reverse transcription and cloning of viral RNAs, it became possible to use the DNA-based methods to determine the sequence of RNA viruses as demonstrated in the early examples of poliovirus (Kitamura et al., 1981; Racaniello and Baltimore, 1981a) and TMV (Goelet et al., 1982). Comparison of the available genomic sequence data from several plant and animal viruses revealed hitherto unsuspected similarities between them suggesting common evolutionary origins (Ahlquist et al., 1985; Franssen et al., 1984; Haseloff et al., 1984)—an early example of the power of bioinformatics.

7. REVERSE GENETICS OF RNA VIRUSES

For many years, detailed molecular genetic studies of RNA viruses were hampered by the lack of a method for efficiently introducing defined mutations into the genome (a reverse genetic system). That such reverse genetic systems were possible was demonstrated by the observations of Taniguchi et al. (1978) and Racaniello and Baltimore (1981b); the introduction of plasmids containing full-length copies of the genomes of bacteriophage Qβ and poliovirus resulted in the production of infectious virus in *Escherichia coli* and mammalian cells, respectively. However, these findings did not appear to be generally applicable. The subsequent studies of Ahlquist and Janda (1984) and Ahlquist et al. (1984) on BMV provided a major breakthrough by providing a generic method for the creation of reverse genetic systems for eukaryotic viruses. These authors created full-length cDNA copies of the three genomic viral RNAs and positioned them downstream of an *E. coli* RNA polymerase promoter and then used in vitro transcription with *E. coli* polymerase to produce transcripts that were able to infect plants. These findings opened the door for the generation of similar systems for a large number of positive-strand viruses of both plants and animals, including TMV (Dawson et al., 1986; Meshi et al., 1986). In later cases transcription by *E. coli* polymerase was replaced by the use of bacteriophage RNA polymerases such as T7 (Janda et al., 1987; van der Werf et al., 1986). Technology has, of course, continued to evolve and nowadays in vitro transcription is less commonly used to initiate virus infections; in the case of plant viruses, agroinfection is now generally the method of choice.

8. GENE SILENCING

Much of the early evidence for the existence of the phenomenon now known as gene silencing came from studies on transgenic plants harboring portions of plant viral genomes. These studies were originally motivated by the desire to create virus-resistant varieties of crops by mimicking the phenomenon of cross-protection (Sherwood and Fulton, 1982) through the transgenic expression of the viral coat (Abel et al., 1986). However, it soon became apparent that other segments of a plant viral genome could also give rise to resistance and, in some cases, this was more absolute and specific than that obtained from the expression of the viral coat protein (Dougherty et al., 1994; Golemboski et al., 1990; Lindbo and Dougherty, 1992). These observations led to the idea that there were two types of phenomenon being observed: protein- and RNA-mediated resistance (reviewed by Baulcombe, 1996; Lomonossoff, 1995). Shortly after, it was shown that RNA-mediated resistance is similar to natural virus resistance in "recovered" plants (Ratcliff et al., 1997) and that both involved the production of specific small RNA fragments (Hamilton and Baulcombe, 1999). At around the same time, similar observations were being made in other organisms, such as nematodes (Fire et al., 1998), and these studies led to the unraveling of the mechanism of what is now known to be an ubiquitous process, RNA interference or RNAi (Lindbo and Dougherty, 2005; Montgomery, 2006). In another twist to the story, it was found that plant viruses encode proteins that can interfere with the silencing pathway, thereby allowing viruses to overcome resistance (Anandalakshmi et al., 1998; Kasschau and Carrington, 1998).

9. BIO- AND NANOTECHNOLOGY

Parts from a number of different plant viruses, including promoters, translational enhancers, and suppressors of silencing, have found use as components of plant-based expression systems (reviewed in Saunders and Lomonossoff, 2013). These applications parallel the use of similar components of viruses of other organisms such as bacteria, insects, and mammals and so will not be discussed in detail here. However, a particular application of plant viruses concerns the use of their particles in bionanotechnology. Though particles of viruses from other organisms have been used, the high yield and stability of plant virus particles have made them particularly attractive.

One of the first uses of plant virus particles was for the display of epitopes on the outer surface of the particles (reviewed in Johnson et al., 1997). This paralleled similar studies with particles such as poliovirus and bacteriophage (Evans et al., 1989; Mastico et al., 1993). Particles of cowpea mosaic virus presenting an epitope from mink enteritis virus protected target animals from challenge with the disease (Dalsgaard et al., 1997), demonstrating that modified plant virus particles could serve as candidate vaccines. The advantage of using plant virus particles, as opposed to other types of particles, for display was demonstrated by the fact that sufficient quantities of material could be obtained to allow crystallographic analysis of the structure adopted by the presented peptides, thus enabling correlations to be made between their structure and immunological properties (Lin et al., 1996; Taylor et al., 2000).

Another major use of plant virus capsids has been their use for the encapsulation of heterologous material (Douglas and Young, 1998; Young et al., 2008). Many of the approaches adopted for this application are based on the ability of the viral particles to self-assemble in vitro and therefore relate back to observations originally made over 60 years ago. The ability to encapsulate foreign material means that plant virus-derived materials are finding an increasing number of applications in biotechnology and biomedicine (reviewed by Lomonossoff and Evans, 2014; Steele et al., 2017).

10. CONCLUSION

In this review, I have attempted to assess the role that the study of plant viruses played in the development of modern virology and molecular biology. Invariably, my choice of "landmarks" is somewhat subjective and reflects my own particular interests. I fully accept that it may be possible to review the same subject and cite a different set of critical references. Indeed, it might also be possible to write a review which concludes that plant viruses played no, or only a minor, role in the development of virology and molecular biology, though I suspect (hope?) that this is not the case.

ACKNOWLEDGMENTS

This work was supported by the BBSRC Institute Strategic Programme Grant "Understanding and Exploiting Plant and Microbial Secondary Metabolism" (BB/J004596/1) and the John Innes Foundation.

REFERENCES

Aach, H.G., Funatsu, G., Nirenberg, N.W., Fraenkel-Conrat, H., 1964. Further attempts to characterize products of TMV-RNA-directed protein synthesis. Biochemistry 3, 1362.

Abad-Zapatero, C., Abdel-Meguid, S.S., Johnson, J.E., Leslie, A.G., Rayment, I., Rossmann, M.G., Suck, D., Tsukihara, T., 1980. Structure of southern bean mosaic virus at 2.8 Å resolution. Nature 286, 33.

Abel, P.P., Nelson, R.S., De, B., Hoffmann, N., Rogers, S.G., Fraley, R.T., Beachy, R.N., 1986. Delay of disease development in transgenic plants that express the tobacco mosaic virus coat protein gene. Science 232, 738.

Ahlquist, P., Janda, M., 1984. cDNA cloning and in vitro transcription of the complete brome mosaic virus genome. Mol. Cell. Biol. 4, 2876.

Ahlquist, P., French, R., Janda, M., Loesch-Fries, L.S., 1984. Multicomponent RNA plant virus infection derived from cloned viral cDNA. Proc. Natl. Acad. Sci. U.S.A. 81, 7066.

Ahlquist, P., Strauss, E.G., Rice, C.M., Strauss, J.H., Haseloff, J., Zimmern, D., 1985. Sindbis virus proteins nsP1 and nsP2 contain homology to nonstructural proteins from several RNA plant viruses. J. Virol. 53, 536.

Anandalakshmi, R., Pruss, G.J., Ge, X., Marathe, R., Mallory, A.C., Smith, T.H., Vance, V.B., 1998. A viral suppressor of gene silencing in plants. Proc. Natl. Acad. Sci. U.S.A. 95, 13079.

Avery, O.T., MacLeod, C.M., McCarty, M., 1944. Studies on the chemical nature of the substance inducing transformation of pneumococcal types: induction of transformation desoxyribonucleic acid fraction isolated from pneumococcus type III. J. Exp. Med. 79, 137.

Baulcombe, D.C., 1996. Mechanisms of pathogen-derived resistance to viruses in transgenic plants. Plant Cell 8, 1833.

Bawden, F.C., Pirie, N.W., Bernal, J.D., Fankuchen, I., 1936. Liquid crystalline substances from virus-infected plants. Nature 138, 1051.

Beckett, D., Uhlenbeck, O.C., 1988. Ribonucleoprotein complexes of R17 coat protein and a translational operator analog. J. Mol. Biol. 204, 927.

Beijerinck, M.W., 1898. Concerning contagium vivum fluidum as a cause of the spot disease of tobacco leaves. English translation, In: Johnson, J. (Ed.), Phytopathological Classics, No. 7. American Phytopathological Society, p. 33.

Bernal, J.D., Fankuchen, I., 1937. Structure types of protein 'crystals' from virus-infected plants. Nature 139, 923.

Bernal, J.D., Fankuchen, I., 1941. X-ray and crystallographic studies of plant virus preparations. III. J. Gen. Physiol. 25, 147.

Bernardi, A., Spahr, P.F., 1972. Nucleotide sequence at the binding site for coat protein on RNA of bacteriophage R17. Proc. Natl. Acad. Sci. U.S.A. 69, 3033.

Bloomer, A.C., Champness, J.N., Bricogne, G., Staden, R., Klug, A., 1978. Protein disk of tobacco mosaic virus at 2.8 Å resolution showing the interactions within and between subunits. Nature 276, 362.

Butler, P.J.G., Klug, A., 1971. Assembly of the particle of tobacco mosaic virus from RNA and disks of protein. Nat. New Biol. 229, 47.

Butler, P.J.G., Finch, J.T., Zimmern, D., 1977. Configuration of tobacco mosaic virus, RNA during virus assembly. Nature 265, 217.

Caspar, D.L.D., Klug, A., 1962. Physical principles in the construction of regular viruses. Cold Spring Harb. Symp. Quant. Biol. 27, 1.

Chen, Z.G., Stauffacher, C., Li, Y., Schmidt, T., Bomu, W., Kamer, G., Shanks, M., Lomonossoff, G., Johnson, J.E., 1989. Protein-RNA interactions in an icosahedral virus at 3.0 Å resolution. Science 245, 154.

Crick, F.H., Watson, J.D., 1956. Structure of small viruses. Nature 177, 473.

Crick, F.H., Barnett, L., Brenner, S., Watts-Tobin, R.J., 1961. General nature of the genetic code for proteins. Nature 192, 1227.

Dai, X., Li, Z., Lai, M., Shu, S., Du, Y., Zhou, Z.H., Sun, R., 2017. In situ structures of the genome and genome-delivery apparatus in a single-stranded RNA virus. Nature 541, 112.

Dalsgaard, K., Uttenthal, A., Jones, T.D., Xu, F., Merryweather, A., Hamilton, W.D.O., Langeveld, J.P., Boshuizen, R.S., Kamstrup, S., Lomonossoff, G.P., Porta, C., Vela, C., Casal, J.I., Meloen, R.H., Rodgers, P.B., 1997. Plant-derived vaccine protects target animals against a viral disease. Nat. Biotechnol. 15, 248.

Dawson, W.O., Beck, D.L., Knorr, D.A., Grantham, G.L., 1986. cDNA cloning of the complete genome of tobacco mosaic virus and production of infectious transcripts. Proc. Natl. Acad. Sci. U.S.A. 83, 1832.

Dougherty, W.G., Lindbo, J.A., Smith, H.A., Parks, T.D., Swaney, S., Proebsting, W.M., 1994. RNA-mediated virus resistance in transgenic plants: exploitation of a cellular pathway possibly involved in RNA degradation. Mol. Plant Microbe Interact. 7, 544.

Douglas, T., Young, M., 1998. Host–guest encapsulation of materials by assembled virus protein cages. Nature 393, 152.

Evans, D.J., McKeating, J., Meredith, J.M., Burke, K.L., Katrak, K., John, A., Ferguson, M., Minor, P.D., Weiss, R.A., Almond, J.W., 1989. An engineered poliovirus chimaera elicits broadly reactive HIV-1 neutralizing antibodies. Nature 339, 385.

Fiers, W., Contreras, R., Duerinck, F., Haegeman, G., Iserentant, D., Merregaert, J., Min Jou, W., Molemans, F., Raeymaekers, A., van den Berghe, A., Volckaert, G., Ysebaert, M., 1976. Complete nucleotide sequence of bacteriophage MS2 RNA: primary and secondary structure of the replicase gene. Nature 260, 500.

Fiers, W., Contreras, R., Haegemann, G., Rogiers, R., van de Voorde, A., van Heuverswyn, H., van Herreweghe, J., Volckaert, G., Ysebaert, M., 1978. Complete nucleotide sequence of SV40 DNA. Nature 273, 113.

Finch, J.T., Klug, A., 1959. Structure of poliomyelitis virus. Nature 183, 1709.

Fire, A., Xu, S., Montgomery, M.K., Kostas, S.A., Driver, S.E., Mello, C.C., 1998. Potent and specific genetic interference by double-stranded RNA in Caenorhabditis elegans. Nature 391, 806.

Fraenkel-Conrat, H., Williams, R.C., 1955. Reconstitution of active tobacco mosaic virus from its inactive protein and nucleic acid components. Proc. Natl. Acad. Sci. U.S.A. 41, 690.

Franck, A., Guilley, H., Jonard, G., Richards, K., Hirth, L., 1980. Nucleotide sequence of cauliflower mosaic virus DNA. Cell 21, 285.

Franklin, R.E., 1956. Location of the ribonucleic acid in the tobacco mosaic virus particle. Nature 177, 928.

Franssen, H., Leunissen, J., Goldbach, R., Lomonossoff, G., Zimmern, D., 1984. Homologous sequences in non-structural proteins from cowpea mosaic virus and picornaviruses. EMBO J. 3, 855.

Gierer, A., Schramm, G., 1956. Infectivity of ribonucleic acid from tobacco mosaic virus. Nature 182, 702.

Goelet, P., Lomonossoff, G.P., Butler, P.J.G., Akam, M.E., Gait, M.J., Karn, J., 1982. Nucleotide sequence of tobacco mosaic virus RNA. Proc. Natl. Acad. Sci. U.S.A. 79, 5818.

Golemboski, D.B., Lomonossoff, G.P., Zaitlin, M., 1990. Plants transformed with a tobacco mosaic virus nonstructural gene sequence are resistant to the virus. Proc. Natl. Acad. Sci. U.S.A. 87, 6311.

Guilley, H., Jonard, G., Hirth, L., 1975. Sequence of 71 nucleotides at the 3'-end of tobacco mosaic virus RNA. Proc. Natl. Acad. Sci. U.S.A. 72, 864.

Hamilton, A.J., Baulcombe, D.C., 1999. A species of small antisense RNA in posttranscriptional gene silencing in plants. Science 286, 950.

Harris, J.I., Knight, C.A., 1952. Action of carboxypeptidase on tobacco mosaic virus. Nature 170, 613.

Harrison, B.D., 1999. The chemical nature of tobacco mosaic virus particles. In: Scholtof, K.-B.G., Shaw, J.G., Zaitlin, M. (Eds.), Tobacco Mosaic Virus: One Hundred Years of Contributions to Virology. APS Press, St. Paul, MN.

Harrison, S.C., Olson, A.J., Schutt, C.E., Winkler, F.K., Bricogne, G., 1978. Tomato bushy stunt virus at 2.9 Å resolution. Nature 276, 368.

Haseloff, J., Goelet, P., Zimmern, D., Ahlquist, P., Dasgupta, R., Kaesberg, P., 1984. Striking similarities in amino acid sequence among nonstructural proteins encoded by RNA viruses that have dissimilar genomic organization. Proc. Natl. Acad. Sci. U.S.A. 81, 4358.

Hershey, A., Chase, M., 1952. Independent functions of viral protein and nucleic acid in growth of bacteriophage. J. Gen. Physiol. 36, 39.

Hunter, T.R., Hunt, T., Knowland, J., Zimmern, D., 1976. Messenger RNA for the coat protein of tobacco mosaic virus. Nature 260, 759.

Ivanowski, D., 1892. Concerning the mosaic disease of the tobacco plant. English translation, In: Johnson, J. (Ed.), Phytopathological Classics, No. 7. American Phytopathological Society, p. 27.

Janda, M., French, R., Ahlquist, P., 1987. High efficiency T7 polymerase synthesis of infectious RNA from cloned brome mosaic virus cDNA and effects of 5' extensions on transcript infectivity. Virology 158, 259.

Johnson, J.E., Lin, T., Lomonossoff, G.P., 1997. Presentation of heterologous peptides on plant viruses: genetics, structure, and function. Annu. Rev. Phytopathol. 35, 67.

Kasschau, K.D., Carrington, J.C., 1998. A counterdefensive strategy of plant viruses: suppression of posttranscriptional gene silencing. Cell 95, 461.

Kausche, G.A., Pflankuch, Ruska, H., 1939. Die Sichtbarmachung von pflanzlichem virus im ubermikroskop. Naturwissenschaften 27, 292.

Kitamura, N., Semler, B.L., Rothberg, P.G., Larsen, G.R., Adler, C.J., Dorner, A.J., Emini, E.A., Hanecak, R., Lee, J.J., van der Werf, S., Anderson, C.W., Wimmer, E., 1981. Primary structure, gene organization and polypeptide expression of poliovirus RNA. Nature 291, 547.

Kruger, D., Schneck, P., Gelderblom, H.R., 2000. Helmut Ruska and the visualisation of viruses. Lancet 355, 1713.

Lebeurier, G., Nicolaieff, A., Richards, K.E., 1977. Inside-out model for self-assembly of tobacco mosaic virus. Proc. Natl. Acad. Sci. U.S.A. 74, 149.

Lin, T., Porta, C., Lomonossoff, G., Johnson, J.E., 1996. Structure-based design of peptide presentation on a viral surface: the crystal structure of a plant/animal virus chimera at 2.8 Å resolution. Fold. Des. 1, 179.

Lindbo, J.A., Dougherty, W.G., 1992. Untranslatable transcripts of the tobacco etch virus coat protein gene sequence can interfere with tobacco etch virus replication in transgenic plants and protoplasts. Virology 189, 725.

Lindbo, J.A., Dougherty, W.G., 2005. Plant pathology and RNAi: a brief history. Annu. Rev. Phytopathol. 43, 191.

Loeffler, F., Frosch, P., 1898. Berichte der Kommission zur Erforschung der Maul- und Klauenseuche bei dem Institut für Infektionskrankheiten in Berlin. Centralblatt für Bakteriologie, Parasitenkunde und Infektionskrankheiten, Abt. I 23, 371.

Lomonossoff, G.P., 1995. Pathogen-derived resistance to plant viruses. Annu. Rev. Phytopathol. 33, 323.

Lomonossoff, G.P., Evans, D.J., 2014. Applications of plant viruses in bio-nanotechnology. Curr. Top. Microbiol. Immunol. 375, 61.

Mastico, R.A., Talbot, S.J., Stockley, P.G., 1993. Multiple presentation of foreign peptides on the surface of an RNA-free spherical bacteriophage capsid. J. Gen. Virol. 74, 541.

Mayer, A., 1886. Concerning the mosaic disease of tobacco. English translation, In: Johnson, J. (Ed.), Phytopathological Classics, No. 7. American Phytopathological Society, p. 11.

Meshi, T., Ishikawa, M., Motoyoshi, F., Semba, K., Okada, Y., 1986. In vitro transcription of infectious RNAs from full-length cDNAs of tobacco mosaic virus. Proc. Natl. Acad. Sci. U.S.A. 83, 5043.

Montgomery, M.K., 2006. RNA interference: unravelling a mystery. Nat. Struct. Mol. Biol. 13, 1039.

Nirenberg, M.W., Matthaei, J.H., 1961. The dependence of cell-free protein synthesis in E. coli upon naturally occurring or synthetic polyribonucleotides. Proc. Natl. Acad. Sci. U.S.A. 47, 1588.

Patel, N., Dykeman, E.C., Coutts, R.H.A., Lomonossoff, G.P., Rowlands, D.J., Phillips, S.E.V., Ranson, N., Twarock, R., Tuma, R., Stockley, P.G., 2015. Revealing the density of encoded functions in a viral RNA. Proc. Natl. Acad. Sci. U.S.A. 112, 2227.

Prusiner, S.B., 2013. Biology and genetics of prions causing neurodegeneration. Annu. Rev. Genet. 47, 601.

Racaniello, V.R., Baltimore, D., 1981a. Molecular cloning of poliovirus cDNA and determination of the complete nucleotide sequence of the viral genome. Proc. Natl. Acad. Sci. U.S.A. 78, 4887.

Racaniello, V.R., Baltimore, D., 1981b. Cloned poliovirus complementary DNA is infectious in mammalian cells. Science 214, 916.

Ratcliff, F., Harrison, B.D., Baulcombe, D.C., 1997. A similarity between viral defense and gene silencing in plants. Science 276, 1558.

Rayment, I., Baker, T.S., Caspar, D.L.D., Murakami, W.T., 1982. Polyoma virus capsid structure at 22.5 Å resolution. Nature 295, 110.

Richards, K., Guilley, H., Jonard, G., Keith, G., 1977. Leader sequence of 71 nucleotides devoid of G in tobacco mosaic virus RNA. Nature 267, 548.

Rossmann, M.G., Johnson, J.E., 1989. Icosahedral RNA virus structure. Annu. Rev. Biochem. 58, 533.

Sanger, F., 1988. Sequences, sequences, and sequences. Annu. Rev. Biochem. 57, 1.

Sanger, F., Air, G.M., Barrell, B.G., Brown, N.L., Coulson, A.R., Fiddes, C.A., Hutchison, C.A., Slocombe, P.M., Smith, M., 1977. Nucleotide sequence of bacteriophage phi X174 DNA. Nature 265, 687.

Saunders, K., Lomonossoff, G.P., 2013. Exploiting plant virus-derived components to achieve in planta expression and for templates for synthetic biology applications. New Phytol. 200, 16.

Sherwood, J.L., Fulton, R.W., 1982. The specific involvement of coat protein in tobacco mosaic virus cross protection. Virology 119, 150.

Shih, D.S., Kaesberg, P., 1973. Translation of brome mosaic viral ribonucleic acid in a cell-free system derived from wheat embryo. Proc. Natl. Acad. Sci. U.S.A. 70, 1799.

Shih, D.S., Lane, L.C., Kaesberg, P., 1972. Origin of the small component of brome mosaic virus RNA. J. Mol. Biol. 64, 353.

Stanley, W.M., 1935. Isolation of a crystalline protein possessing the properties of tobacco mosaic virus. Science 81, 644.

Steele, J.F.C., Peyret, H., Saunders, K., Castells-Graells, R., Marsian, J., Meshcheriakova, Y., Lomonossoff, G.P., 2017. Synthetic plant virology for nanobiotechnology and nanomedicine. Wiley Interdiscip. Rev. Nanomed. Nanobiotechnol. 9, e1447. https://doi.org/10.1002/wnan.1447.

Stockley, P.G., Twarock, R., Bakker, S.E., Barker, A.M., Borodavka, A., Dykeman, E., Ford, R.J., Pearson, A.R., Phillips, S.E., Ranson, N.A., Tuma, R., 2013. Packaging signals in single-stranded RNA viruses: nature's alternative to a purely electrostatic assembly mechanism. J. Biol. Phys. 39, 277.

Stubbs, G., Warren, S., Holmes, K., 1977. Structure of RNA and RNA binding site in tobacco mosaic virus from 4-Å map calculated from X-ray fibre diagrams. Nature 267, 216.

Taniguchi, T., Palmieri, M., Weissmann, C., 1978. Qβ DNA-containing hybrid plasmids giving rise to Qβ phage formation in the bacterial host. Nature 274, 223.

Taylor, K.M., Lin, T., Porta, C., Mosser, A.G., Giesing, H.A., Lomonossoff, G.P., Johnson, J.E., 2000. Influence of three-dimensional structure on the immunogenicity of a peptide expressed on the surface of a plant virus. J. Mol. Recognit. 13, 71.

Tsugita, A., Fraenkel-conrat, H., Nirenberg, M.W., Matthaei, J.H., 1962. Demonstration of the messenger role of viral RNA. Proc. Natl. Acad. Sci. U.S.A. 48, 846.

Twort, F.W., 1915. An investigation on the nature of ultra-microscopic viruses. Lancet 186, 1241.

van der Werf, S., Bradley, J., Wimmer, E., Studier, F.W., Dunn, J.J., 1986. Synthesis of infectious poliovirus RNA by purified T7 RNA polymerase. Proc. Natl. Acad. Sci. U.S.A. 83, 2330.

Watson, J.D., 1954. The structure of tobacco mosaic virus. I. X-ray evidence of a helical arrangement of sub-units around the longitudinal axis. Biochim. Biophys. Acta 3, 10.

Wittmann, H.G., Wittmann-Liebold, B., 1963. Tobacco mosaic virus mutants and the genetic coding problem. Cold Spring Harb. Symp. Quant. Biol. 28, 589.

Wittmann, H.G., Wittmann-Liebold, B., 1966. Protein chemical studies of two RNA viruses and their mutants. Cold Spring Harb. Symp. Quant. Biol. 31, 163.

Wu, X., Shaw, J.G., 1996. Bidirectional uncoating of the genomic RNA of a helical virus. Proc. Natl. Acad. Sci. U.S.A. 93, 2981.

Young, M., Willits, D., Uchida, M., Douglas, T., 2008. Plant viruses as biotemplates for materials and their use in nanotechnology. Annu. Rev. Phytopathol. 46, 361.

Zimmern, D., 1977. The nucleotide sequence at the origin for assembly on tobacco mosaic virus RNA. Cell 11, 463.

Zimmern, D., Butler, P.J.G., 1977. The isolation of tobacco mosaic virus RNA fragments containing the origin for viral assembly. Cell 11, 455.

Zimmern, D., Wilson, T.M.A., 1976. Location of the origin for viral reassembly on tobacco mosaic virus RNA and its relation to stable fragment. FEBS Lett. 71, 294.

CHAPTER EIGHT

Hosts and Sources of Endemic Human Coronaviruses

Victor M. Corman*,†, Doreen Muth*,†, Daniela Niemeyer*, Christian Drosten*,†,1

*Charité–Universitätsmedizin Berlin, corporate member of Freie Universität Berlin, Humboldt-Universität zu Berlin, and Berlin Institute of Health, Institute of Virology, Berlin, Germany
†German Center for Infection Research (DZIF), Berlin, Germany
1Corresponding author: e-mail address: christian.drosten@charite.de

Contents

Abstract

The four endemic human coronaviruses HCoV-229E, -NL63, -OC43, and -HKU1 contribute a considerable share of upper and lower respiratory tract infections in adults and children. While their clinical representation resembles that of many other agents of the common cold, their evolutionary histories, and host associations could provide important insights into the natural history of past human pandemics. For two of these viruses, we have strong evidence suggesting an origin in major livestock species while primordial associations for all four viruses may have existed with bats and rodents. HCoV-NL63 and -229E may originate from bat reservoirs as assumed for many other coronaviruses, but HCoV-OC43 and -HKU1 seem more likely to have speciated from rodent-associated viruses. HCoV-OC43 is thought to have emerged from ancestors in domestic animals such as cattle or swine. The bovine coronavirus has been suggested to be a possible ancestor, from which HCoV-OC43 may have emerged in the context of a pandemic recorded historically at the end of the 19th century. New data suggest that HCoV-229E may actually be transferred from dromedary camels similar to Middle East respiratory syndrome (MERS) coronavirus. This scenario provides important ecological parallels to the present prepandemic pattern of host associations of the MERS coronavirus.

Advances in Virus Research, Volume 100
ISSN 0065-3527
https://doi.org/10.1016/bs.aivir.2018.01.001

1. INTRODUCTION

Coronaviruses (CoV) (order *Nidovirales*, family *Coronaviridae*, subfamily *Coronavirinae*) are enveloped, positive stranded RNA viruses. The subfamily *Coronavirinae* contains the four genera *Alpha-*, *Beta-*, *Gamma-*, and *Deltacoronavirus*. Coronaviruses infect birds (gamma- and deltacoronaviruses) and several mammalian species (mainly alpha- and betacoronaviruses), including humans. Animal CoVs, which include important livestock pathogens such as transmissible gastroenteritis virus (TGEV) of swine, bovine CoV (BCoV), and feline coronavirus (FCoV) have been known for more than 80 years (Saif, 2004). Six different CoVs have been identified in humans. The earliest reports of *endemic human CoV (HCoV)* date back to the 1960s, when HCoV-OC43 and -229E were described (Hamre and Procknow, 1966; McIntosh et al., 1967). HCoV-NL63 and -HKU1 were discovered only in 2004 and 2005, respectively (van der Hoek et al., 2004; Woo et al., 2005). In addition to these four endemic HCoVs, two epidemic CoVs have emerged in humans in the last 2 decades, severe acute respiratory syndrome (SARS)-CoV and the Middle East respiratory syndrome (MERS)-CoV discovered in 2003 and 2012, respectively (Drosten et al., 2003; Zaki et al., 2012). Both viruses belong to the genus *Betacoronavirus* and were responsible for outbreaks involving high case fatality rates. SARS-CoV was responsible for an outbreak of viral pneumonia in 2002/2003. This outbreak affected at least 8000 individuals and was characterized by a case fatality rate of approximately 10% (Cheng et al., 2007; Drosten et al., 2003). The epidemic lineage of SARS-CoV is believed to have been acquired by humans from carnivorous wild game such as civet cats, which in turn are thought to have acquired the virus from rhinolophid bats (Drexler et al., 2010; Drosten et al., 2003; Ge et al., 2013; Peiris et al., 2003; Poon et al., 2005; Yang et al., 2015). Since 2004, no human SARS-CoV cases have been reported, but SARS-CoV or closely related viruses carried by bats may still be able to cause human disease after spillover infection (Ge et al., 2012, 2013).

The other highly pathogenic CoV infecting humans—the MERS-CoV—was incidentally discovered in a fatal human case of pneumonia in Saudi Arabia in 2012 (Zaki et al., 2012). A large body of subsequent work suggests that humans regularly and frequently acquire MERS-CoV as a zoonotic infection from dromedary camels, a major livestock species in the Middle East. Dromedary camels across their habitats in Africa, the Middle East, and Asia are now known to be seropositive for MERS-CoV at very high proportions (Chu et al., 2014, 2015; Corman et al., 2014b; Muller et al., 2014; Reusken et al., 2013; Saqib et al., 2017). Conspecific viruses in coancestral relationship to dromedary-associated viruses were found in bats. However, these bat-associated MERS-related CoVs are far more genetically distant from their human-infecting counterpart than bat-associated viruses related to SARS-CoV (Annan et al., 2013; Corman et al., 2014a; de Groot et al., 2013; Ithete et al., 2013; van Boheemen et al., 2012). Since the discovery of MERS-CoV, more than 2000 human cases were reported. The case fatality rate in hospital-associated clusters ranged around 35% (WHO, 2017). Hospital-based outbreaks are known to have involved up to four consecutive steps of human-to-human transmission before further spread could be halted by intensified measures of infection control (Drosten et al., 2015; Kim et al., 2017; Oboho et al., 2015). Owing to the role of dromedaries as a major livestock species in the Middle East, MERS-CoV represents a serious zoonotic threat involving an unknown epidemic and pandemic potential.

In extension of our knowledge on origins of MERS- and SARS-CoV in bats, it has been proposed that all HCoVs may be of zoonotic origin, and may indeed originate from bats (Drexler et al., 2014; Vijaykrishna et al., 2007; Woo et al., 2009a, b). The common scenario of CoV evolution then involves past transitions into intermediate hosts such as livestock that have closer interaction with humans, and that may carry a diversity of viruses including variants directly related to ancestral strains. Discovering intermediary viruses may enable comparisons between original and current viral characteristics in humans, elucidating the process of human adaptation. However, there is still a gross lack of comprehensive data on the evolutionary history of most HCoVs. Only for HCoV-OC43, which belongs to the species *Betacoronavirus 1* (BetaCoV 1), a zoonotic acquisition from ungulate livestock is widely accepted (de Groot et al., 2012a, b; Vijgen et al., 2005, 2006). Recently, a number of studies of CoV in wildlife and livestock have advanced our knowledge of origins of the other HCoVs. In this text, we will provide definitions that are important to correctly describe the process of host transition during emergence of HCoVs, and continue to summarize what is known and thought about the natural histories of emergence of HCoVs.

1.1 Endemic Human Coronavirus Disease

The alphacoronaviruses HCoV-NL63 and -229E and the betacoronaviruses HCoV-OC43 and -HKU1 are established human pathogens. They are responsible for episodes of common cold in humans worldwide (Annan et al., 2016; Graat et al., 2003; Mackay et al., 2012; Owusu et al., 2014; van Elden et al., 2004). Depending on the study setting, up to 20% of tests in individuals with respiratory disease yielded evidence of acute infection with these viruses (Annan et al., 2016; Arden et al., 2005; Bastien et al., 2005; Berkley et al., 2010; Dijkman et al., 2012; Fielding, 2011; Gaunt et al., 2010; Larson et al., 1980; Walsh et al., 2013). HCoV-229E was first isolated in 1967 and shares only 65% nucleotide identity with the other human alphacoronavirus, HCoV-NL63. The latter was first isolated in 2003 from a 7-months-old child suffering from bronchiolitis and conjunctivitis (Hamre and Procknow, 1966; van der Hoek et al., 2004). HCoV-OC43 is already known since the 1960s, whereas HCoV-HKU1 was discovered only in 2005 in a 71-year-old man with pneumonia treated in Hong Kong (McIntosh et al., 1967; Woo et al., 2005).

Although the majority of infections with HCoVs cause only mild respiratory tract illness, all HCoVs can also induce fulminant courses of disease, especially but not exclusively in immunosuppressed patients and infants (Konca et al., 2017; Mayer et al., 2016; Oosterhof et al., 2010; van der Hoek, 2007). Beside the occurrence in the respiratory tract, all endemic CoVs can also be detected in stool samples but they do not seem to be a major cause of gastroenteritis (Esper et al., 2010; Paloniemi et al., 2015; Risku et al., 2010). In particular, HCoV-OC43 has been suspected to play a role in neurological diseases such as chronic demyelinating disease and acute encephalomyelitis (Morfopoulou et al., 2016; Murray et al., 1992; Yeh et al., 2004).

1.2 Definitions and Concepts
1.2.1 Virus Species
The International Committee for the Taxonomy of Viruses (ICTV) endorsed the following definition for a virus species in 1991: "A virus species is a polythetic class of viruses that constitute a replicating lineage and occupy a particular ecological niche". In spite of this comprehensive definition, the delineation of specific viral species is often not well defined. For CoVs, the ICTV coronavirus study group has suggested a species criterion based on rooted phylogenies and pair wise amino acid distances in seven concatenated domains of the nonstructural part of the CoV genome (de Groot et al., 2013). While the group is presently working on a comprehensive revision of the present CoV classification, we use the above-described classification and current taxonomic virus designations for this overview.

ICTV classifies HCoV-NL63, -229E, and -HKU1 as independent viral species, whereas HCoV-OC43 is part of a virus species named *Betacoronavirus 1* (BetaCoV 1). Beside HCoV-OC43, BetaCoV1 comprises BCoV and several closely related viruses found in odd- and even-toed ungulates, carnivores, and lagomorphs (Alekseev et al., 2008; Guy et al., 2000; Hasoksuz et al., 2007; Lau et al., 2012; Lim et al., 2013; Majhdi et al., 1997).

1.2.2 Application of Niche- vs Genetic Distance Criteria in Species Classification

The ICTV species definition includes a general recognition of the role of habitat in the process of speciation. It also implicates genetic restrictions separating species by referring to a species as "a replicating lineage." However, only for some virus groups have the genetic basis of speciation—limited fitness of recombinants—been used to systematically delimit species. Habitat or niche separation leads to physical, but not necessarily genetic reproductive isolation. In classical approaches to species definition in animals, populations living in disconnected habitats continue to belong to one same species as long as they can generate fit and fertile progeny. In some viral taxa including the CoVs, genetic distance criteria have been established, using data that at least partly consider the empirical capability of viral lineages to form viable recombinants (de Groot et al., 2012a, b). Genetic species delimitation criteria enable us to discover cases in which viral species exist over several host systems. We can then identify those host species that contain a higher genetic viral diversity, and thereupon derive source attributions in zoonotic or evolutionary scenarios. Adequate comparisons of genetic diversity can only be conducted as long as the compared viruses belong to one same species. This is because the biology of separated species—even if they belong to closely related phylogenetic clades—may be so different that genetic diversity could have developed at considerably different pace. Consequently, information on ecological niche—often a particular host species—should not be used as a leading criterion for the classification of viral species.

1.2.3 Natural Hosts

As ICTV's general view on species involves the concept of niche, we have to reflect on the implications for multihost species of viruses. For the purpose of the present text, we will define a *natural host* as the long-term ecological niche (resembling a habitat) of a viral population or metapopulation, whereas *dead-end host* is a niche in which the maintenance of populations is routinely unsuccessful (and success may lead to a pandemic). It should be noted that "host" in this context does not necessarily mean a species of animals but can extend over wider taxonomic groups (such as a genus). The host niche can also be restricted by nontaxonomic properties such as geographic range.

Natural hosts are expected to show typical common characteristics related to infection patterns: First, they should contain a higher genetic virus diversity than other host species. Second, they should harbor the virus continuously, at least on the level of social groups. And third, they should be naturally infected beyond the geographic range of present social groups (Drexler et al., 2012; Greger, 2007; Haydon et al., 2002). For some viral species all of these criteria are met, and consensus regarding natural host associations can be reached. For instance, virologists agree on the association of rabies virus with dogs and related carnivores, as well as influenza A virus with several species of waterfowl.

In many studies, the concept of natural host is used with an evolutionary connotation. To discriminate evolutionary concepts from epidemiological concepts, we will hereafter use the term *primordial host* when we imply animal taxa in (or from which) the virus of interest is thought to have speciated. Primordial hosts are crown group taxa, meaning that they can contain extinct species.

1.2.4 Zoonotic Sources
Several zoonotic spillover infections or epidemics in humans are explained by the involvement of *intermediate hosts*, creating additional complexity when analyzing multihost species of viruses. In cases in which the virus establishes long-term endemicity in intermediate hosts, intermediate hosts can become natural hosts according to the above definition. The viruses existing in the primordial host and the intermediate host can both belong to the same species, but the viral source population involved in zoonotic transmission may be disconnected from that in the primordial host. For clarity of source implications, we will therefore refer to source species in zoonotic transmission processes as *zoonotic sources*, irrespective of whether they also fulfill all criteria of natural hosts. A prominent example is rabies virus that has highly diversified conspecifics in bats but is enzootic in dogs to such a degree that dogs are considered zoonotic sources and natural hosts at the same time, but not primordial hosts. The transmission of Nipah and Hendra virus (belonging to the family *Paramyxoviridae*) from bats to humans involves swine or horses that act as zoonotic sources but are not considered natural

hosts because they are only accidentally infected (Eaton et al., 2006). Intermediate hosts may act as zoonotic sources for dead-end hosts not only because they close gaps of contact between species, but also because they could make the virus transmissible by intermediary adaptation (Caron et al., 2015; Plowright et al., 2015). Intermediary adaptation was strongly suspected for the SARS-CoV whose zoonotic source is in carnivores, in which the virus would have evolved human-compatible receptor tropism (Graham and Baric, 2010; Guan et al., 2003; Song et al., 2005; Wang et al., 2005; Xu et al., 2004). However, viruses directly infecting human cells have later been found in rhinolophid bats, the primordial natural host of the species SARS-related CoV (Drexler et al., 2014; Ge et al., 2013; Yang et al., 2015). Of note, these viruses are conspecific with SARS-CoV but do not fall into the viral clade that was transferred from carnivores to humans and initiated the epidemic. The actual ancestors of the SARS-CoV may continue to exist in the natural reservoir, as new virus variants are continuously formed in the reservoir. If the natural host (e.g., a bat species) harbors different virus populations of the same species, recombination contributes new variants. The proofreading and repair mechanisms typical in CoVs may aid the survival and selection of recombinant viruses in populations (Eckerle et al., 2010; Hanada et al., 2004; Minskaia et al., 2006). Indeed, recombination between the S1 and S2 subunits of the spike gene has been discussed as one of the major mechanism involved in the emergence of human SARS-CoV strains from bat and civet ancestors (Eckerle et al., 2010). On the other hand, ongoing recombination maintains stability of the gene pool of a defined virus species by shuffling sequences and thus limiting divergence processes (Lukashev, 2010).

The ubiquitous occurrence and the vast diversity of bat-associated CoVs have led to the assumption that bats are the primordial hosts of CoVs (Vijaykrishna et al., 2007). Whereas it seems possible that all mammalian CoVs may have originated in bats (Drexler et al., 2014; Woo et al., 2009a, b), this hypothesis should be reevaluated after more complete data on the diversity in other, similarly complex groups of mammalian hosts are available.

1.2.5 Tropism Changes During Emergence

After host transition, fidelity-associated mutation and selection in the novel host environment may gradually optimize virus–host interactions maintained from the former host environment, for instance regarding interactions between spike protein and receptor (Eckerle et al., 2010). Provided that receptor distribution is similar in donor and recipient host, these gradual changes are not expected to cause general changes of disease pattern. Nevertheless, the emergence of coronaviral diseases has also involved drastic changes including switches in tissue tropism by combinations of gene deletion and recombination. For instance, in TEGV of swine, deletions in the spike protein have been associated with changed tropism. TEGV with a full-length spike gene has tropism for both the respiratory and the enteric tracts, whereas strains with deletions (termed PRCV for porcine respiratory coronavirus) mainly replicate in and are transmitted via the respiratory tract (Kim et al., 2000; Sanchez et al., 1992). PRCV outcompeted TGEV in pig populations in spite of its virtual identical antigen composition (Openshaw, 2009). As respiratory viruses do not require direct contact for transmission, they are naturally more contagious irrespective of antigen variation and escape of population immunity. Because of increased prevalence in zoonotic sources, such viruses may then undergo onward host transition.

In humans, infections with CoVs are thought to cause mainly respiratory tract infections, while many (but not all) livestock CoVs cause infections of the gastrointestinal tract. Although many studies examining human intestinal specimens reported that coronaviral RNA can be detected in stool samples (Risku et al., 2010; Zhang et al., 1994), it seems that this detection is most likely explained by the presence of ingested virus particles from the respiratory tract, than resulting from productive replication in intestinal tissue (Jevsnik et al., 2013). It is worth mentioning that viruses in coancestral relationship to human CoVs are well known in bats. As these viruses are almost universally detected in feces, this suggests a primordial tropism for the intestinal tract before emergence as human respiratory pathogens (Smith et al., 2016).

1.3 Natural Hosts and Zoonotic Sources of Human Coronaviruses

To elucidate natural hosts and potential zoonotic sources of HCoVs, it is helpful to review the virus diversity and genome characteristics of related viruses. Fig. 1 provides a schematic overview of animal groups that may have played a role in the evolution and emergence of HCoVs.

2. HCoV-NL63

HCoV-NL63 was discovered by Dutch researchers in the supernatant of tertiary monkey kidney cells used to screen patients with respiratory

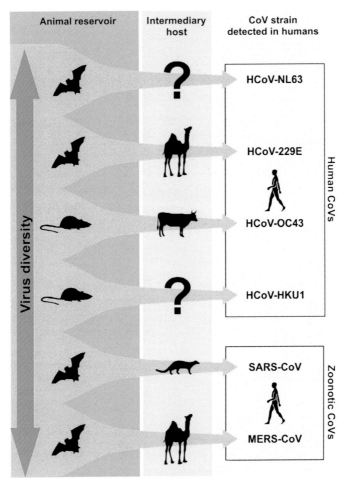

Fig. 1 Summary diagram of the animal groups representing natural hosts and the putative intermediate hosts for the six CoVs found in humans.

disease (van der Hoek et al., 2004). An independent study, also from the Netherlands, found the same virus in blind cell culture isolate that had been stored for many years before final characterization (Fouchier et al., 2004). American researchers identified the same virus, then termed HCoV-NH (for New Haven), by RT-PCR (Esper et al., 2005). The first bat CoVs related to HCoV-NL63 were found in feces of European and African bats belonging to the family *Vespertilionidae* (Drexler et al., 2010; Gloza-Rausch et al., 2008; Pfefferle et al., 2009). While these viruses are related to HCoV-NL63, they are not conspecific. The same applies to another virus found in the American tricolored bat (*Perimyotis subflavus*, also a vespertilionid species), termed ARCoV.2, which is also not conspecific with HCoV-NL63 by definition (Donaldson et al., 2010). Nevertheless, this study provides functional data that bat cells can support HCoV-NL63 replication by conducting infection experiments in an immortalized lung cell line from the American tricolored bat (Donaldson et al., 2010; Huynh et al., 2012). The cell line was infected with HCoV-NL63 and virus replication was confirmed by the detection of subgenomic RNA and the production of nucleocapsid protein. Foci of infected cells appeared to increase when observed under a fluorescence microscope. Interestingly, the number of infectious particles as determined by plaque assay remained low, which was explained by a potential block in viral egress (Huynh et al., 2012). It was proposed that the functional and genetic findings for American tricolored bats and ARCoV.2 have implications on origins of HCoV-NL63 (Huynh et al., 2012).

More recently, other researchers presented three different sequences of CoVs in *Triaenops afer* (family *Hipposideridae*) from Kenya that are more closely related to HCoV-NL63 (Tao et al., 2017). These bats are not closely related to vespertilionids. The report by Tao et al. included one strain (BtKYNL63-9a, GenBank ACC no. KY073744) that exceeded the 90% amino acid sequence identity threshold applicable for species typing in three of the seven conserved gene domains (Tao et al., 2017). The genome organization of the NL63-related bat CoV was similar to that of HCoV-NL63 (ORF1ab-S-ORF3-*E*-M-N) with the exception that the bat CoV genomes coded for an additional open reading frame (ORF *X*) downstream of the N gene. Even if distance-based typing did not allow to formally classify the virus as conspecific with HCoV-NL63, there was evidence for recombination between ancestral lineages of BtKYNL63-9a and bat-associated HCoV-229E-related viruses (Tao et al., 2017). This is important as HCoV-NL63 and -229E form sister species. The recombination processes involved the spike gene via two breakpoints, one located near the gene's 5′-end and the second around 200 nucleotides upstream of the 3′-end (Tao et al., 2017). Similar recombination breakpoints were also reported for SARS- and SARS-like CoV and HCoV-OC43 (Hon et al., 2008; Lau et al., 2010, 2011). Because the existence of viable recombinants could indicate incomplete speciation, the existence of BtKYNL63-9a should be regarded as a hint toward the primordial host of HCoV-NL63. Its ancestors may well have existed in hipposiderid or rhinolophid bats.

We have no knowledge about zoonotic sources of HCoV-NL63.

3. HCoV-229E

The human respiratory agent HCoV-229E was first described in 1966 (Hamre and Procknow, 1966). It was isolated in cell cultures inoculated with samples from diseased student volunteers. In 2007, sequences related to HCoV-229E were detected in captive Alpacas (*Vicugna pacos*) during a trade fair in California. The single virus strain, termed Alpaca coronavirus (ACoV), was fully sequenced and found to be highly related to known HCoV-229E strains. Epidemiological records suggested that the virus had caused a small outbreak of respiratory disease in exposed alpacas (Crossley et al., 2010, 2012), but it was never observed in feral animals. As no knowledge existed on related viruses other than HCoV-229E at that time, the finding was difficult to interpret as the strain could simply have been acquired from humans.

Around the same time, studies of CoV diversity in bats revealed viruses in close and conspecific relationship to HCoV-229E in hipposiderid bats in Africa (Corman et al., 2015; Pfefferle et al., 2009). Phylogenetic analysis identified lineages closely related to HCoV-229E and Alpaca-CoV, as well as novel sister and cousin groups that altogether showed a much larger viral diversity in hipposiderid bats, than in humans and alpaca together. Epidemiological findings and physiological data suggested long-term endemicity and absence of disease in infected bats, which provides further support for a natural host relationship (Corman et al., 2015; Pfefferle et al., 2009). While humans can come in contact with hipposiderid bats in their natural habitats, the existence of the alpaca virus remained difficult to explain except by human-derived infection; hipposiderid bats and alpaca do not share habitats (Old World vs New World species) (Corman et al., 2015).

In studies on MERS-CoV in dromedary camels, we and others found 229E-related CoVs in dromedary camels in the Arabian Peninsula and Africa (Corman et al., 2016; Sabir et al., 2016). Phylogenetic analyses of complete genomes placed the dromedary-associated viruses in sister relationship to HCoV-229E, while the Alpaca-CoV clustered with dromedary camel viruses. Alpaca is a species in the genus *Vicugna* of the family *Camelidae*. The monophyletic clade formed by human and camelid viruses has an immediate sister lineage within bat-associated viruses (Fig. 2A). Whereas the novel finding does not challenge the assumption of bats acting as natural hosts of HCoV-229E, the virus could have been acquired by humans or camels in either direction of transmission, and could also have been acquired

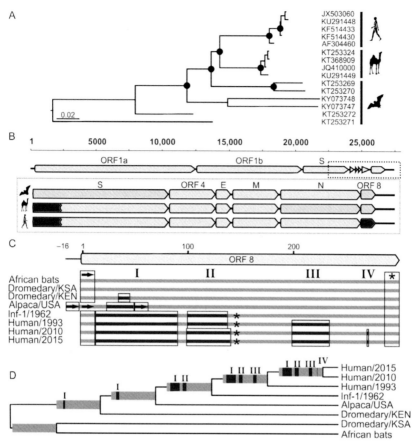

Fig. 2 Genome characteristics and mutation patterns of HCoV-229E and related viruses from animals. (A) Maximum-likelihood phylogeny of complete genomes of representative HCoV-229E-related coronaviruses from humans, camelids, and bats. *Filled circles* at nodes indicate bootstrap supports of 100% (200 replicates). HCoV-NL63 GenBank (accession no. NC_005831) was used as an outgroup (*branch truncated*). (B) Genomic organization of 229E-related coronaviruses. Regions with deletions are given in *red*. (C and D) Deletion patterns in ORF 8 homologs of 229E-related coronaviruses regions with deletions are given in *red* (numbered I–IV). *Asterisks* represent triplets that would act as in-frame stop codons; *arrows* represent possible start codons. *Figure was adapted from Corman, V.M., Eckerle, I., Memish, Z.A., Liljander, A.M., Dijkman, R., Jonsdottir, H., Juma Ngeiywa, K.J., Kamau, E., Younan, M., Al Masri, M., Assiri, A., Gluecks, I., Musa, B.E., Meyer, B., Muller, M.A., Hilali, M., Bornstein, S., Wernery, U., Thiel, V., Jores, J., Drexler, J.F., Drosten, C. 2016. Link of a ubiquitous human coronavirus to dromedary camels, Proc. Natl. Acad. Sci. U. S. A., 113, 9864–9869.*

by both from an unknown source including bats. However, more detailed analyses suggest HCoV-229E to have evolved toward the human genotype in camelids, thereby identifying the latter as a zoonotic source of human infection, and creating a scenario of emergence that is congruent with the present prepandemic pattern of MERS-CoV infection (Corman et al., 2015, 2016).

In particular, the spike genes of all HCoV-229E and camelid-associated 229E viruses contain deletions as compared to bat-associated viruses (Fig. 2B). Moreover, all 229E viruses from camels and all strains from bats showed an additional gene (termed ORF 8) downstream of the nucleocapsid gene (Fig. 2C). HCoV-229E has retained the transcription regulatory sequence upstream of a remnant ORF 8 (Corman et al., 2016). Interestingly, a process of gradual deletion of ORF 8 sequence can be traced from the camelid-associated viruses via early human isolates to contemporary human strains, defining hallmarks in genome evolution that provide additional topological information to the phylogenetic tree (Fig. 2D).

The deletions in the spike gene of bat-associated 229E viruses could have played a role in host switching by enabling an altered organ tropism in recipient hosts (Corman et al., 2015). This is because camelid- and human strains, in contrast to bat-associated viruses, replicate primarily in the respiratory tract (Corman et al., 2016; Crossley et al., 2010). Loss of spike gene content could have occurred by recombination, as recombination breakpoints were identified in bat-associated viruses within the ORF1ab gene upstream of the spike gene, as well as at the border of the S1 and S2 domains. This is consistent with previous evidence of major recombination events which in part lead to changes in tropism or host association in other CoVs (Corman et al., 2014a; Eckerle et al., 2010; Sabir et al., 2016; Tao et al., 2017).

It should be mentioned that the identification of a wide diversity of 229E-related viruses in dromedary camels provides an interesting possibility to explain the occurrence of Alpaca-CoV; dromedaries are often displayed in alpaca trade fairs and are sometimes kept along with alpacas in husbandries and zoological gardens. Routine testing of dromedaries for 229E-related viruses may be an option to prevent similar outbreaks.

4. HCoV-OC43

The human endemic pathogen HCoV-OC43 is part of the virus species BetaCoV1. It was first isolated in the 1960s based on human tracheal explants kept in organ culture, hence the "OC" in the virus name. Other bona fide human CoVs were isolated the same way but were not followed up upon and forgotten (McIntosh, 2005; McIntosh et al., 1967; Tyrrell and Bynoe, 1965).

BetaCoV 1 differs from many other CoV species in that it comprises strains detected in highly divergent host species. The bovine CoV (BCoV) is the best-studied representative, whereas essentially the same virus is present in other ungulates whose common names are often identified in virus designations (e.g., Giraffe-CoV; Hasoksuz et al., 2007). The recently described camel CoV HKU23 is a BCoV variant previously known to exist in camels (Corman et al., 2016; Reusken et al., 2013; Sabir et al., 2016; Woo et al., 2016; Wunschmann et al., 2002). All of these viruses belong to BetaCoV1, whose hosts comprise primates, lagomorphs, artiodactyls, and perissodactyls, as well as carnivores (Alekseev et al., 2008; Drexler et al., 2014; Erles et al., 2003; Guy et al., 2000; Hasoksuz et al., 2007; Lau et al., 2012; Lim et al., 2013; Majhdi et al., 1997; Tsunemitsu et al., 1995; Woo et al., 2014) (Fig. 3).

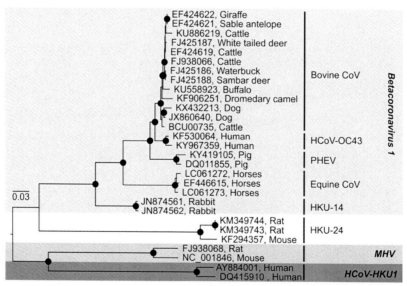

Fig. 3 Maximum-likelihood phylogeny of complete genomes of representatives of *Betacoronavirus 1*, *Mouse Hepatitis virus* (MHV), and *HCoV-HKU1* strains from humans and animals. Virus designations include GenBank accession numbers and host information. ICTV species are given to the right of clade designations. *Filled circles* at nodes indicate bootstrap supports of 100% (200 replicates). SARS-CoV (accession no. NC_004718) was used as an outgroup (*branch truncated*). PHEV; porcine hemagglutinating encephalomyelitis virus.

The emergence of HCoV-OC43 in humans was proposed to be linked to a host-switching event around the year 1890, a time that coincides with a pandemic of respiratory disease recorded in humans (Vijgen et al., 2005, 2006). Whether the zoonotic sources for this host transition were cattle, pigs, or other animals are not definitely resolved. However, the high diversity of related BetaCoV1 strains recently described in livestock species support their role as zoonotic sources in the emergence of HCoV-OC43 in humans. Why BetaCoV1 strains are found in many host species is not understood, but like for other CoVs recombination and deletion events likely played a role in these host-transition or adaptation processes. A deletion downstream of the spike gene of HCoV-OC43 was proposed to reflect adaptation to humans (Vijgen et al., 2005, 2006). Recombination within the species seems to promote the emergence of variants. For instance, Lu et al. recently described a novel canine respiratory coronavirus strain, which likely resulted from recombination between a Chinese canine respiratory coronavirus and BCoV (Lu et al., 2017).

Unlike other alpha- and betacoronavirus species, BetaCoV1 and the related mouse hepatitis virus (MHV) and HCoV-HKU1 do not seem to have ancestral links to bats. Several recent descriptions of novel BetaCoV1 members or relatives in rodents suggest them as primordial hosts (Hu et al., 2017; Lau et al., 2015; Wang et al., 2015). HCoV-OC43 was found to have tropism for neural cells in vitro and in experimentally infected mice, resembling MHV (Arbour et al., 1999; Jacomy et al., 2006). Presence of virus in the central nervous system was reported in patients with chronic demyelinating disease and acute encephalomyelitis (Morfopoulou et al., 2016; Murray et al., 1992; Yeh et al., 2004). The mechanisms that enable neurotropism are not fully understood, but once again mutations within the spike gene may play a role (St-Jean et al., 2004).

There is a single study reporting the isolation of BCoV from a 6-year-old child with watery diarrhea (Zhang et al., 1994). Although the report does not provide information on the patient's disease and immune status, it reminds us of the potential of BetaCoV1 members to cause spillover infections upon contact with zoonotic sources.

5. HCoV-HKU1

Human coronavirus HKU1 (for Hong Kong University) was detected in 2004 in a patient with viral pneumonia (Woo et al., 2005). The virus has subsequently been isolated in tissue cultures and is now recognized as a human respiratory agent (Pyrc et al., 2010; Woo et al., 2006, 2009b). There are no conspecific virus sequences from any other animal species. However, as HCoV-HKU1 is a sister taxon to MHV and rat sialodacryoadenitis virus, and together with these stands in sister relationship to BetaCoV1 with its basal rodent-associated viruses, a primordial association with rodent hosts may be considered (Hu et al., 2017; Lau et al., 2015; Wang et al., 2015; Woo et al., 2005).

5.1 Perspectives

There is a growing trend in the field of molecular epidemiology to conduct studies of host associations guided by taxonomy. Comprehensive studies suggest that the large lineages in the mammalian CoV phylogeny have primordial links to small mammals, focused but not limited to bats (Drexler et al., 2014; Vijaykrishna et al., 2007; Woo et al., 2009a, b). The enormous effort behind field studies can cause biases in the spectrum of potential host associations studied. The increased attention toward bats triggered by the discovery of natural host relationships for the SARS-CoV will continue to influence the current interpretations of CoV host associations (Guan et al., 2003). Already we sense that rodents, the largest group of mammals, seem to be underrepresented in studies of CoV hosts. The important role of rodents is highlighted by the recent findings of rodent CoVs that hint at primordial host relationships for the BetaCoV1 species. Data bias is further exemplified by the very few studies on CoVs in shrews and hedgehogs, belonging to the order *Eulipotyphla*. The 450 species in the order suggest a smaller genetic diversity as compared to the orders *Rodentia* and *Chiroptera* with 2269 and 1241 species, respectively. Nevertheless, surprisingly diverse alpha- and betacoronaviruses were detected in *Eulipotyphla*, including viruses clustering with important CoV clades such as MERS-CoV (Corman et al., 2014c; Tsoleridis et al., 2016; Wang et al., 2017). Other CoVs in shrews and hedgehogs are genetically equidistant and represent relatively deep lineages in the phylogenetic tree. It seems possible that Eulipotyphla may provide missing links in the evolutionary history of some major CoV groups.

Despite a clear role for intermediate hosts in the transmission of viruses from their natural hosts to humans, we have little information on adaptive processes that contributed by passage through these intermediate hosts. For instance, while it has long been assumed that adaptive changes happened in the SARS-CoV spike protein during passage in civets, there are now reports suggesting direct infectivity, for humans, of some but not all virus variants existing in the natural host (Eckerle et al., 2010; Guan et al., 2003; Wang et al., 2005). Has the virus evolved in civets to become more compatible to humans? Or was it selected from a wider spectrum of variants that have different fitness upon host switching? Understanding (and eventually predicting) the process of host switching will have to be based on functional comparison of natural host-associated viruses with their epidemic counterparts.

Similarly, the ubiquitous presence of MERS-CoV and the high diversity of HCoV-229E-related strains in camels suggests that these animals may be an important zoonotic source for pandemic CoVs in humans—including the prepandemic MERS-CoV (Anthony et al., 2017; Corman et al., 2014a, 2015, 2016). Understanding the past natural history of endemic HCoVs may help to recognize early signs of emergence from highly exposed hosts such as livestock species. We have ideas regarding the emergence of HCoV-OC43 that can potentially be refined (Vijgen et al., 2006). It seems peculiar that there is a complete absence of host-specific CoVs in great apes and other primates. This absence provides further support to the suspicion that contact with domestic animals may have been essential in human acquisition of most or all endemic CoV. For HCoV-HKU1 and HCoV-NL63, we therefore should study more of the virus diversity in livestock including closely related wildlife species to find footprints of their evolution and emergence. Finally, humans and domestic animals may have carried evolutionary intermediates that explain the emergence of major viral taxa, but that are extinct today.

ACKNOWLEDGMENT

This contribution was supported by a grant from Deutsche Forschungsgemeinschaft (DR 772/7-2).

REFERENCES

Alekseev, K.P., Vlasova, A.N., Jung, K., Hasoksuz, M., Zhang, X., Halpin, R., Wang, S., Ghedin, E., Spiro, D., Saif, L.J., 2008. Bovine-like coronaviruses isolated from four species of captive wild ruminants are homologous to bovine coronaviruses, based on complete genomic sequences. J. Virol. 82, 12422–12431.

Annan, A., Baldwin, H.J., Corman, V.M., Klose, S.M., Owusu, M., Nkrumah, E.E., Badu, E.K., Anti, P., Agbenyega, O., Meyer, B., Oppong, S., Sarkodie, Y.A., Kalko, E.K.V., Lina, P.H.C., Godlevska, E.V., Reusken, C., Seebens, A., Gloza-Rausch, F., Vallo, P., Tschapka, M., Drosten, C., Drexler, J.F., 2013. Human betacoronavirus 2c EMC/2012-related viruses in bats, Ghana and Europe. Emerg. Infect. Dis. 19, 456–459.

Annan, A., Ebach, F., Corman, V.M., Krumkamp, R., Adu-Sarkodie, Y., Eis-Hubinger, A.M., Kruppa, T., Simon, A., May, J., Evans, J., Panning, M., Drosten, C.,

Drexler, J.F., 2016. Similar virus spectra and seasonality in paediatric patients with acute respiratory disease, Ghana and Germany. Clin. Microbiol. Infect. 22, 340–346.

Anthony, S.J., Gilardi, K., Menachery, V.D., Goldstein, T., Ssebide, B., Mbabazi, R., Navarrete-Macias, I., Liang, E., Wells, H., Hicks, A., Petrosov, A., Byarugaba, D.K., Debbink, K., Dinnon, K.H., Scobey, T., Randell, S.H., Yount, B.L., Cranfield, M., Johnson, C.K., Baric, R.S., Lipkin, W.I., Mazet, J.A., 2017. Further evidence for bats as the evolutionary source of Middle East respiratory syndrome coronavirus. mBio 8 (2) e00373-17.

Arbour, N., Cote, G., Lachance, C., Tardieu, M., Cashman, N.R., Talbot, P.J., 1999. Acute and persistent infection of human neural cell lines by human coronavirus OC43. J. Virol. 73, 3338–3350.

Arden, K.E., Nissen, M.D., Sloots, T.P., Mackay, I.M., 2005. New human coronavirus, HCoV-NL63, associated with severe lower respiratory tract disease in Australia. J. Med. Virol. 75, 455–462.

Bastien, N., Anderson, K., Hart, L., Van Caeseele, P., Brandt, K., Milley, D., Hatchette, T., Weiss, E.C., Li, Y., 2005. Human coronavirus NL63 infection in Canada. J. Infect. Dis. 191, 503–506.

Berkley, J.A., Munywoki, P., Ngama, M., Kazungu, S., Abwao, J., Bett, A., Lassauniere, R., Kresfelder, T., Cane, P.A., Venter, M., Scott, J.A., Nokes, D.J., 2010. Viral etiology of severe pneumonia among Kenyan infants and children. JAMA 303, 2051–2057.

Caron, A., Cappelle, J., Cumming, G.S., de Garine-Wichatitsky, M., Gaidet, N., 2015. Bridge hosts, a missing link for disease ecology in multi-host systems. Vet. Res. 46 (83).

Cheng, V.C., Lau, S.K., Woo, P.C., Yuen, K.Y., 2007. Severe acute respiratory syndrome coronavirus as an agent of emerging and reemerging infection. Clin. Microbiol. Rev. 20, 660–694.

Chu, D.K., Poon, L.L., Gomaa, M.M., Shehata, M.M., Perera, R.A., Abu Zeid, D., El Rifay, A.S., Siu, L.Y., Guan, Y., Webby, R.J., Ali, M.A., Peiris, M., Kayali, G., 2014. MERS coronaviruses in dromedary camels, Egypt. Emerg. Infect. Dis. 20, 1049–1053.

Chu, D.K., Oladipo, J.O., Perera, R.A., Kuranga, S.A., Chan, S.M., Poon, L.L., Peiris, M., 2015. Middle East respiratory syndrome coronavirus (MERS-CoV) in dromedary camels in Nigeria, 2015. Euro Surveill. 20 (49). https://doi.org/10.2807/1560-7917.

Corman, V.M., Ithete, N.L., Richards, L.R., Schoeman, M.C., Preiser, W., Drosten, C., Drexler, J.F., 2014a. Rooting the phylogenetic tree of Middle East respiratory syndrome coronavirus by characterization of a conspecific virus from an African bat. J. Virol. 88, 11297–11303.

Corman, V.M., Jores, J., Meyer, B., Younan, M., Liljander, A., Said, M.Y., Gluecks, I., Lattwein, E., Bosch, B.J., Drexler, J.F., Bornstein, S., Drosten, C., Muller, M.A., 2014b. Antibodies against MERS coronavirus in dromedary camels, Kenya, 1992–2013. Emerg. Infect. Dis. 20, 1319–1322.

Corman, V.M., Kallies, R., Philipps, H., Gopner, G., Muller, M.A., Eckerle, I., Brunink, S., Drosten, C., Drexler, J.F., 2014c. Characterization of a novel betacoronavirus related to Middle East respiratory syndrome coronavirus in European hedgehogs. J. Virol. 88, 717–724.

Corman, V.M., Baldwin, H.J., Tateno, A.F., Zerbinati, R.M., Annan, A., Owusu, M., Nkrumah, E.E., Maganga, G.D., Oppong, S., Adu-Sarkodie, Y., Vallo, P., da Silva Filho, L.V., Leroy, E.M., Thiel, V., van der Hoek, L., Poon, L.L., Tschapka, M., Drosten, C., Drexler, J.F., 2015. Evidence for an ancestral association of human coronavirus 229E with bats. J. Virol. 89, 11858–11870.

Corman, V.M., Eckerle, I., Memish, Z.A., Liljander, A.M., Dijkman, R., Jonsdottir, H., Juma Ngeiywa, K.J., Kamau, E., Younan, M., Al Masri, M., Assiri, A., Gluecks, I., Musa, B.E., Meyer, B., Muller, M.A., Hilali, M., Bornstein, S., Wernery, U.,

Thiel, V., Jores, J., Drexler, J.F., Drosten, C., 2016. Link of a ubiquitous human coronavirus to dromedary camels. Proc. Natl. Acad. Sci. U. S. A. 113, 9864–9869.

Crossley, B.M., Barr, B.C., Magdesian, K.G., Ing, M., Mora, D., Jensen, D., Loretti, A.P., McConnell, T., Mock, R., 2010. Identification of a novel coronavirus possibly associated with acute respiratory syndrome in alpacas (Vicugna pacos) in California, 2007. J. Vet. Diagn. Invest. 22, 94–97.

Crossley, B.M., Mock, R.E., Callison, S.A., Hietala, S.K., 2012. Identification and characterization of a novel alpaca respiratory coronavirus most closely related to the human coronavirus 229E. Virus 4, 3689–3700.

de Groot, R.J., Baker, S.C., Baric, R., Enjuanes, L., Gorbalenya, A.E., Holmes, K.V., Perlman, S., Poon, L., Rottier, P.J.M., Talbot, P.J., Woo, P.C.Y., Ziebuhr, J., 2012a. Family coronaviridae. In: AMQ, K., Adams, M.J., Carstens, E.B., Lefkowitz, E.J. (Eds.), Virus Taxonomy: Classification and Nomenclature of Viruses. Ninth Report of the International Committee on Taxonomy of Viruses. Academic Press, London, pp. 806–820.

de Groot, R.J., Baker, S.C., Baric, R., Enjuanes, L., Gorbalenya, A.E., Holmes, K.V., Perlman, S., Poon, L., Rottier, P.J.M., Talbot, P.J., Woo, P.C.Y., Ziebuhr, J., 2012b. Family coronaviridae. In: King, A.M.Q., Adams, M.J., Carstens, E.B., Lefkowitz, E.J. (Eds.), Virus Taxonomy: Classification and Nomenclature of Viruses: Ninth Report of the International Committee on Taxonomy of Viruses. Elsevier/Academic Press, Amsterdam/Boston.

de Groot, R.J., Baker, S.C., Baric, R.S., Brown, C.S., Drosten, C., Enjuanes, L., Fouchier, R.A., Galiano, M., Gorbalenya, A.E., Memish, Z., Perlman, S., Poon, L.L., Snijder, E.J., Stephens, G.M., Woo, P.C., Zaki, A.M., Zambon, M., Ziebuhr, J., 2013. Middle East respiratory syndrome coronavirus (MERS-CoV); announcement of the coronavirus study group. J. Virol. 87 (14), 7790–7792.

Dijkman, R., Jebbink, M.F., Gaunt, E., Rossen, J.W., Templeton, K.E., Kuijpers, T.W., van der Hoek, L., 2012. The dominance of human coronavirus OC43 and NL63 infections in infants. J. Clin. Virol. 53, 135–139.

Donaldson, E.F., Haskew, A.N., Gates, J.E., Huynh, J., Moore, C.J., Frieman, M.B., 2010. Metagenomic analysis of the Viromes of three north American bat species: viral diversity among different bat species that share a common habitat. J. Virol. 84, 13004–13018.

Drexler, J.F., Gloza-Rausch, F., Glende, J., Corman, V.M., Muth, D., Goettsche, M., Seebens, A., Niedrig, M., Pfefferle, S., Yordanov, S., Zhelyazkov, L., Hermanns, U., Vallo, P., Lukashev, A., Muller, M.A., Deng, H., Herrler, G., Drosten, C., 2010. Genomic characterization of severe acute respiratory syndrome-related coronavirus in European bats and classification of coronaviruses based on partial RNA-dependent RNA polymerase gene sequences. J. Virol. 84, 11336–11349.

Drexler, J.F., Corman, V.M., Muller, M.A., Maganga, G.D., Vallo, P., Binger, T., Gloza-Rausch, F., Cottontail, V.M., Rasche, A., Yordanov, S., Seebens, A., Knornschild, M., Oppong, S., Adu Sarkodie, Y., Pongombo, C., Lukashev, A.N., Schmidt-Chanasit, J., Stocker, A., Carneiro, A.J., Erbar, S., Maisner, A., Fronhoffs, F., Buettner, R., Kalko, E.K., Kruppa, T., Franke, C.R., Kallies, R., Yandoko, E.R., Herrler, G., Reusken, C., Hassanin, A., Kruger, D.H., Matthee, S., Ulrich, R.G., Leroy, E.M., Drosten, C., 2012. Bats host major mammalian paramyxoviruses. Nat. Commun. 3, 796.

Drexler, J.F., Corman, V.M., Drosten, C., 2014. Ecology, evolution and classification of bat coronaviruses in the aftermath of SARS. Antiviral Res. 101, 45–56.

Drosten, C., Gunther, W., Preiser, W., van der Werf, S., Brodt, H.R., Becker, S., Rabenau, H., Panning, M., Kolesnikova, L., Fouchier, R.A., Berger, A., Burguiere, A.M., Cinatl, J., Eickmann, M., Escriou, N., Grywna, K., Kramme, S., Manuguerra, J.C., Muller, S., Rickerts, V., Sturmer, M., Vieth, S., Klenk, H.D.,

Osterhaus, A.D., Schmitz, H., Doerr, H.W., 2003. Identification of a novel coronavirus in patients with severe acute respiratory syndrome. N. Engl. J. Med. 348, 1967–1976.

Drosten, C., Muth, D., Corman, V.M., Hussain, R., Al Masri, M., HajOmar, W., Landt, O., Assiri, A., Eckerle, I., Al Shangiti, A., Al-Tawfiq, J.A., Albarrak, A., Zumla, A., Rambaut, A., Memish, Z.A., 2015. An observational, laboratory-based study of out-breaks of Middle East respiratory syndrome coronavirus in Jeddah and Riyadh, kingdom of Saudi Arabia, 2014. Clin. Infect. Dis. 60, 369–377.

Eaton, B.T., Broder, C.C., Middleton, D., Wang, L.F., 2006. Hendra and Nipah viruses: different and dangerous. Nat. Rev. Microbiol. 4, 23–35.

Eckerle, L.D., Becker, M.M., Halpin, R.A., Li, K., Venter, E., Lu, X., Scherbakova, S., Graham, R.L., Baric, R.S., Stockwell, T.B., Spiro, D.J., Denison, M.R., 2010. Infidelity of SARS-CoV Nsp14-exonuclease mutant virus replication is revealed by complete genome sequencing. PLoS Pathog. 6, e1000896.

Erles, K., Toomey, C., Brooks, H.W., Brownlie, J., 2003. Detection of a group 2 corona-virus in dogs with canine infectious respiratory disease. Virology 310, 216–223.

Esper, F., Weibel, C., Ferguson, D., Landry, M.L., Kahn, J.S., 2005. Evidence of a novel human coronavirus that is associated with respiratory tract disease in infants and young children. J. Infect. Dis. 191, 492–498.

Esper, F., Ou, Z., Huang, Y.T., 2010. Human coronaviruses are uncommon in patients with gastrointestinal illness. J. Clin. Virol. 48, 131–133.

Fielding, B.C., 2011. Human coronavirus NL63: a clinically important virus? Future Microbiol. 6, 153–159.

Fouchier, R.A., Hartwig, N.G., Bestebroer, T.M., Niemeyer, B., de Jong, J.C., Simon, J.H., Osterhaus, A.D., 2004. A previously undescribed coronavirus associated with respiratory disease in humans. Proc. Natl. Acad. Sci. U. S. A. 101, 6212–6216.

Gaunt, E.R., Hardie, A., Claas, E.C., Simmonds, P., Templeton, K.E., 2010. Epidemiology and clinical presentations of the four human coronaviruses 229E, HKU1, NL63, and OC43 detected over 3 years using a novel multiplex real-time PCR method. J. Clin. Microbiol. 48, 2940–2947.

Ge, X., Li, Y., Yang, X., Zhang, H., Zhou, P., Zhang, Y., Shi, Z., 2012. Metagenomic anal-ysis of viruses from bat fecal samples reveals many novel viruses in insectivorous bats in China. J. Virol. 86, 4620–4630.

Ge, X.Y., Li, J.L., Yang, X.L., Chmura, A.A., Zhu, G., Epstein, J.H., Mazet, J.K., Hu, B., Zhang, W., Peng, C., Zhang, Y.J., Luo, C.M., Tan, B., Wang, N., Zhu, Y., Crameri, G., Zhang, S.Y., Wang, L.F., Daszak, P., Shi, Z.L., 2013. Isolation and char-acterization of a bat SARS-like coronavirus that uses the ACE2 receptor. Nature 503, 535–538.

Gloza-Rausch, F., Ipsen, A., Seebens, A., Gottsche, M., Panning, M., Felix Drexler, J., Petersen, N., Annan, A., Grywna, K., Muller, M., Pfefferle, S., Drosten, C., 2008. Detection and prevalence patterns of group I coronaviruses in bats, northern Germany. Emerg. Infect. Dis. 14, 626–631.

Graat, J.M., Schouten, E.G., Heijnen, M.L., Kok, F.J., Pallast, E.G., de Greeff, S.C., Dorigo-Zetsma, J.W., 2003. A prospective, community-based study on virologic assessment among elderly people with and without symptoms of acute respiratory infection. J. Clin. Epidemiol. 56, 1218–1223.

Graham, R.L., Baric, R.S., 2010. Recombination, reservoirs, and the modular spike: mech-anisms of coronavirus cross-species transmission. J. Virol. 84, 3134–3146.

Greger, M., 2007. The human/animal interface: emergence and resurgence of zoonotic infectious diseases. Crit. Rev. Microbiol. 33, 243–299.

Guan, Y., Zheng, B.J., He, Y.Q., Liu, X.L., Zhuang, Z.X., Cheung, C.L., Luo, S.W., Li, P.H., Zhang, L.J., Guan, Y.J., Butt, K.M., Wong, K.L., Chan, K.W., Lim, W., Shortridge, K.F., Yuen, K.Y., Peiris, J.S., Poon, L.L., 2003. Isolation and characterization of viruses related to the SARS coronavirus from animals in southern China. Science 302, 276–278.

Guy, J.S., Breslin, J.J., Breuhaus, B., Vivrette, S., Smith, L.G., 2000. Characterization of a coronavirus isolated from a diarrheic foal. J. Clin. Microbiol. 38, 4523–4526.

Hamre, D., Procknow, J.J., 1966. A new virus isolated from the human respiratory tract. Proc. Soc. Exp. Biol. Med. 121, 190–193.

Hanada, K., Suzuki, Y., Gojobori, T., 2004. A large variation in the rates of synonymous substitution for RNA viruses and its relationship to a diversity of viral infection and transmission modes. Mol. Biol. Evol. 21, 1074–1080.

Hasoksuz, M., Alekseev, K., Vlasova, A., Zhang, X., Spiro, D., Halpin, R., Wang, S., Ghedin, E., Saif, L.J., 2007. Biologic, antigenic, and full-length genomic characterization of a bovine-like coronavirus isolated from a giraffe. J. Virol. 81, 4981–4990.

Haydon, D.T., Cleaveland, S., Taylor, L.H., Laurenson, M.K., 2002. Identifying reservoirs of infection: a conceptual and practical challenge. Emerg. Infect. Dis. 8, 1468–1473.

Hon, C.C., Lam, T.Y., Shi, Z.L., Drummond, A.J., Yip, C.W., Zeng, F., Lam, P.Y., Leung, F.C., 2008. Evidence of the recombinant origin of a bat severe acute respiratory syndrome (SARS)-like coronavirus and its implications on the direct ancestor of SARS coronavirus. J. Virol. 82, 1819–1826.

Hu, B., Zeng, L.P., Yang, X.L., Ge, X.Y., Zhang, W., Li, B., Xie, J.Z., Shen, X.R., Zhang, Y.Z., Wang, N., Luo, D.S., Zheng, X.S., Wang, M.N., Daszak, P., Wang, L.F., Cui, J., Shi, Z.L., 2017. Discovery of a rich gene pool of bat SARS-related coronaviruses provides new insights into the origin of SARS coronavirus. PLoS Pathog. 13 (11), e1006698.

Huynh, J., Li, S., Yount, B., Smith, A., Sturges, L., Olsen, J.C., Nagel, J., Johnson, J.B., Agnihothram, S., Gates, J.E., Frieman, M.B., Baric, R.S., Donaldson, E.F., 2012. Evidence supporting a zoonotic origin of human coronavirus strain NL63. J. Virol. 86, 12816–12825.

Ithete, N.L., Stoffberg, S., Corman, V.M., Cottontail, V.M., Richards, L.R., Schoeman, M.C., Drosten, C., Drexler, J.F., Preiser, W., 2013. Close relative of human Middle East respiratory syndrome coronavirus in bat, South Africa. Emerg. Infect. Dis. 19, 1697–1699.

Jacomy, H., Fragoso, G., Almazan, G., Mushynski, W.E., Talbot, P.J., 2006. Human coronavirus OC43 infection induces chronic encephalitis leading to disabilities in BALB/C mice. Virology 349, 335–346.

Jevsnik, M., Steyer, A., Zrim, T., Pokorn, M., Mrvic, T., Grosek, S., Strle, F., Lusa, L., Petrovec, M., 2013. Detection of human coronaviruses in simultaneously collected stool samples and nasopharyngeal swabs from hospitalized children with acute gastroenteritis. Virol. J. 10, 46.

Kim, L., Hayes, J., Lewis, P., Parwani, A.V., Chang, K.O., Saif, L.J., 2000. Molecular characterization and pathogenesis of transmissible gastroenteritis coronavirus (TGEV) and porcine respiratory coronavirus (PRCV) field isolates co-circulating in a swine herd. Arch. Virol. 145, 1133–1147.

Kim, S.W., Park, J.W., Jung, H.D., Yang, J.S., Park, Y.S., Lee, C., Kim, K.M., Lee, K.J., Kwon, D., Hur, Y.J., Choi, B.Y., Ki, M., 2017. Risk factors for transmission of Middle East respiratory syndrome coronavirus infection during the 2015 outbreak in South Korea. Clin. Infect. Dis. 64, 551–557.

Konca, C., Korukluoglu, G., Tekin, M., Almis, H., Bucak, I.H., Uygun, H., Altas, A.B., Bayrakdar, F., 2017. The first infant death associated with human coronavirus NL63 infection. Pediatr. Infect. Dis. J. 36, 231–233.

Larson, H.E., Reed, S.E., Tyrrell, D.A., 1980. Isolation of rhinoviruses and coronaviruses from 38 colds in adults. J. Med. Virol. 5, 221–229.

Lau, S.K., Li, K.S., Huang, Y., Shek, C.T., Tse, H., Wang, M., Choi, G.K., Xu, H., Lam, C.S., Guo, R., Chan, K.H., Zheng, B.J., Woo, P.C., Yuen, K.Y., 2010. Ecoepidemiology and complete genome comparison of different strains of severe acute respiratory syndrome-related Rhinolophus bat coronavirus in China reveal bats as a reservoir for acute, self-limiting infection that allows recombination events. J. Virol. 84, 2808–2819.

Lau, S.K., Lee, P., Tsang, A.K., Yip, C.C., Tse, H., Lee, R.A., So, L.Y., Lau, Y.L., Chan, K.H., Woo, P.C., Yuen, K.Y., 2011. Molecular epidemiology of human coronavirus OC43 reveals evolution of different genotypes over time and recent emergence of a novel genotype due to natural recombination. J. Virol. 85, 11325–11337.

Lau, S.K., Woo, P.C., Yip, C.C., Fan, R.Y., Huang, Y., Wang, M., Guo, R., Lam, C.S., Tsang, A.K., Lai, K.K., Chan, K.H., Che, X.Y., Zheng, B.J., Yuen, K.Y., 2012. Isolation and characterization of a novel Betacoronavirus subgroup A coronavirus, rabbit coronavirus HKU14, from domestic rabbits. J. Virol. 86, 5481–5496.

Lau, S.K., Woo, P.C., Li, K.S., Tsang, A.K., Fan, R.Y., Luk, H.K., Cai, J.P., Chan, K.H., Zheng, B.J., Wang, M., Yuen, K.Y., 2015. Discovery of a novel coronavirus, China Rattus coronavirus HKU24, from Norway rats supports the murine origin of Betacoronavirus 1 and has implications for the ancestor of Betacoronavirus lineage A. J. Virol. 89, 3076–3092.

Lim, S.I., Choi, S., Lim, J.A., Jeoung, H.Y., Song, J.Y., Dela Pena, R.C., An, D.J., 2013. Complete genome analysis of canine respiratory coronavirus. Genome Announc. 1 (1), e00093-12.

Lu, S., Wang, Y., Chen, Y., Wu, B., Qin, K., Zhao, J., Lou, Y., Tan, W., 2017. Discovery of a novel canine respiratory coronavirus support genetic recombination among betacoronavirus1. Virus Res. 237, 7–13.

Lukashev, A.N., 2010. Recombination among picornaviruses. Rev. Med. Virol. 20, 327–337.

Mackay, I.M., Arden, K.E., Speicher, D.J., O'Neil, N.T., McErlean, P.K., Greer, R.M., Nissen, M.D., Sloots, T.P., 2012. Co-circulation of four human coronaviruses (HCoVs) in Queensland children with acute respiratory tract illnesses in 2004. Virus 4, 637–653.

Majhdi, F., Minocha, H.C., Kapil, S., 1997. Isolation and characterization of a coronavirus from elk calves with diarrhea. J. Clin. Microbiol. 35, 2937–2942.

Mayer, K., Nellessen, C., Hahn-Ast, C., Schumacher, M., Pietzonka, S., Eis-Hubinger, A.M., Drosten, C., Brossart, P., Wolf, D., 2016. Fatal outcome of human coronavirus NL63 infection despite successful viral elimination by IFN-alpha in a patient with newly diagnosed ALL. Eur. J. Haematol. 97, 208–210.

McIntosh, K., 2005. Coronaviruses in the limelight. J. Infect. Dis. 191, 489–491.

McIntosh, K., Dees, J.H., Becker, W.B., Kapikian, A.Z., Chanock, R.M., 1967. Recovery in tracheal organ cultures of novel viruses from patients with respiratory disease. Proc. Natl. Acad. Sci. U. S. A. 57, 933–940.

Minskaia, E., Hertzig, T., Gorbalenya, A.E., Campanacci, V., Cambillau, C., Canard, B., Ziebuhr, J., 2006. Discovery of an RNA virus $3'->5'$ exoribonuclease that is critically involved in coronavirus RNA synthesis. Proc. Natl. Acad. Sci. U. S. A. 103 (13), 5108.

Morfopoulou, S., Brown, J.R., Davies, E.G., Anderson, G., Virasami, A., Qasim, W., Chong, W.K., Hubank, M., Plagnol, V., Desforges, M., Jacques, T.S., Talbot, P.J., Breuer, J., 2016. Human coronavirus OC43 associated with fatal encephalitis. N. Engl. J. Med. 375, 497–498.

Muller, M.A., Corman, V.M., Jores, J., Meyer, B., Younan, M., Liljander, A., Bosch, B.J., Lattwein, E., Hilali, M., Musa, B.E., Bornstein, S., Drosten, C., 2014. MERS coronavirus neutralizing antibodies in camels, Eastern Africa, 1983–1997. Emerg. Infect. Dis. 20, 2093–2095.

Murray, R.S., Brown, B., Brian, D., Cabirac, G.F., 1992. Detection of coronavirus RNA and antigen in multiple sclerosis brain. Ann. Neurol. 31, 525–533.

Oboho, I.K., Tomczyk, S.M., Al-Asmari, A.M., Banjar, A.A., Al-Mugti, H., Aloraini, M.S., Alkhaldi, K.Z., Almohammadi, E.L., Alraddadi, B.M., Gerber, S.I., Swerdlow, D.L., Watson, J.T., Madani, T.A., 2015. 2014 MERS-CoV outbreak in Jeddah—a link to health care facilities. N. Engl. J. Med. 372, 846–854.

Oosterhof, L., Christensen, C.B., Sengelov, H., 2010. Fatal lower respiratory tract disease with human corona virus NL63 in an adult haematopoietic cell transplant recipient. Bone Marrow Transplant. 45 (6), 1115.

Openshaw, P.J., 2009. Crossing barriers: infections of the lung and the gut. Mucosal Immunol. 2 (2), 100.

Owusu, M., Annan, A., Corman, V.M., Larbi, R., Anti, P., Drexler, J.F., Agbenyega, O., Adu-Sarkodie, Y., Drosten, C., 2014. Human coronaviruses associated with upper respiratory tract infections in three rural areas of Ghana. PLoS One 9, e99782.

Paloniemi, M., Lappalainen, S., Vesikari, T., 2015. Commonly circulating human coronaviruses do not have a significant role in the etiology of gastrointestinal infections in hospitalized children. J. Clin. Virol. 62, 114–117.

Peiris, J.S., Yuen, K.Y., Osterhaus, A.D., Stohr, K., 2003. The severe acute respiratory syndrome. N. Engl. J. Med. 349, 2431–2441.

Pfefferle, S., Oppong, S., Drexler, J.F., Gloza-Rausch, F., Ipsen, A., Seebens, A., Muller, M.A., Annan, A., Vallo, P., Adu-Sarkodie, Y., Kruppa, T.F., Drosten, C., 2009. Distant relatives of severe acute respiratory syndrome coronavirus and close relatives of human coronavirus 229E in bats, Ghana. Emerg. Infect. Dis. 15, 1377–1384.

Plowright, R.K., Eby, P., Hudson, P.J., Smith, I.L., Westcott, D., Bryden, W.L., Middleton, D., Reid, P.A., McFarlane, R.A., Martin, G., Tabor, G.M., Skerratt, L.F., Anderson, D.L., Crameri, G., Quammen, D., Jordan, D., Freeman, P., Wang, L.F., Epstein, J.H., Marsh, G.A., Kung, N.Y., McCallum, H., 2015. Ecological dynamics of emerging bat virus spillover. Proc. Biol. Sci. 282, 20142124.

Poon, L.L., Chu, D.K., Chan, K.H., Wong, O.K., Ellis, T.M., Leung, Y.H., Lau, S.K., Woo, P.C., Suen, K.Y., Yuen, K.Y., Guan, Y., Peiris, J.S., 2005. Identification of a novel coronavirus in bats. J. Virol. 79, 2001–2009.

Pyrc, K., Sims, A.C., Dijkman, R., Jebbink, M., Long, C., Deming, D., Donaldson, E., Vabret, A., Baric, R., van der Hoek, L., Pickles, R., 2010. Culturing the unculturable: human coronavirus HKU1 infects, replicates, and produces progeny virions in human ciliated airway epithelial cell cultures. J. Virol. 84, 11255–11263.

Reusken, C.B., Haagmans, B.L., Muller, M.A., Gutierrez, C., Godeke, G.J., Meyer, B., Muth, D., Raj, V.S., Smits-De Vries, L., Corman, V.M., Drexler, J.F., Smits, S.L., El Tahir, Y.E., De Sousa, R., van Beek, J., Nowotny, N., van Maanen, K., Hidalgo-Hermoso, E., Bosch, B.J., Rottier, P., Osterhaus, A., Gortazar-Schmidt, C., Drosten, C., Koopmans, M.P., 2013. Middle East respiratory syndrome coronavirus neutralising serum antibodies in dromedary camels: a comparative serological study. Lancet Infect. Dis. 13, 859–866.

Risku, M., Lappalainen, S., Rasanen, S., Vesikari, T., 2010. Detection of human coronaviruses in children with acute gastroenteritis. J. Clin. Virol. 48, 27–30.

Sabir, J.S., Lam, T.T., Ahmed, M.M., Li, L., Shen, Y., Abo-Aba, S.E., Qureshi, M.I., Abu-Zeid, M., Zhang, Y., Khiyami, M.A., Alharbi, N.S., Hajrah, N.H., Sabir, M.J., Mutwakil, M.H., Kabli, S.A., Alsulaimany, F.A., Obaid, A.Y., Zhou, B., Smith, D.K., Holmes, E.C., Zhu, H., Guan, Y., 2016. Co-circulation of three camel coronavirus species and recombination of MERS-CoVs in Saudi Arabia. Science 351, 81–84.

Saif, L.J., 2004. Animal coronaviruses: what can they teach us about the severe acute respiratory syndrome? Rev. Sci. Tech. 23, 643–660.

Sanchez, C.M., Gebauer, F., Sune, C., Mendez, A., Dopazo, J., Enjuanes, L., 1992. Genetic evolution and tropism of transmissible gastroenteritis coronaviruses. Virology 190, 92–105.

Saqib, M., Sieberg, A., Hussain, M.H., Mansoor, M.K., Zohaib, A., Lattwein, E., Muller, M.A., Drosten, C., Corman, V.M., 2017. Serologic evidence for MERS-CoV infection in dromedary camels, Punjab, Pakistan, 2012–2015. Emerg. Infect. Dis. 23, 550–551.

Smith, C.S., de Jong, C.E., Meers, J., Henning, J., Wang, L., Field, H.E., 2016. Coronavirus infection and diversity in bats in the Australasian region. Ecohealth 13, 72–82.

Song, H.D., Tu, C.C., Zhang, G.W., Wang, S.Y., Zheng, K., Lei, L.C., Chen, Q.X., Gao, Y.W., Zhou, H.Q., Xiang, H., Zheng, H.J., Chern, S.W., Cheng, F., Pan, C.M., Xuan, H., Chen, S.J., Luo, H.M., Zhou, D.H., Liu, Y.F., He, J.F., Qin, P.Z., Li, L.H., Ren, Y.Q., Liang, W.J., Yu, Y.D., Anderson, L., Wang, M., Xu, R.H., Wu, X.W., Zheng, H.Y., Chen, J.D., Liang, G., Gao, Y., Liao, M., Fang, L., Jiang, L.Y., Li, H., Chen, F., Di, B., He, L.J., Lin, J.Y., Tong, S., Kong, X., Du, L., Hao, P., Tang, H., Bernini, A., Yu, X.J., Spiga, O., Guo, Z.M., Pan, H.Y., He, W.Z., Manuguerra, J.C., Fontanet, A., Danchin, A., Niccolai, N., Li, Y.X., Wu, C.I., Zhao, G.P., 2005. Cross-host evolution of severe acute respiratory syndrome coronavirus in palm civet and human. Proc. Natl. Acad. Sci. U. S. A. 102, 2430–2435.

St-Jean, J.R., Jacomy, H., Desforges, M., Vabret, A., Freymuth, F., Talbot, P.J., 2004. Human respiratory coronavirus OC43: genetic stability and neuroinvasion. J. Virol. 78, 8824–8834.

Tao, Y., Shi, M., Chommanard, C., Queen, K., Zhang, J., Markotter, W., Kuzmin, I.V., Holmes, E.C., Tong, S., 2017. Surveillance of bat coronaviruses in Kenya identifies relatives of human coronaviruses NL63 and 229E and their recombination history. J. Virol. 91 (5), pii: e01953-16.

Tsoleridis, T., Onianwa, O., Horncastle, E., Dayman, E., Zhu, M., Danjittrong, T., Wachtl, M., Behnke, J.M., Chapman, S., Strong, V., Dobbs, P., Ball, J.K., Tarlinton, R.E., McClure, C.P., 2016. Discovery of novel alphacoronaviruses in European rodents and shrews. Virus 8, 84.

Tsunemitsu, H., el-Kanawati, Z.R., Smith, D.R., Reed, H.H., Saif, L.J., 1995. Isolation of coronaviruses antigenically indistinguishable from bovine coronavirus from wild ruminants with diarrhea. J. Clin. Microbiol. 33, 3264–3269.

Tyrrell, D.A., Bynoe, M.L., 1965. Cultivation of a novel type of common-cold virus in organ cultures. Br. Med. J. 1, 1467–1470.

van Boheemen, S., de Graaf, M., Lauber, C., Bestebroer, T.M., Raj, V.S., Zaki, A.M., Osterhaus, A.D., Haagmans, B.L., Gorbalenya, A.E., Snijder, E.J., Fouchier, R.A., 2012. Genomic characterization of a newly discovered coronavirus associated with acute respiratory distress syndrome in humans. MBio 3 (6), e00473-12.

van der Hoek, L., 2007. Human coronaviruses: what do they cause? Antivir. Ther. 12, 651–658.

van der Hoek, L., Pyrc, K., Jebbink, M.F., Vermeulen-Oost, W., Berkhout, R.J., Wolthers, K.C., Wertheim-van Dillen, P.M., Kaandorp, J., Spaargaren, J., Berkhout, B., 2004. Identification of a new human coronavirus. Nat. Med. 10, 368–373.

van Elden, L.J., van Loon, A.M., van Alphen, F., Hendriksen, K.A., Hoepelman, A.I., van Kraaij, M.G., Oosterheert, J.J., Schipper, P., Schuurman, R., Nijhuis, M., 2004. Frequent detection of human coronaviruses in clinical specimens from patients with respiratory tract infection by use of a novel real-time reverse-transcriptase polymerase chain reaction. J. Infect. Dis. 189, 652–657.

Vijaykrishna, D., Smith, G.J., Zhang, J.X., Peiris, J.S., Chen, H., Guan, Y., 2007. Evolutionary insights into the ecology of coronaviruses. J. Virol. 81, 4012–4020.

Vijgen, L., Keyaerts, E., Moes, E., Thoelen, I., Wollants, E., Lemey, P., Vandamme, A.M., Van Ranst, M., 2005. Complete genomic sequence of human coronavirus OC43: molecular clock analysis suggests a relatively recent zoonotic coronavirus transmission event. J. Virol. 79, 1595–1604.

Vijgen, L., Keyaerts, E., Lemey, P., Maes, P., Van Reeth, K., Nauwynck, H., Pensaert, M., Van Ranst, M., 2006. Evolutionary history of the closely related group 2 coronaviruses: porcine hemagglutinating encephalomyelitis virus, bovine coronavirus, and human coronavirus OC43. J. Virol. 80, 7270–7274.

Walsh, E.E., Shin, J.H., Falsey, A.R., 2013. Clinical impact of human coronaviruses 229E and OC43 infection in diverse adult populations. J. Infect. Dis. 208, 1634–1642.

Wang, M., Yan, M., Xu, H., Liang, W., Kan, B., Zheng, B., Chen, H., Zheng, H., Xu, Y., Zhang, E., Wang, H., Ye, J., Li, G., Li, M., Cui, Z., Liu, Y.F., Guo, R.T., Liu, X.N., Zhan, L.H., Zhou, D.H., Zhao, A., Hai, R., Yu, D., Guan, Y., Xu, J., 2005. SARS-CoV infection in a restaurant from palm civet. Emerg. Infect. Dis. 11, 1860–1865.

Wang, W., Lin, X.D., Guo, W.P., Zhou, R.H., Wang, M.R., Wang, C.Q., Ge, S., Mei, S.H., Li, M.H., Shi, M., Holmes, E.C., Zhang, Y.Z., 2015. Discovery, diversity and evolution of novel coronaviruses sampled from rodents in China. Virology 474, 19–27.

Wang, W., Lin, X.D., Liao, Y., Guan, X.Q., Guo, W.P., Xing, J.G., Holmes, E.C., Zhang, Y.Z., 2017. Discovery of a highly divergent coronavirus in the Asian house shrew from China illuminates the origin of the alphacoronaviruses. J. Virol. 91, e00764–17.

WHO, 2017. Middle East Respiratory Syndrome Coronavirus (MERS-CoV)—Disease Outbreak News: 21 September 2017. accessed 03.10.2017.

Woo, P.C., Lau, S.K., Chu, C.M., Chan, K.H., Tsoi, H.W., Huang, Y., Wong, B.H., Poon, R.W., Cai, J.J., Luk, W.K., Poon, L.L., Wong, S.S., Guan, Y., Peiris, J.S., Yuen, K.Y., 2005. Characterization and complete genome sequence of a novel coronavirus, coronavirus HKU1, from patients with pneumonia. J. Virol. 79, 884–895.

Woo, P.C., Lau, S.K., Yip, C.C., Huang, Y., Tsoi, H.W., Chan, K.H., Yuen, K.Y., 2006. Comparative analysis of 22 coronavirus HKU1 genomes reveals a novel genotype and evidence of natural recombination in coronavirus HKU1. J. Virol. 80, 7136–7145.

Woo, P.C., Lau, S.K., Huang, Y., Yuen, K.Y., 2009a. Coronavirus diversity, phylogeny and interspecies jumping. Exp. Biol. Med. (Maywood) 234, 1117–1127.

Woo, P.C., Lau, S.K., Yuen, K.Y., 2009b. Clinical features and molecular epidemiology of coronavirus-HKU1-associated community-acquired pneumonia. Hong Kong Med. J. 15 (Suppl. 9), 46–47.

Woo, P.C., Lau, S.K., Wernery, U., Wong, E.Y., Tsang, A.K., Johnson, B., Yip, C.C., Lau, C.C., Sivakumar, S., Cai, J.P., Fan, R.Y., Chan, K.H., Mareena, R., Yuen, K.Y., 2014. Novel betacoronavirus in dromedaries of the Middle East, 2013. Emerg. Infect. Dis. 20, 560–572.

Woo, P.C., Lau, S.K., Fan, R.Y., Lau, C.C., Wong, E.Y., Joseph, S., Tsang, A.K., Wernery, R., Yip, C.C., Tsang, C.C., Wernery, U., Yuen, K.Y., 2016. Isolation and characterization of dromedary camel coronavirus UAE-HKU23 from dromedaries of the Middle East: minimal serological cross-reactivity between MERS coronavirus and dromedary camel coronavirus UAE-HKU23. Int. J. Mol. Sci. 17 (5), pii: E691.

Wunschmann, A., Frank, R., Pomeroy, K., Kapil, S., 2002. Enteric coronavirus infection in a juvenile dromedary (Camelus dromedarius). J. Vet. Diagn. Invest. 14, 441–444.

Xu, R.H., He, J.F., Evans, M.R., Peng, G.W., Field, H.E., Yu, D.W., Lee, C.K., Luo, H.M., Lin, W.S., Lin, P., Li, L.H., Liang, W.J., Lin, J.Y., Schnur, A., 2004. Epidemiologic clues to SARS origin in China. Emerg. Infect. Dis. 10, 1030–1037.

Yang, X.L., Hu, B., Wang, B., Wang, M.N., Zhang, Q., Zhang, W., Wu, L.J., Ge, X.Y., Zhang, Y.Z., Daszak, P., Wang, L.F., Shi, Z.L., 2015. Isolation and characterization of a novel bat coronavirus closely related to the direct progenitor of severe acute respiratory syndrome coronavirus. J. Virol. 90 (6), 3253.

Yeh, E.A., Collins, A., Cohen, M.E., Duffner, P.K., Faden, H., 2004. Detection of coronavirus in the central nervous system of a child with acute disseminated encephalomyelitis. Pediatrics 113, e73–6.

Zaki, A.M., van Boheemen, S., Bestebroer, T.M., Osterhaus, A.D., Fouchier, R.A., 2012. Isolation of a novel coronavirus from a man with pneumonia in Saudi Arabia. N. Engl. J. Med. 367, 1814–1820.

Zhang, X.M., Herbst, W., Kousoulas, K.G., Storz, J., 1994. Biological and genetic characterization of a hemagglutinating coronavirus isolated from a diarrhoeic child. J. Med. Virol. 44, 152–161.

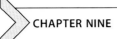

CHAPTER NINE

Filoviruses: Ecology, Molecular Biology, and Evolution

Jackson Emanuel, Andrea Marzi, Heinz Feldmann[1]
Laboratory of Virology, National Institute of Allergy and Infectious Diseases, National Institutes of Health, Hamilton, MT, United States
[1]Corresponding author: e-mail address: feldmannh@niaid.nih.gov

Contents

Abstract

The *Filoviridae* are a family of negative-strand RNA viruses that include several important human pathogens. Ebola virus (EBOV) and Marburg virus are well-known filoviruses which cause life-threatening viral hemorrhagic fever in human and nonhuman primates. In addition to severe pathogenesis, filoviruses also exhibit a propensity for human-to-human transmission by close contact, posing challenges to containment and crisis management. Past outbreaks, in particular the recent West African EBOV epidemic, have been responsible for thousands of deaths and vaulted the filoviruses into public consciousness. Both national and international health agencies continue to

Advances in Virus Research, Volume 100
ISSN 0065-3527
https://doi.org/10.1016/bs.aivir.2017.12.002

regard potential filovirus outbreaks as critical threats to global public health. To develop effective countermeasures, a basic understanding of filovirus biology is needed. This review encompasses the epidemiology, ecology, molecular biology, and evolution of the filoviruses.

1. INTRODUCTION

The discovery of filoviruses dates back five decades when cases with a hemorrhagic fever syndrome were investigated in Marburg, Germany and Belgrade, Yugoslavia (now Serbia). The source of infection was associated with handling African green monkeys imported from Uganda. This outbreak resulted in a total of 32 human cases and 7 fatalities across Europe. The etiologic agent was subsequently identified and characterized; it was named Marburg virus (MARV) after the location of the first cases (Siegert et al., 1967; Slenczka, 1999). Nine years later two outbreaks of hemorrhagic fever occurred almost simultaneously in southern Sudan (now the Republic of South Sudan) and northern Zaire (now the Democratic Republic of the Congo, DRC). Studies revealed a new virus which was named Ebola virus (EBOV) after a nearby river in northern Zaire. The virus was related but distinct from MARV (WHO, 1978a,b). A few years later, molecular characterization revealed distinct ebolaviruses as the causative agents for the two outbreaks with EBOV causing disease in northern Zaire and the Sudan virus (SUDV) being responsible for disease in southern Sudan (Richman et al., 1983).

Despite infrequent smaller outbreaks and episodes of viral hemorrhagic fevers caused by the above-described filoviruses throughout sub-Saharan Africa, the next discovery of a new ebolavirus dates to 1989 in Reston, Virginia, USA. Macaques imported from the Philippines showed signs of hemorrhagic fever during quarantine and a new filovirus, named Reston virus (RESTV) after the geographic location of first isolation, was coisolated from these macaques together with simian hemorrhagic fever virus (Jahrling et al., 1990). Despite verified human infections, today RESTV is considered apathogenic for humans and epizootic in the Philippines and perhaps greater Southeast Asia (Miranda and Miranda, 2011).

In 1994, another different ebolavirus, Taï Forest virus (TAFV), was discovered in a single nonfatal case of viral hemorrhagic fever in Côte d'Ivoire. Until today, this remains the only described human TAFV case. A massive, years-long ecological investigation in the Taï Forest did not reveal the reservoir for TAFV (Formenty et al., 1999; Le Guenno et al., 1995). The newest ebolavirus to be discovered was Bundibugyo virus (BDBV) in Uganda in 2007 (Towner et al., 2008; Wamala et al., 2010) where it caused an outbreak of hemorrhagic fever in humans.

All known marburgviruses as well as EBOV, SUDV, and BDBV are considered pathogens of significant public health importance in Africa. Outbreaks are especially notable for their high case fatality rates, commonly ranging from 25% to 90%, depending on the virus species (Muyembe-Tamfum et al., 2012). The recent West African EBOV epidemic has dramatically emphasized the public health relevance of these pathogens with unprecedented case numbers and fatalities (approximately 30,000 cases and 11,000 fatalities) (WHO, 2016). For the first time, it has added a global public health perspective to filoviruses with multiple introductions of exposed people and confirmed cases through returning travelers and evacuations of health care workers from West Africa (WHO, 2016).

In 2011, sequences of a novel filovirus, related but distinct from ebolaviruses and marburgviruses, were detected in specimens derived from dying bats in Spain (Negredo et al., 2011). An isolate is missing, but the putative virus was named Lloviu virus (LLOV) and is classified in its own genus *Cuevavirus* within the *Filoviridae*. LLOV has not been associated with human infections.

2. TAXONOMY

The *Filoviridae* family is grouped within the order *Mononegavirales*, a diverse taxon of unsegmented negative-sense single-stranded RNA viruses. Other virus families within this order include *Bornaviridae*, *Mymonaviridae*, *Nyamiviridae*, *Paramyxoviridae*, *Pneumoviridae*, *Rhabdoviridae*, and *Sunviridae*. The taxonomy of filoviruses was substantially changed in 2010 to reflect advances in the field and has since been revised (Bukreyev et al., 2014; Kuhn et al., 2010). Filoviruses share a long, filamentous morphology and comprise three distinct genera: *Ebolavirus*, *Marburgvirus*, and *Cuevavirus* (Fig. 1). The *Ebolavirus* genus is the most diverse, consisting of five recognized species: *Zaire ebolavirus*, *Sudan ebolavirus*, *Reston ebolavirus*, *Taï Forest ebolavirus*, and *Bundibugyo ebolavirus* (represented by EBOV, SUDV, RESTV, TAFV, and BDBV, respectively). The *Marburgvirus* genus consists of only a single species, *Marburg marburgvirus*, that has been further delineated into the variants MARV and Ravn virus (RAVV). The relatively new *Cuevavirus* genus also consists of a single species, *Lloviu cuevavirus*

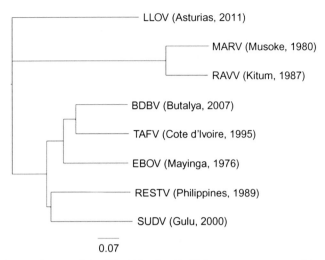

0.07

Fig. 1 Phylogenetic tree of the *Filoviridae* family. This tree was generated based on the nucleotide sequences for the GP gene coding regions. All sequences were acquired from GenBank (LLOV, NC_016144.1; MARV, NC_001608; SUDV, NC_006432.1; RESTV, NC_004161.1; EBOV, NC_002549; TAFV, NC_014372.1; BDBV, NC_014373.1; RAVV, NC_024781).

(represented by LLOV). This putative classification of LLOV is based on genomic sequence data only as a virus isolate could not be obtained (Negredo et al., 2011). In 2015, novel filovirus sequences were detected in Chinese fruit bats, but a virus has not been isolated and a whole-genome alignment has yet to be obtained (He et al., 2015). A basic phylogeny of the family *Filoviridae* is provided in Fig. 1.

3. VIRUS ECOLOGY

Filoviruses only sporadically infect human and nonhuman primates but principally circulate in nonhuman hosts. The exact mechanism of zoonotic transmission is unknown, but unprotected exposure to the reservoir, handling contaminated bushmeat, and receiving bites from an infected animal are possible routes (Azarian et al., 2015; Chippaux, 2014). MARV, RAVV, BDBV, TAFV, EBOV, and SUDV circulate in the tropical regions of sub-Saharan Africa, whereas RESTV has been identified in the Philippines and sequences of LLOV in Spain. Although EBOV has not been isolated outside Africa, filovirus-specific antibodies cross-reactive with EBOV have been found in *Rousettus leschenaulti* bats in Bangladesh and in *Pongo pygmaeus orangutans* on Borneo (Nidom et al., 2012; Olival et al., 2013).

Furthermore, in China, new filovirus sequences with phylogenetic identities intermediate between EBOV, RESTV, and LLOV have been detected (He et al., 2015). These findings suggest that there are hitherto unidentified filovirus species circulating in Asia. At present, all filoviruses are considered serious human pathogens apart from RESTV, which is thought to be apathogenic although unambiguous evidence for human infection is lacking, and the nonisolated LLOV and Chinese filoviruses, for which pathogenicity in humans is unknown.

Over the past few decades, there has been an increasing effort to identify the zoonotic origin of filoviruses. This task has been complicated by the remote and ecologically rich jungle habitats where outbreaks are known to occur, as the diverse number of mammalian species in these regions makes it difficult to identify putative reservoir hosts. One commonly accepted view is that animal-to-human transmission events are exceedingly rare, but virus spread between humans after an initial introduction is efficient. Recent evidence from the 2013 to 2016 EBOV epidemic supports this hypothesis, as genomic surveillance data postulate that a single animal-to-human transmission was responsible for the epidemic, even though an increased rate of human-to-human transmission gave rise to an accumulation of largely nonsynonymous mutations (Gire et al., 2014). The 1995 Kikwit EBOV outbreak is also thought to be caused by a single reservoir-to-host introduction, but in contrast to the 2013–2016 epidemic, no sequence variation in the EBOV glycoprotein (GP) gene was found possibly due to a more limited number of transmission chains in humans (Rodriguez et al., 1999). Other outbreaks, including a series of recurrent outbreaks in Gabon and the Republic of the Congo (RC), were also characterized by shorter transmission chains of multiple EBOV lineages that affected both human and nonhuman primates with little or no evidence of mutations in the end host (Leroy et al., 2004). Lastly, the MARV outbreak in Durba/Watsa in 1998–2000 was characterized by multiple simultaneous introductions of distinct genetic MARV lineages into the human population with shorter transmission chains in the end host (Bausch et al., 2006).

3.1 Ebolaviruses

It is well known that EBOV, and perhaps also other ebolaviruses, affect other primates besides humans. Wild gorilla (*Gorilla gorilla*) and chimpanzee (*Pan troglodytes*) populations have experienced significant declines as a result of EBOV outbreaks (Bermejo et al., 2006; Formenty et al., 1999; Rouquet et al., 2005). The severe pathogenicity of EBOV in nonhuman primates and the sporadic nature of infection suggest that primates are dead-end hosts like humans. Beginning with the detection of EBOV genomic material in several Old-World fruit and insectivorous bat species, bats have come under increasing suspicion as filovirus carriers (Hayman et al., 2010, 2012; Leroy et al., 2005; Ogawa et al., 2015; Pourrut et al., 2009). However, ebolaviruses have yet to be isolated from any wild bat or animal species. Table 1 summarizes evidence and proof for the detection of filoviruses in bats. Evidence of EBOV and RESTV has been found in numerous bat species spanning a wide geographical area, including Ghana, Gabon, RC, DRC, Zambia, Bangladesh, Philippines, and China. In contrast, BDBV, SUDV, and TAFV have not been surveyed to the same degree (Table 1). An overview of EBOV transmission is proposed in Fig. 2.

RESTV was isolated from domesticated pigs (*Sus scrofa*) in the Philippines in 2008 (Barrette et al., 2009). More recently, RESTV RNA has been found in pigs near Shanghai, China (Pan et al., 2014), but domesticated swine are more likely to serve as intermediate or amplifying hosts rather than as the reservoir (Barrette et al., 2009; Pan et al., 2014). Pigs experimentally infected with RESTV remain asymptomatic (Marsh et al., 2011). This stands in contrast to experimental EBOV infection in pigs, which can cause severe respiratory symptoms and viral shedding (Kobinger et al., 2011). RESTV causes severe disease in nonhuman primates (Jahrling et al., 1996), but is not known to cause serious disease in humans (CDC, 1990a,b). As with EBOV, there is evidence that RESTV is also present in bats (Jayme et al., 2015; Taniguchi et al., 2011; Yuan et al., 2012) (Table 1).

3.2 Marburgviruses

Like EBOV and SUDV, members of the *Marburgvirus* genus cause disease with high rates of lethality in human and nonhuman primates. MARV and RAVV variants have been isolated from Egyptian fruit bats (*Rousettus aegypticus*), appearing to be a major natural reservoir for marburgviruses (Amman et al., 2014; Pourrut et al., 2009; Towner et al., 2009) (Table 1). This is supported by the observation that seasonal changes in MARV circulation among *R. aegypticus* correlate with the risk of human infection (Amman et al., 2012). *R. aegypticus* have also been shown to orally shed MARV when experimentally infected, despite showing no signs of overt morbidity (Amman et al., 2015). This may indicate that MARV has evolved to proliferate in *Rousettus* host populations and that bat bites may

Table 1 Overview of Filovirus Detection in Wild Bat Species

Virus/Bat Species	Location	Detection Method	References
BDBV/			
Eidolon helvum	Zambia	Antibodies	Ogawa et al. (2015)
EBOV/			
Eidolon helvum	Ghana, Zambia	Antibodies	Hayman et al. (2010); Ogawa et al. (2015)
Epomops franqueti	Gabon, RC	Antibodies	Leroy et al. (2005); Pourrut et al. (2009)
Epomophorus gambianus	Ghana	Antibodies	Hayman et al. (2012)
Hypsignathus monstrosus	Gabon, RC	Antibodies	Leroy et al. (2005); Pourrut et al. (2009)
Micropteropus pusillus	Gabon, RC	Antibodies	Pourrut et al. (2009)
Mops condylurus	Gabon, RC	Antibodies	Pourrut et al. (2009)
Myonycteris torquata	Gabon, RC	Antibodies	Leroy et al. (2005); Pourrut et al. (2009)
Rousettus aegyptiacus	Gabon, RC	Antibodies	Pourrut et al. (2009)
R. leschenaultia	Bangladesh	Antibodies	Olival et al. (2013)
RESTV/			
Acerodon jubatus	Philippines	Antibodies	Jayme et al. (2015)
Miniopterus schreibersii	China, Philippines	Antibodies, RNA	Jayme et al. (2015); Yuan et al. (2012)
Chaerephon plicata	Philippines	RNA	Jayme et al. (2015)
Cynopterus brachyotis	Philippines	RNA	Jayme et al. (2015)
Cynopterus sphinx	China	Antibodies	Yuan et al. (2012)
Eidolon helvum	Zambia	Antibodies	Ogawa et al. (2015)

Continued

Table 1 Overview of Filovirus Detection in Wild Bat Species—cont'd

Virus/Bat Species	Location	Detection Method	References
Hipposideros Pomona	China	Antibodies	Yuan et al. (2012)
Miniopterus australis	Philippines	RNA	Jayme et al. (2015)
Myotis ricketti	China	Antibodies	Yuan et al. (2012)
Pipistrellus pipistrellus	China	Antibodies	Yuan et al. (2012)
Rousettus amplexicaudatus	Philippines	Antibodies	Taniguchi et al. (2011)
R. leschenaultia	China, Bangladesh	Antibodies	Olival et al. (2013); Yuan et al. (2012)
SUDV/			
Eidolon helvum	Zambia	Antibodies	Ogawa et al. (2015)
TAFV/			
Eidolon helvum	Zambia	Antibodies	Ogawa et al. (2015)
MARV and RAVV/[a]			
Eidolon helvum	Zambia	Antibodies	Ogawa et al. (2015)
Epomops franqueti	Gabon, RC	Antibodies	Pourrut et al. (2009)
Hypsignathus monstrosus	Gabon, RC	Antibodies	Pourrut et al. (2009)
Miniopterus inflatus	DRC	RNA	Swanepoel et al. (2007)
Rhinolophus eloquens	DRC	Antibodies, RNA	Swanepoel et al. (2007)
Rousettus aegyptiacus	DRC, Gabon, RC, Uganda	Virus isolation, antibodies, RNA	Amman et al. (2014); Pourrut et al. (2009); Swanepoel et al. (2007); Towner et al. (2009)
LLOV/			
Miniopterus schreibersii	Spain	Antibodies, whole-genome sequencing	Negredo et al. (2011)

[a]N.B.: Both MARV and RAVV variants have been detected by Swanepoel et al. (2007) via PCR, but in cases where antibodies were used, due to antibody cross-reactivity, the subspecies variant is not always possible to determine

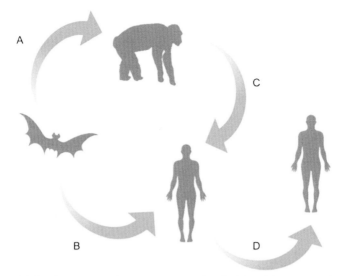

Fig. 2 Model for the proposed transmission cycle of EBOV. (A) Reservoir bat species are thought to infect nonhuman primates such as *Gorilla gorilla* and *Pan troglodytes*. (B) It has been widely hypothesized that bats directly infect humans through an unknown mechanism, although bites may be a possible route of transmission. (C) Consumption of nonhuman primate bushmeat has been well documented as a source of past EBOV outbreaks. (D) Human-to-human transmission occurs via direct contact with bodily fluids and through airborne droplets. Fomites and aerosols are thought to be less probable routes of transmission.

be a route of zoonotic infection. Besides fruit bats, insectivorous bats, such as *Miniopterus inflatus* and *Rhinolophus eloquens*, have also been implicated as carriers (Swanepoel et al., 2007). Like the ebolaviruses, marburgviruses have also been identified in the urban-dwelling straw-colored bat (*Eidolon helvum*) (Ogawa et al., 2015).

3.3 Cuevaviruses

LLOV, the only known cuevavirus, was first identified after a spate of bat die-offs on the Iberian Peninsula. In the Lloviu Cave in Northern Spain, colonies of Schreiber's bats (*Miniopterus schreibersii*) and greater mouse-eared bats (*Myotis myotis*) yielded numerous carcasses available for microbiological and toxicological analysis (Table 1). Although no gross pathology was observed, histopathological signs of viral pneumonia were present. All the dead *M. schreibersii* were positive for LLOV RNA, whereas no LLOV was detected in healthy *M. schreibersii* taken from the same location (Negredo et al., 2011). Although little else is known about LLOV, its pathogenicity in *M. schreibersii* may suggest the existence of an alternative reservoir host.

4. FILOVIRAL PARTICLES

4.1 Morphology

Filovirus particles are long and filamentous. The particles may form elongated rods or curve one or more times, giving them a string or torus-like appearance (Fig. 3B). These distinctive shapes originally gave rise to the name *Filoviridae*, after the Latin *filum*, meaning thread. Although the virion filaments have a consistent diameter of about 80 nm, the length of particles is variable. The median virion length for an infectious particle has been determined to be about 800 and 1000 nm for MARV and EBOV, respectively

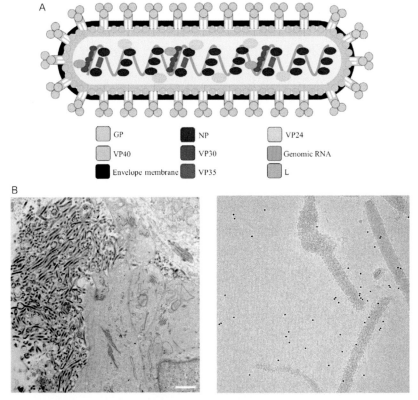

Fig. 3 The filovirus particle. (A) Schematic of filovirus particle. GP trimers are embedded in the membrane, projecting spike-like structures away from the virion. The matrix underneath the membrane is composed primarily of VP40. The ribonucleoprotein complex (RNP) is composed of L, NP, VP30, and VP35. (B) EBOV electron micrographs. The *left panel* is a TEM image of EBOV. The virus is budding from the cellular membrane, forming pleiomorphic virions outside the cell (scale bar = 1 μm). The *right panel* is a 2D cryo-EM image of EBOV. Note the thread-like turns characteristic of filovirus morphology (scale bar = 100 nm).

(Geisbert and Jahrling, 1995). All seven structural filovirus proteins are incorporated into the virion as shown in Fig. 3A. Only the soluble glyco-protein (sGP) and the small soluble glycoprotein (ssGP) of ebolaviruses are entirely nonstructural and are discussed in further detail later. From these protein–protein, protein–RNA, and protein–membrane interactions, the complex filovirus morphology is generated. The nucleoprotein (NP) and virion protein (VP) 30 interact strongly with RNA; this complex together with the polymerase L and VP35 forms the ribonucleoprotein complex (RNP). This, in turn, is enclosed by an outer envelope derived from the host-cell plasma membrane, lined with the matrix protein VP40. Protruding from the envelope surface are membrane-anchored glycoprotein trimers, studded across the virion. A brief summary of protein function is provided in Table 2.

Table 2 Overview of Filovirus Proteins

Genome Position	Protein	Protein Functions	Molecular Weight (kDa)
1	Nucleoprotein (NP)	Major nucleoprotein, component of the RNP	90–104
2	Virion protein 35 (VP35)	Polymerase cofactor, component of the RNP, interferon antagonist	35
3	Virion protein 40 (VP40)	Matrix protein, virion assembly, budding, interferon antagonist for MARV only	35–40
4	Glycoprotein (GP)	Viral entry, receptor binding, membrane fusion	150–170
	Soluble glycoprotein (sGP) (EBOV only)	Antigenic subversion, restores endothelial barrier function	50–55
	Small soluble glycoprotein (ssGP) (EBOV only)	Unknown	50–55
5	Virion protein 30 (VP30)	Minor nucleoprotein, component of the RNP	27–30
6	Virion protein 24 (VP24)	Nucleocapsid condensation, virion assembly, interferon antagonist for EBOV only	24–25
7	RNA polymerase (L)	RNA-dependent RNA polymerase, component of the RNP	~270

4.2 Genome Structure

All filovirus genomes comprise a negative-sense single-stranded RNA molecule, approximately 19 kilobases (kb) in length. Filoviruses generally encode seven genes, arranged in a consistent order: NP, VP35, VP40, glycoprotein (GP), VP30, VP24, and RNA-dependent RNA polymerase (L) (Sanchez et al., 1993). An exception is LLOV, which is believed to encode only six mRNA transcripts, including one bicistronic transcript that expresses both VP24 and L (Negredo et al., 2011). Each gene is flanked by conserved transcription initiation and termination sites with minimal variation (Bukreyev et al., 1995; Feldmann et al., 1992; Groseth et al., 2002; Ikegami et al., 2001; Sanchez et al., 1993). A single long intergenic region has been noted in both the *Ebolavirus* genus (between VP30 and VP24) and the *Marburgvirus* genus (between GP and VP30) (Crary et al., 2003; Mühlberger et al., 1992; Sanchez and Rollin, 2005). Other genes are either separated by short intergenic regions, comprising four to seven highly conserved nucleotides, or overlap (Bukreyev et al., 1995; Feldmann et al., 1992; Groseth et al., 2002). The overlapping genes vary between virus species and may be used to identify specific isolates (Sanchez et al., 1993). A schematic representation of various filovirus genome structures is provided in Fig. 4.

In addition to intergenic regions, there are also extragenic regions located on the 3' and 5' ends of all filovirus genomes. The 3' end contains a leader sequence that is approximately 60 bp in length. The 5' end contains a trailer sequence that varies in length between species, but may be as large as 676 bp in the case of EBOV. The terminal ends of the genome have conserved sequences with high complementarity that form stem-loop structures (Crary et al., 2003; Mühlberger et al., 1992; Sanchez and Rollin, 2005). RNA secondary structure in the 3'-leader region mediates binding specificity of the viral transcription factor VP30 and is required in EBOV for activating transcription (Biedenkopf et al., 2016; Schlereth et al., 2016).

Each gene contains a single open reading frame (ORF) apart from LLOV VP24/L, which is bicistronic, and GP of the ebolaviruses, which contain three overlapping ORFs (Ikegami et al., 2001; Mehedi et al., 2011; Negredo et al., 2011). Filovirus ORFs are flanked by untranslated regions, ranging in length from 57 to 684 nucleotides (Groseth et al., 2002; Ikegami et al., 2001; Sanchez and Rollin, 2005; Towner et al., 2006). The presence of long untranslated regions is an unusual characteristic of the filovirus genome, a feature that is only shared by the henipaviruses of the *Paramyxoviridae* family (Wang et al., 2001). The precise importance of these

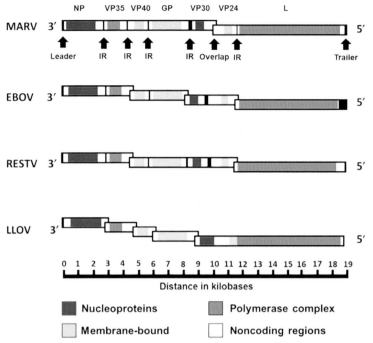

Fig. 4 Filovirus genome organization. This schematic of four representative filovirus genomes depicts the arrangement of genes and intergenic regions. Notably, there is an appreciable diversity with regard to the number of gene overlaps. MARV exhibits only a single-gene overlap between VP30 and VP24, whereas LLOV exhibits four gene overlaps. SUDV, BDBV, and TAFV (not shown) have three overlaps, arranged in a pattern similar to EBOV. The sizes of the overlaps have been slightly exaggerated for clarity.

untranslated elements is currently unknown, but their considerable size and distribution across all filoviruses may suggest a functional role.

4.3 Protein Structure and Function

4.3.1 Nucleoprotein Complex

Filoviruses contain major (NP) and minor (VP30) nucleoproteins which interact with viral genomic RNA to form the primary structure of the RNP (Elliott et al., 1985) (Fig. 3). When expressed in mammalian cells, recombinant NP forms cytoplasmic inclusion bodies and nonspecifically associates with host-cell RNA, forming helices (Noda et al., 2010). Moreover, 450 amino acids located on the N-terminus of EBOV NP have been shown to facilitate spontaneous assembly of NP tubes that may form a type of scaffolding for the RNP (Noda et al., 2010; Watanabe et al., 2006).

VP30 also directly binds RNA and preferentially binds viral genomic RNA at a stem-loop structure near the leader sequence. VP30 has two homo-oligomerization domains and forms hexamers via an N-terminal domain (Hartlieb et al., 2003). The crystal structure of the C-terminal region has been solved, showing a role in transcription and nucleocapsid association (Hartlieb et al., 2007). VP30 also possesses a zinc-finger motif that is highly conserved across all filoviruses and binds to RNA more readily in the presence of Zn^{2+} (Modrof et al., 2003). In terms of structural importance, it has been suggested that VP30 acts as a bridge between NP and L in the RNP (Groseth et al., 2009). In vitro studies using an artificial replication system originally showed that coexpression of NP, VP35, and L is necessary and sufficient for transcription and genome replication of MARV, whereas VP30 was additionally required for EBOV transcription (Mühlberger et al., 1998, 1999). More recently, the crystal structure of the NP–VP30 complex has been solved and the complex was shown to be essential for the transcription of EBOV genomic RNA with the binding strength modulating the rate of RNA synthesis (Kirchdoerfer et al., 2016). When expressed alone in mammalian cells, VP30 does not form inclusions like NP, but is distributed throughout the cytoplasm (Groseth et al., 2009). EBOV VP30 also serves as a *trans*-acting factor for RNA editing of the GP gene (Mehedi et al., 2013). EBOV VP30 has been shown to act as a phosphorylation-dependent transcription activator and replication inhibitor (Biedenkopf et al., 2013), whereas MARV VP30 appears to lack this property (Mühlberger et al., 1998).

4.3.2 Polymerase Complex

The L protein, an RNA-dependent RNA polymerase, is the enzymatic component of the RNP, for which VP35 is an essential cofactor (Mühlberger et al., 1992). When expressed alone in mammalians cells, the L protein forms small perinuclear inclusions. L does not directly interact with NP, and VP35 has been identified as the bridging factor between these two RNP components in vitro (Groseth et al., 2009). Both the template binding and catalytic sites of the polymerase complex have been identified (Feldmann et al., 1992). As might be expected, the enzymatically active portions of the L protein are highly conserved to maintain appropriate polymerase functions. However, certain portions of the sequence, especially near the C-terminus, exhibit some interspecies variation. For instance, the length of the MARV L gene (about 7.7 kb) is substantially longer than the EBOV (6.8 kb) or LLOV L gene (6.6 kb) (Fig. 4).

4.3.3 Matrix Protein

The matrix protein VP40 is the most abundant protein in the filovirus particle (Han et al., 2003). VP40 does not possess transmembrane domains, but exhibits a strong affinity for membranes and associates with the viral envelope. VP40 directly facilitates the envelopment of the RNP by the cellular membrane and is essential for viral budding (Jasenosky and Kawaoka, 2004). VP40 is the primary structural component of the matrix and forms hexameric and octameric ring structures in vitro (Jasenosky et al., 2001; Timmins et al., 2003). Oligomerization has been shown to be a prerequisite for the budding activity of VP40 (Hoenen et al., 2010b). Recently, biochemical and biophysical studies have demonstrated an intrinsic ability of VP40 to penetrate into lipid bilayers and initiate membrane curvature leading to virus particle formation (Adu-Gyamfi et al., 2012; Soni et al., 2013).

4.3.4 Viral Surface Spike

All filoviruses express the trimeric structural GP on the particle surface that is integral to viral entry and pathogenesis. GP is the best characterized of all the filovirus proteins, in part because of its functional importance and high immunogenic potential. To assemble into the functional GP, a series of processing steps must occur. First, ebolavirus GP transcripts must undergo transcriptional editing resulting in what is called the "8A" or "full-length" transcript (Sanchez et al., 1996; Volchkov et al., 1995). This unique feature is not present in marburgviruses. For all filovirus GPs, this full-length transcript gets translated into an ~680 amino acid (aa) long protein, representing the uncleaved precursor GP0. While in the ER, the N-terminal signal peptide is cleaved off cotranslationally and intramolecular disulfide binding occurs at key cysteine residues. As GP is transported through the ER and Golgi, it gets heavily glycosylated with N-linked and O-linked glycans that potentially mask antigenic epitopes in particular in the mucin-like domain (Reynard et al., 2009; Volchkov et al., 1998b). Next, GP0 is moved to the *trans* Golgi, where the cellular protease furin (or furin-like proteases) cleaves GP0 at a conserved cleavage site into the amino-terminal GP1 (approx. 470 aa) and carboxyl-terminal GP2 (approx. 175 aa) (Volchkov et al., 1998a,b). Interestingly, this cleavage event is not essential for virus replication or viral entry (Neumann et al., 2002; Wool-Lewis and Bates, 1999). GP1 contains a divergent mucin-like domain near the C-terminus and a region with several conserved cysteine residues near the N-terminus; it also contains the receptor-binding domain. GP2 also contains conserved cysteine residues, as well as a fusion peptide, heptad repeats, a Type 1 transmembrane domain

(Feldmann et al., 1991; Volchkov et al., 1998b), and a pattern homologous to the conserved immunosuppressive motif found in oncogenic retroviruses (Volchkov et al., 1992). In vitro studies have shown that for pathogenic filoviruses (but not RESTV) this motif inhibits human CD4 and CD8 T cell cycle progression and suppresses the host cytokine response (Yaddanapudi et al., 2006). Postcleavage, the polypeptides are oriented such that the N-terminus ends appose one another, comprising GP1,2 heterodimers connected by means of a disulfide bridge (Malashkevich et al., 1999). Three GP1,2 heterodimers trimerize to form a GP peplomer, the spiked protrusions on the surface of the virion. This trimerization is facilitated by the coiled coils of heptad repeat sequences present on GP2, and the trimeric GP is embedded in the envelope membrane via the transmembrane domain in GP2 (Weissenhorn et al., 1998a,b). While the majority of GP is membrane bound, it has been shown that shed forms of GP exist: shed GP1 due to disulfide bond instability (Volchkov et al., 1998a) and GP1,2ΔTM, the trimeric GP without the transmembrane domain due to cleavage by the metalloprotease TACE (Dolnik et al., 2004). Although all filovirus GPs are presumed to undergo the processing described earlier, little data exist for LLOV GP (Maruyama et al., 2014). In recent years, much has been learned about the role of GP, particularly regarding EBOV entry, which is discussed further in Section 5.

4.3.5 Nonstructural Glycoproteins

One distinct feature of ebolaviruses that is lacking with all marburgviruses is transcriptional editing of the GP ORF and the resulting production of three different proteins: full-length GP (8A), soluble GP (sGP, 7A), and small, soluble GP (ssGP, 6A, or 9A). The N-terminal region (approx. 300 aa) including the signal peptide of all three proteins is identical; however, the C-terminal sequences are unique. Like GP0, pre-sGP is cleaved at the furin cleavage site resulting in sGP and delta-peptide (Volchkov et al., 1999; Volchkova et al., 1999). For delta-peptide a modulatory role has been proposed by inhibiting virus entry into target cells (Radoshitzky et al., 2011). Both sGP and ssGP form parallel homodimers via disulfide bonding at cysteine residues (Barrientos et al., 2004; Mehedi et al., 2011). Regarding protein function, sGP is thought to play a role in pathogenesis through multiple mechanisms. First, sGP has the antiinflammatory property of restoring endothelial barrier function, which is antagonized by GP1,2 and VP40 (Wahl-Jensen et al., 2005). Second, epitopes common to both sGP and structural GP allow sGP to competitively bind host antibodies in a process termed "antigenic subversion" (Cook and Lee, 2013; Mohan et al., 2012). This potential evasion of the host immune response may, in part, be responsible for the severity of disease, as patients with acute infection have large amounts of sGP circulating in the blood (Sanchez et al., 1999). However, in the guinea pig animal model, elimination of sGP expression using reverse genetics did not significantly attenuate virulence and lethality of EBOV infection (Hoenen et al., 2015b). The function of ssGP is not understood, but unlike sGP, ssGP does not restore endothelial barrier function (Mehedi et al., 2011).

4.3.6 Interferon Antagonists

Both ebolaviruses and marburgviruses have been found to potently antagonize the host interferon (IFN) response through similar as well as distinct mechanisms. VP35 and VP24 have been identified to interfere with the host innate immune response during EBOV infection; VP35 and VP40 have been associated with this function for MARV.

EBOV and MARV VP35 antagonize the host innate immune response by actively blocking IFN through interaction with IFN regulatory factor 3 (IRF3) and IRF7 (Basler et al., 2003; Prins et al., 2009). Cocrystal structures of the EBOV VP35 RNA-binding domain and double-stranded (ds)RNA revealed that VP35 coats the dsRNA during replication, thereby circumventing pattern recognition receptors such as those found in the RIG-I pathway (Bale et al., 2013; Leung et al., 2010). Interestingly, VP35 is analogous to the phosphoprotein present in *Pneumoviridae* and *Paramyxoviridae*, but VP35 seems only weakly phosphorylated (Becker et al., 1998; Elliott et al., 1985). EBOV VP35 is distributed throughout the cytoplasm and forms a bridge structure, connecting NP and L, when expressed in vitro (Groseth et al., 2009).

EBOV VP24 is associated with the outside of RNPs in the virus particle and blocks the nuclear accumulation of tyrosine-phosphorylated STAT1 by binding to karyopherin $\alpha 1$, the nuclear localization signal for STAT1 (Leung et al., 2006). Additionally, VP24 is able to inhibit IFN-stimulated phosphorylation of p38-α in certain cell lines, an immunosuppressive mechanism found in other viruses (Halfmann et al., 2011; Ishida et al., 2004). Furthermore, VP24 has been shown to localize near the cellular membrane and perinuclear region where it regulates viral RNA synthesis. An N-terminal domain confers the ability of VP24 to oligomerize in vitro (Han et al., 2003). It has been demonstrated that a knockdown of VP24 hinders nucleocapsid assembly (Mateo et al., 2011). More recently, VP24 was described to play a role in genome packaging (Watt et al., 2014) likely through interaction with NP (Banadyga et al., 2017).

MARV VP40 directly inhibits Jak1 and STAT tyrosine phosphorylation and, therefore, blocks efficiently IFN and interleukin 6 signaling (Valmas et al., 2010).

5. VIRAL LIFE CYCLE

5.1 Entry and Uncoating

The entry mechanism for filoviruses has been studied for several decades mainly using EBOV. While the GP is essential for the attachment, uptake, and receptor binding, this process does not follow a classical entry mechanism. Over the last decade, light has been shed on the rather complicated sequence of events critical for EBOV entry into target cells (Fig. 5). However, some steps remain controversial among filovirus researchers.

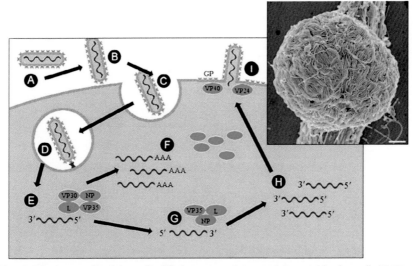

Fig. 5 Filovirus replication cycle. (A) A mature virus particle outside the cell. (B) Virus attaches to the cell via GP binding to attachment factors, e.g., C-type lectins. (C) The virus is subsumed by the cell largely via macropinocytosis. (D) An endosome forms. GP is cleaved by cysteine proteases and engages its receptor NPC1 (*purple*), initiating membrane fusion. (E) The genome is deposited into the cytosol. Positive-sense transcripts and antigenomes are generated via the polymerase complex. (F) Viral RNA transcripts are translated by host ribosomes. (G) The replication complex uses the antigenomes as a template for progeny genomes. (H) Progeny genomes are formed. (I) VP40 and VP24 facilitate virion assembly and budding from the cell. Filovirus GP expressed on the cellular surface is incorporated into the virus envelope and the mature virus is released from the cell. The SEM image is of a Vero E6 cell with large amounts of EBOV budding from its cellular membrane (scale bar = 2 μm).

In a first step the virus particle attaches to the cell surface binding to C-type lectins like DC-SIGN (Alvarez et al., 2002; Simmons et al., 2003) and other proteins in the past mistakenly proposed as universal EBOV receptors. Binding to these molecules enhances viral entry at least in certain cell types, but they do not function as the EBOV receptor. After the virus particle is attached to the cell surface, it is taken up mainly via macropinocytosis (Aleksandrowicz et al., 2011; Nanbo et al., 2010; Saeed et al., 2010), although some studies demonstrated that other pathways contribute to virus uptake and propose that multiple pathways may be used together (Aleksandrowicz et al., 2011; Hunt et al., 2012; Sanchez, 2007). Regardless, the virus particle ends up in the acidic environment of endosomes. There, it has been shown that proteolysis of the EBOV GP1 is required for viral entry. Specifically, a role for cathepsin B and a likely accessory role for cathepsin L (both endosomal host cysteine proteases) have been established in vitro (Chandran et al., 2005). In vivo experiments have shown that neither cathepsin B nor L knockout mice displayed a delayed disease phenotype (Marzi et al., 2012), indicating that in the absence of these specific proteases other, functionally similar proteases like thermolysin could cleave GP1 (Brecher et al., 2012). However, this cleavage event is essential to the entry mechanism as it exposes the structurally buried fusion loop which can now engage the filovirus receptor, the cholesterol transporter Niemann-Pick C1 (NPC1) (Carette et al., 2011; Côté et al., 2011). Specific sequences in the luminal domain C of NPC1 have been identified as essential for GP binding and viral entry (Krishnan et al., 2012). The crystal structure of the NPC1–GP binding complex has highlighted several regions of interest, such as the area of interaction between NPC1 and the GP α1 helix (Wang et al., 2016). This is in line with the finding that variations surrounding the GP α1 helix sequence have been shown to contribute to differences in host species tropism (Martinez et al., 2013; Ng et al., 2015; Urbanowicz et al., 2016).

Finally, cleaved GP1 binds to NPC1 and triggers fusion between the viral and endosomal membrane. Subsequently the viral RNP is released into the cytoplasm and production of progeny virus is initiated. It is believed that all filoviruses follow the entry mechanism described for EBOV as shown by Davey et al. (2017).

5.2 Transcription and Replication

The mechanism of filovirus replication has been studied in detail using artificial replication systems such as minigenomes (Mühlberger et al., 1998, 1999). All filoviruses encode the proteins required to form an RNA-dependent RNA polymerase complex, which produces a positive-sense antigenome that serves as a template for replication of the negative-sense genome. In both MARV and EBOV, it has been shown that NP, VP35, and L are necessary and sufficient to support genome replication. This is similar to paramyxovirus and rhabdovirus replication, which require only NP, P, and L proteins to be replication competent (Conzelmann, 2004; Whelan et al., 2004). Key protein interactions such as NP–VP35 and VP35–L have been established, highlighting the important structural role VP35 plays in the viral polymerase complex (Becker et al., 1998; Groseth et al., 2009). It has been shown that the proteins involved in genome replication change localization over the course of cellular infection: first they are distributed in cytoplasmic inclusions that are enlarged near the nucleus, then broken into smaller pieces, and subsequently localized near the plasma membrane (Nanbo et al., 2013). In EBOV, replication begins at a bipartite promoter region that obeys the rule of six and flanks the transcription initiation sequence for the NP gene (Weik et al., 2005).

Filoviruses encode seven monocistronic transcriptional units (genes), except for LLOV, which is thought to possess only six including one bicistronic unit. Each unit is associated with a corresponding transcriptional promoter region. As stated previously, filoviruses have overlapping ORFs. There is a surprising difference in the protein requirement for transcription in MARV and EBOV. For MARV, NP, VP35, and L are sufficient to initiate transcription (Mühlberger et al., 1998). In EBOV, however, a fourth protein, VP30, is an essential cofactor that acts to circumvent a hairpin loop in the noncoding 3' region of the genome (Weik et al., 2002).

Over the past decade, much has been learned about the mechanisms responsible for regulating transcription and genome replication, specifically regarding VP30 and VP24. It is known that VP30 stabilizes VP35–L RNA binding. As a result, it has been hypothesized that the phosphorylation state of VP30 modulates the conformation of the RNP to form either a transcriptase or a replicase complex (Biedenkopf et al., 2013). VP24 is also believed to regulate RNA synthesis by affecting the conformation of RNP. Electron microscopy analysis of VP24 shows that it associates with the exterior surface of the RNP and that this association condenses RNP into the form found in viral particles (Beniac et al., 2012; Bharat et al., 2012). In vitro systems with overexpression of VP24 show inhibition of RNA synthesis (Hoenen et al., 2010b; Watanabe et al., 2007). Thus, it is believed that the presence of VP24 changes the RNP from a form compatible with transcription/replication to a packaging-competent form (Banadyga et al., 2017; Watt et al., 2014).

5.3 Virion Assembly

While viral RNA synthesis occurs in inclusion bodies (Hoenen et al., 2012; Nanbo et al., 2013), virion assembly occurs in the cytosol. When expressed in vitro, VP40 alone forms virus-like particles (VLPs). These VLPs exhibit smaller diameters (53–80 nm) than infectious particles (about 80 nm), indicating that other viral proteins contribute to virus morphology (Kolesnikova et al., 2004; Noda et al., 2002). VP40 is formed as a monomer and is subsequently oligomerized into hexameric and octameric rings by means of an N-terminal domain (Ruigrok et al., 2000; Timmins et al., 2003). The conformation of the metastable monomeric form of VP40 is determined by interactions with the lipid membrane, as mediated by the C-terminal domain (Jasenosky et al., 2001; Scianimanico et al., 2000). The hexameric form of VP40 results when the C-terminal domain extends via a flexible linker from the ring structure, allowing stable binding of VP40 (Dessen et al., 2000; Scianimanico et al., 2000). The octameric form depends on four homodimers binding RNA trinucleotides of the sequence 5′-UGA-3′ and cannot form in the absence of RNA (Gomis-Rüth et al., 2003; Timmins et al., 2003). In EBOV, VP40 octamerization is essential for infectivity (Hoenen et al., 2005, 2010a).

VP24 is also important for proper assembly as it plays a role regulating viral RNA synthesis. While VP24 was early on suggested to function as a minor matrix protein due to its location in the matrix space (Becker et al., 1998), recent electron microscopy studies have shown that VP24 is indeed associated with the outside of viral RNPs resulting in rigid RNP forms as observed in EBOV particles (Beniac et al., 2012; Bharat et al., 2012). These and other findings suggest that VP24 is essential for RNP production capable of replication, as it controls RNP condensation from a flexible form which can undergo transcription and replication to a rigid form that is packaged into virus particles (Banadyga et al., 2017; Bharat et al., 2012; Hoenen et al., 2006).

5.4 Budding

Several studies have identified the actin cytoskeleton to be important for the transport of virus particle components to the site of virus budding. Progeny RNPs travel from the inclusion bodies to the sites of budding using the actin fibers (Schudt et al., 2015). Actin has also been shown to direct the transport of VP40 to the budding sites (Adu-Gyamfi et al., 2012). The mature GP trimers are already embedded in the plasma membrane. VP40, the major driver for particle formation and membrane deformation, needs to oligomerize in order to form the proper particle matrix (Hoenen et al., 2010a). VP40 has the intrinsic ability to penetrate into lipid bilayers and initiate membrane curvature which is consistent with virus particle formation (Adu-Gyamfi et al., 2012; Soni and Stahelin, 2014).

6. EVOLUTION

The evolutionary origin of filoviruses is a matter of some controversy, as the timescale of viral evolution is widely disputed (Holmes, 2003; Patel et al., 2011; Sharp and Simmonds, 2011; Wertheim and Kosakovsky Pond, 2011). Some analyses estimate that the filoviruses emerged several thousand years ago (Carroll et al., 2013; Suzuki and Gojobori, 1997). Other estimates propose a much older emergence event on the order of several million years ago, as evidenced by filovirus-like elements incorporated into mammalian genomes, with *Ebolavirus* and *Cuevavirus* genera diverging from the *Marburgvirus* genus since the early Miocene (Taylor et al., 2010, 2011, 2014). If true, it remains unknown what effects filoviruses may have had on mammalian evolution in the distant past. A long-term coevolutionary relationship with bats has been hypothesized on the basis of selective pressure on NPC1 and the presence of endogenous viral elements (Ng et al., 2015; Taylor et al., 2011). Differences in the intraspecies diversity of the filoviruses have also been noted as measured by the time estimates for the most recent common ancestor (MRCA). Members of the *Marburgvirus marburgvirus* species exhibit considerable sequence diversity and are thought to have an MRCA about 700 years ago. This stands in contrast to *Zaire ebolavirus* and *Reston ebolavirus*, which are believed to have undergone genetic bottlenecks within the past several decades (Carroll et al., 2013). In any case, the modern evolutionary rate of filoviruses ranges from approximately 4.6×10^{-5} nucleotide substitutions/site/year for *Sudan ebolavirus* to 8.2×10^{-4} nucleotide substitutions/site/year for *Reston ebolavirus* (Carroll et al., 2013). The variation in this rate of change reflects a difference in selective pressure as it relates to the ecological niche of each virus species.

Regarding the pathogenic filoviruses, spillover events into human populations seem to occur infrequently. A genetically diverse filovirus population circulates in largely unknown natural reservoirs and seems to fluctuate over time (Amman et al., 2012; Ogawa et al., 2015). Some human outbreaks, such as the MARV outbreaks in Durba (1998–2000) and the EBOV outbreaks in Gabon and RC (2000–2004), have been characterized by multiple incursion events occurring simultaneously or over a relatively short period of time, respectively (Bausch et al., 2006; Leroy et al., 2004). Other outbreaks, such as the MARV outbreak in Angola, the EBOV outbreak in Kikwit (1995), and the SUDV outbreak in Gulu (2000 – 2001), yielded clinical samples that showed a surprisingly low amount of genetic diversity throughout the entire course of the outbreak (Rodriguez et al., 1999; Towner et al., 2004, 2006). This suggests that the outbreaks were due to a single zoonotic transmission, followed by low rates of viral evolution during limited transmission chains in humans.

The recent EBOV epidemic in West Africa (2013–2016) is also thought to be derived from a single zoonotic incursion followed by an unfamiliar sustained human-to-human transmission. The index case is believed to be a young boy living in Guéckédou, Guinea who is thought to have acquired EBOV from a local bat in December 2013 (Baize et al., 2014). Although the exact timeline and geographic distribution remain uncertain, it is believed that the West African strain diverged from Central African strains around 2004 (Gire et al., 2014). As a result of improved sequencing technology, it is increasingly feasible to monitor changes in viral genomes over the course of a single outbreak (Carroll et al., 2015). This makes it possible to easily identify species-specific adaptations and raises the question of whether filoviruses adapt or attenuate to humans over time. Regarding host adaptation, it has been shown in vitro that amino acid substitutions observed during the West African outbreak altered EBOV GP to increase tropism for human cells and reduce tropism for bat cells by effecting changes in N-glycosylation, the GP signal peptide, NPC1 binding, and various epistatic interactions (Bedford and Malik, 2016; Diehl et al., 2016; Urbanowicz et al., 2016). Regarding human-to-human transmission, some investigators have indicated that the specific changes in the EBOV Makona genome reflect adaptive evolution (Liu et al., 2015), whereas other groups have found no evidence for human adaptation (Azarian et al., 2015; Hoenen et al., 2015a; Olabode et al., 2015). Despite some initial concerns about an increased rate of mutation (Gire et al., 2014), extended analyses have suggested that the mutation rate of West African EBOV isolate Makona displays a similar mutation rate than those isolates causing previous Central African outbreaks (Hoenen et al., 2015a). Extensive human-to-human transmission, however, resulted in an accumulation of synonymous and nonsynonymous mutations with hitherto unknown importance.

7. FUTURE PERSPECTIVES

Although much has been learned about filoviruses over the past two decades, many important gaps in our knowledge remain. Filovirus ecology is still poorly understood and, with the exception of marburgviruses, no natural reservoirs have been identified. Therefore, selection of the appropriate species for surveillance is consequently challenging. Greater effort should be directed toward identifying the precise mechanism of zoonotic transmission, so public health practices to reduce potential exposure can be established. Thanks to an improved understanding of how GP affects immunogenicity and cellular tropism, vaccines and therapeutics may be specifically tailored to viral targets to lend the greatest efficacy. Similar studies need to be intensified to better understand the functions of other viral proteins for virus life cycle and pathogenicity to define new targets for intervention. Comparative analyses of pathogenic and nonpathogenic filoviruses will also be valuable for the purposes of evaluating isolate-specific health risks. Moving forward, it will also be important to continue the search for novel filoviruses, especially in East Asia, to evaluate their pathogenic potential. Understanding the broad evolutionary forces driving changes in filovirus sequence and host distribution will be instrumental in identifying optimal regions for filovirus surveillance.

ACKNOWLEDGMENTS

The authors would like to thank Elizabeth Fischer and Vinod Nair of the Electron Microscopy Core (NIAID) for providing the images for Figs. 3 and 5. Work on filoviruses in the Laboratory of Virology, NIAID is funded by the Intramural Research Program.

REFERENCES

Adu-Gyamfi, E., Digman, M.A., Gratton, E., Stahelin, R.V., 2012. Investigation of Ebola VP40 assembly and oligomerization in live cells using number and brightness analysis. Biophys. J. 102, 2517.

Aleksandrowicz, P., Marzi, A., Biedenkopf, N., Beimforde, N., Becker, S., Hoenen, T., Feldmann, H., Schnittler, H.-J., 2011. Ebola virus enters host cells by macropinocytosis and clathrin-mediated endocytosis. J. Infect. Dis. 204, S957.

Alvarez, C.P., Lasala, F., Carrillo, J., Muñiz, O., Corbí, A.L., Delgado, R., 2002. C-type lectins DC-SIGN and L-SIGN mediate cellular entry by Ebola virus in cis and in trans. J. Virol. 76, 6841.

Amman, B.R., Carroll, S.A., Reed, Z.D., Sealy, T.K., Balinandi, S., Swanepoel, R., Kemp, A., Erickson, B.R., Comer, J.A., Campbell, S., 2012. Seasonal pulses of Marburg virus circulation in juvenile Rousettus aegyptiacus bats coincide with periods of increased risk of human infection. PLoS Pathog. 8, e1002877.

Amman, B.R., Nyakarahuka, L., McElroy, A.K., Dodd, K.A., Sealy, T.K., Schuh, A.J., Shoemaker, T.R., Balinandi, S., Atimnedi, P., Kaboyo, W., 2014. Marburgvirus resurgence in Kitaka mine bat population after extermination attempts, Uganda. Emerg. Infect. Dis. 20, 1761.

Amman, B.R., Jones, M.E., Sealy, T.K., Uebelhoer, L.S., Schuh, A.J., Bird, B.H., Coleman-McCray, J.D., Martin, B.E., Nichol, S.T., Towner, J.S., 2015. Oral shedding of Marburg virus in experimentally infected Egyptian fruit bats (Rousettus aegyptiacus). J. Wildl. Dis. 51, 113.

Azarian, T., Presti, A.L., Giovanetti, M., Cella, E., Rife, B., Lai, A., Zehender, G., Ciccozzi, M., Salemi, M., 2015. Impact of spatial dispersion, evolution, and selection on Ebola Zaire Virus epidemic waves. Sci. Rep. 5, 10170.

Baize, S., Pannetier, D., Oestereich, L., Rieger, T., Koivogui, L., Magassouba, N.F., Soropogui, B., Sow, M.S., Keïta, S., De Clerck, H., 2014. Emergence of Zaire Ebola virus disease in Guinea. N. Engl. J. Med. 371, 1418.

Bale, S., Julien, J.-P., Bornholdt, Z.A., Krois, A.S., Wilson, I.A., Saphire, E.O., 2013. Ebolavirus VP35 coats the backbone of double-stranded RNA for interferon antagonism. J. Virol. 87, 10385.

Banadyga, L., Hoenen, T., Ambroggio, X., Dunham, E., Groseth, A., Ebihara, H., 2017. Ebola virus VP24 interacts with NP to facilitate nucleocapsid assembly and genome packaging. Sci. Rep. 7, 7698.

Barrette, R.W., Metwally, S.A., Rowland, J.M., Xu, L., Zaki, S.R., Nichol, S.T., Rollin, P.E., Towner, J.S., Shieh, W.-J., Batten, B., 2009. Discovery of swine as a host for the Reston ebolavirus. Science 325, 204.

Barrientos, L.G., Martin, A.M., Rollin, P.E., Sanchez, A., 2004. Disulfide bond assignment of the Ebola virus secreted glycoprotein SGP. Biochem. Biophys. Res. Commun. 323, 696.

Basler, C.F., Mikulasova, A., Martinez-Sobrido, L., Paragas, J., Mühlberger, E., Bray, M., Klenk, H.-D., Palese, P., García-Sastre, A., 2003. The Ebola virus VP35 protein inhibits activation of interferon regulatory factor 3. J. Virol. 77, 7945.

Bausch, D.G., Nichol, S.T., Muyembe-Tamfum, J.J., Borchert, M., Rollin, P.E., Sleurs, H., Campbell, P., Tshioko, F.K., Roth, C., Colebunders, R., 2006. Marburg hemorrhagic fever associated with multiple genetic lineages of virus. N. Engl. J. Med. 355, 909.

Becker, S., Rinne, C., Hofsäss, U., Klenk, H.-D., Mühlberger, E., 1998. Interactions of Marburg virus nucleocapsid proteins. Virology 249, 406.

Bedford, T., Malik, H.S., 2016. Did a single amino acid change make Ebola virus more virulent? Cell 167, 892.

Beniac, D.R., Melito, P.L., Hiebert, S.L., Rabb, M.J., Lamboo, L.L., Jones, S.M., Booth, T.F., 2012. The organisation of Ebola virus reveals a capacity for extensive, modular polyploidy. PLoS One 7, e29608.

Bermejo, M., Rodríguez-Teijeiro, J.D., Illera, G., Barroso, A., Vilà, C., Walsh, P.D., 2006. Ebola outbreak killed 5000 gorillas. Science 314, 1564.

Bharat, T.A., Noda, T., Riches, J.D., Kraehling, V., Kolesnikova, L., Becker, S., Kawaoka, Y., Briggs, J.A., 2012. Structural dissection of Ebola virus and its assembly determinants using cryo-electron tomography. Proc. Natl. Acad. Sci. U.S.A. 109, 4275.

Biedenkopf, N., Hartlieb, B., Hoenen, T., Becker, S., 2013. Phosphorylation of Ebola virus VP30 influences the composition of the viral nucleocapsid complex impact on viral transcription and replication. J. Biol. Chem. 288, 11165.

Biedenkopf, N., Schlereth, J., Grünweller, A., Becker, S., Hartmann, R.K., 2016. RNA binding of Ebola virus VP30 is essential for activating viral transcription. J. Virol. 90, 7481.

Brecher, M., Schornberg, K.L., Delos, S.E., Fusco, M.L., Saphire, E.O., White, J.M., 2012. Cathepsin cleavage potentiates the Ebola virus glycoprotein to undergo a subsequent fusion-relevant conformational change. J. Virol. 86, 364.

Bukreyev, A., Volchkov, V., Blinov, V., Dryga, S., Netesov, S., 1995. The complete nucleotide sequence of the Popp (1967) strain of Marburg virus: a comparison with the
Musoke (1980) strain. Arch. Virol. 140, 1589.

Bukreyev, A.A., Chandran, K., Dolnik, O., Dye, J.M., Ebihara, H., Leroy, E.M.,
Mühlberger, E., Netesov, S.V., Patterson, J.L., Paweska, J.T., 2014. Discussions and
decisions of the 2012–2014 International Committee on Taxonomy of Viruses
(ICTV) Filoviridae study group, January 2012–June 2013. Arch. Virol. 159, 821.

Carette, J.E., Raaben, M., Wong, A.C., Herbert, A.S., Obernosterer, G., Mulherkar, N.,
Kuehne, A.I., Kranzusch, P.J., Griffin, A.M., Ruthel, G., 2011. Ebola virus entry
requires the cholesterol transporter Niemann-Pick C1. Nature 477, 340.

Carroll, S.A., Towner, J.S., Sealy, T.K., McMullan, L.K., Khristova, M.L., Burt, F.J.,
Swanepoel, R., Rollin, P.E., Nichol, S.T., 2013. Molecular evolution of viruses of
the family Filoviridae based on 97 whole-genome sequences. J. Virol. 87, 2608.

Carroll, M.W., Matthews, D.A., Hiscox, J.A., Elmore, M.J., Pollakis, G., Rambaut, A.,
Hewson, R., García-Dorival, I., Bore, J.A., Koundouno, R., 2015. Temporal and spatial
analysis of the 2014-2015 Ebola virus outbreak in West Africa. Nature 524, 97.

CDC, 1990a. Epidemiologic notes and reports updates: filovirus infection in animal handlers.
MMWR Morb. Mortal. Wkly. Rep. 39, 221.

CDC, 1990b. Update: filovirus infections among persons with occupational exposure to
nonhuman primates. MMWR Morb. Mortal. Wkly. Rep. 39, 266.

Chandran, K., Sullivan, N.J., Felbor, U., Whelan, S.P., Cunningham, J.M., 2005.
Endosomal proteolysis of the Ebola virus glycoprotein is necessary for infection.
Science 308, 1643.

Chippaux, J.-P., 2014. Outbreaks of Ebola virus disease in Africa: the beginnings of a tragic
saga. J. Venom. Anim. Toxins Incl. Trop Dis. 20, 44.

Conzelmann, K., 2004. Reverse genetics of mononegavirales. In: Kawaoka, Y. (Ed.), Biology of Negative Strand RNA Viruses: The Power of Reverse Genetics. Springer, p. 1.

Cook, J.D., Lee, J.E., 2013. The secret life of viral entry glycoproteins: moonlighting in
immune evasion. PLoS Pathog. 9 . e1003258.

Côté, M., Misasi, J., Ren, T., Bruchez, A., Lee, K., Filone, C.M., Hensley, L., Li, Q.,
Ory, D., Chandran, K., 2011. Small molecule inhibitors reveal Niemann-Pick C1 is
essential for Ebola virus infection. Nature 477, 344.

Crary, S.M., Towner, J.S., Honig, J.E., Shoemaker, T.R., Nichol, S.T., 2003. Analysis of the
role of predicted RNA secondary structures in Ebola virus replication. Virology
306, 210.

Davey, R., Shtanko, O., Anantpadma, M., Sakurai, Y., Chandran, K., Maury, W., 2017.
Mechanisms of filovirus entry. In: Mühlberger, E., Hensley, L.L., Towner, J.S. (Eds.),
Marburg and Ebola Viruses. Curr. Top. Microbiol. Immunol. 323–352.

Dessen, A., Volchkov, V., Dolnik, O., Klenk, H.D., Weissenhorn, W., 2000. Crystal structure of the matrix protein VP40 from Ebola virus. EMBO J. 19, 4228.

Diehl, W.E., Lin, A.E., Grubaugh, N.D., Carvalho, L.M., Kim, K., Kyawe, P.P.,
McCauley, S.M., Donnard, E., Kucukural, A., McDonel, P., 2016. Ebola virus glycoprotein with increased infectivity dominated the 2013–2016 epidemic. Cell 167, 1088.

Dolnik, O., Volchkova, V., Garten, W., Carbonnelle, C., Becker, S., Kahnt, J., Ströher, U.,
Klenk, H.D., Volchkov, V., 2004. Ectodomain shedding of the glycoprotein GP of
Ebola virus. EMBO J. 23, 2175.

Elliott, L.H., Kiley, M.P., McCormick, J.B., 1985. Descriptive analysis of Ebola virus proteins. Virology 147, 169.

Feldmann, H., Will, C., Schikore, M., Slenczka, W., Klenk, H.-D., 1991. Glycosylation and
oligomerization of the spike protein of Marburg virus. Virology 182, 353.

Feldmann, H., Mühlberger, E., Randolf, A., Will, C., Kiley, M.P., Sanchez, A., Klenk, H.-
D., 1992. Marburg virus, a filovirus: messenger RNAs, gene order, and regulatory elements of the replication cycle. Virus Res. 24, 1.

Formenty, P., Boesch, C., Wyers, M., Steiner, C., Donati, F., Dind, F., Walker, F., Le Guenno, B., 1999. Ebola virus outbreak among wild chimpanzees living in a rain forest of Cote d'Ivoire. J. Infect. Dis. 179, S120.

Geisbert, T., Jahrling, P., 1995. Differentiation of filoviruses by electron microscopy. Virus Res. 39, 129.

Gire, S.K., Goba, A., Andersen, K.G., Sealfon, R.S., Park, D.J., Kanneh, L., Jalloh, S., Momoh, M., Fullah, M., Dudas, G., 2014. Genomic surveillance elucidates Ebola virus origin and transmission during the 2014 outbreak. Science 345, 1369.

Gomis-Rüth, F.X., Dessen, A., Timmins, J., Bracher, A., Kolesnikowa, L., Becker, S., Klenk, H.-D., Weissenhorn, W., 2003. The matrix protein VP40 from Ebola virus octamerizes into pore-like structures with specific RNA binding properties. Structure 11, 423.

Groseth, A., Ströher, U., Theriault, S., Feldmann, H., 2002. Molecular characterization of an isolate from the 1989/90 epizootic of Ebola virus Reston among macaques imported into the United States. Virus Res. 87, 155.

Groseth, A., Charton, J., Sauerborn, M., Feldmann, F., Jones, S., Hoenen, T., Feldmann, H., 2009. The Ebola virus ribonucleoprotein complex: a novel VP30–L interaction identified. Virus Res. 140, 8.

Halfmann, P., Neumann, G., Kawaoka, Y., 2011. The ebolavirus VP24 protein blocks phosphorylation of p38 mitogen-activated protein kinase. J. Infect. Dis. 204, S953.

Han, Z., Boshra, H., Sunyer, J.O., Zwiers, S.H., Paragas, J., Harty, R.N., 2003. Biochemical and functional characterization of the Ebola virus VP24 protein: implications for a role in virus assembly and budding. J. Virol. 77, 1793.

Hartlieb, B., Modrof, J., Mühlberger, E., Klenk, H.-D., Becker, S., 2003. Oligomerization of Ebola virus VP30 is essential for viral transcription and can be inhibited by a synthetic peptide. J. Biol. Chem. 278, 41830.

Hartlieb, B., Muziol, T., Weissenhorn, W., Becker, S., 2007. Crystal structure of the C-terminal domain of Ebola virus VP30 reveals a role in transcription and nucleocapsid association. Proc. Natl. Acad. Sci. U.S.A. 104, 624.

Hayman, D.T., Emmerich, P., Yu, M., Wang, L.-F., Suu-Ire, R., Fooks, A.R., Cunningham, A.A., Wood, J.L., 2010. Long-term survival of an urban fruit bat seropositive for Ebola and Lagos bat viruses. PLoS One 5, e11978.

Hayman, D.T., Yu, M., Crameri, G., Wang, L.-F., Suu-Ire, R., Wood, J.L., Cunningham, A.A., 2012. Ebola virus antibodies in fruit bats, Ghana, West Africa. Emerg. Infect. Dis. 18, 1207.

He, B., Feng, Y., Zhang, H., Xu, L., Yang, W., Zhang, Y., Li, X., Tu, C., 2015. Filovirus RNA in fruit bats, China. Emerg. Infect. Dis. 21, 1675.

Hoenen, T., Volchkov, V., Kolesnikova, L., Mittler, E., Timmins, J., Ottmann, M., Reynard, O., Becker, S., Weissenhorn, W., 2005. VP40 octamers are essential for Ebola virus replication. J. Virol. 79, 1898.

Hoenen, T., Groseth, A., Kolesnikova, L., Theriault, S., Ebihara, H., Hartlieb, B., Bamberg, S., Feldmann, H., Ströher, U., Becker, S., 2006. Infection of naive target cells with virus-like particles: implications for the function of Ebola virus VP24. J. Virol. 80, 7260.

Hoenen, T., Biedenkopf, N., Zielecki, F., Jung, S., Groseth, A., Feldmann, H., Becker, S., 2010a. Oligomerization of Ebola virus VP40 is essential for particle morphogenesis and regulation of viral transcription. J. Virol. 84, 7053.

Hoenen, T., Jung, S., Herwig, A., Groseth, A., Becker, S., 2010b. Both matrix proteins of Ebola virus contribute to the regulation of viral genome replication and transcription. Virology 403, 56.

Hoenen, T., Shabman, R.S., Groseth, A., Herwig, A., Weber, M., Schudt, G., Dolnik, O., Basler, C.F., Becker, S., Feldmann, H., 2012. Inclusion bodies are a site of ebolavirus replication. J. Virol. 86, 11779.

Hoenen, T., Safronetz, D., Groseth, A., Wollenberg, K., Koita, O., Diarra, B., Fall, I., Haidara, F., Diallo, F., Sanogo, M., 2015a. Mutation rate and genotype variation of Ebola virus from Mali case sequences. Science 348, 117.

Hoenen, T., Marzi, A., Scott, D.P., Feldmann, F., Callison, J., Safronetz, D., Ebihara, H., Feldmann, H., 2015b. Soluble glycoprotein is not required for Ebola virus virulence in guinea pigs. J. Infect. Dis. 212, S242.

Holmes, E.C., 2003. Molecular clocks and the puzzle of RNA virus origins. J. Virol. 77, 3893.

Hunt, C.L., Lennemann, N.J., Maury, W., 2012. Filovirus entry: a novelty in the viral fusion world. Viruses 4, 258.

Ikegami, T., Calaor, A., Miranda, M., Niikura, M., Saijo, M., Kurane, I., Yoshikawa, Y., Morikawa, S., 2001. Genome structure of Ebola virus subtype Reston: differences among Ebola subtypes. Arch. Virol. 146, 2021.

Ishida, H., Ohkawa, K., Hosui, A., Hiramatsu, N., Kanto, T., Ueda, K., Takehara, T., Hayashi, N., 2004. Involvement of p38 signaling pathway in interferon-α-mediated antiviral activity toward hepatitis C virus. Biochem. Biophys. Res. Commun. 321, 722.

Jahrling, P., Geisbert, T., Johnson, E., Peters, C., Dalgard, D., Hall, W., 1990. Preliminary report: isolation of Ebola virus from monkeys imported to USA. Lancet 335, 502.

Jahrling, P., Geisbert, T., Jaax, N., Hanes, M., Ksiazek, T., Peters, C., 1996. Experimental infection of cynomolgus macaques with Ebola-Reston filoviruses from the 1989-1990 U.S. epizootic. Arch. Virol. Suppl. 11, 115–134.

Jasenosky, L.D., Kawaoka, Y., 2004. Filovirus budding. Virus Res. 106, 181.

Jasenosky, L.D., Neumann, G., Lukashevich, I., Kawaoka, Y., 2001. Ebola virus VP40-induced particle formation and association with the lipid bilayer. J. Virol. 75, 5205.

Jayme, S.I., Field, H.E., de Jong, C., Olival, K.J., Marsh, G., Tagtag, A.M., Hughes, T., Bucad, A.C., Barr, J., Azul, R.R., 2015. Molecular evidence of Ebola Reston virus infection in Philippine bats. Virol. J. 12, 107.

Kirchdoerfer, R.N., Moyer, C.L., Abelson, D.M., Saphire, E.O., 2016. The Ebola virus VP30-NP interaction is a regulator of viral RNA synthesis. PLoS Pathog. 12, e1005937.

Kobinger, G.P., Leung, A., Neufeld, J., Richardson, J.S., Falzarano, D., Smith, G., Tierney, K., Patel, A., Weingartl, H.M., 2011. Replication, pathogenicity, shedding, and transmission of Zaire ebolavirus in pigs. J. Infect. Dis. 204, 200.

Kolesnikova, L., Berghöfer, B., Bamberg, S., Becker, S., 2004. Multivesicular bodies as a platform for formation of the Marburg virus envelope. J. Virol. 78, 12277.

Krishnan, A., Miller, E.H., Herbert, A.S., Ng, M., Ndungo, E., Whelan, S.P., Dye, J.M., Chandran, K., 2012. Niemann-Pick C1 (NPC1)/NPC1-like1 chimeras define sequences critical for NPC1's function as a filovirus entry receptor. Virus 4, 2471.

Kuhn, J.H., Becker, S., Ebihara, H., Geisbert, T.W., Johnson, K.M., Kawaoka, Y., Lipkin, W.I., Negredo, A.I., Netesov, S.V., Nichol, S.T., 2010. Proposal for a revised taxonomy of the family Filoviridae: classification, names of taxa and viruses, and virus abbreviations. Arch. Virol. 155, 2083.

Le Guenno, B., Formenty, P., Wyers, M., Gounon, P., Walker, F., Boesch, C., 1995. Isolation and partial characterisation of a new strain of Ebola virus. Lancet 345, 1271.

Leroy, E.M., Rouquet, P., Formenty, P., Souquière, S., Kilbourne, A., Froment, J.-M., Bermejo, M., Smit, S., Karesh, W., Swanepoel, R., 2004. Multiple Ebola virus transmission events and rapid decline of central African wildlife. Science 303, 387.

Leroy, E.M., Kumulungui, B., Pourrut, X., Rouquet, P., Hassanin, A., Yaba, P., Délicat, A., Paweska, J.T., Gonzalez, J.-P., Swanepoel, R., 2005. Fruit bats as reservoirs of Ebola virus. Nature 438, 575.

Leung, L.W., Hartman, A.L., Martinez, O., Shaw, M.L., Carbonnelle, C., Volchkov, V.E., Nichol, S.T., Basler, C.F., 2006. Ebola virus VP24 binds karyopherin α1 and blocks STAT1 nuclear accumulation. J. Virol. 80, 5156.

Leung, D.W., Prins, K.C., Borek, D.M., Farahbakhsh, M., Tufariello, J.M., Ramanan, P., Nix, J.C., Helgeson, L.A., Otwinowski, Z., Honzatko, R.B., 2010. Structural basis for dsRNA recognition and interferon antagonism by Ebola VP35. Nat. Struct. Mol. Biol. 17, 165.

Liu, S.-Q., Deng, C.-L., Yuan, Z.-M., Rayner, S., Zhang, B., 2015. Identifying the pattern of molecular evolution for Zaire ebolavirus in the 2014 outbreak in West Africa. Infect. Genet. Evol. 32, 51.

Malashkevich, V.N., Schneider, B.J., McNally, M.L., Milhollen, M.A., Pang, J.X., Kim, P.S., 1999. Core structure of the envelope glycoprotein GP2 from Ebola virus at 1.9-Å resolution. Proc. Natl. Acad. Sci. U.S.A. 96, 2662.

Marsh, G.A., Haining, J., Robinson, R., Foord, A., Yamada, M., Barr, J.A., Payne, J., White, J., Yu, M., Bingham, J., 2011. Ebola Reston virus infection of pigs: clinical significance and transmission potential. J. Infect. Dis. 204, S804.

Martinez, O., Ndungo, E., Tantral, L., Miller, E.H., Leung, L.W., Chandran, K., Basler, C.F., 2013. A mutation in the Ebola virus envelope glycoprotein restricts viral entry in a host species-and cell-type-specific manner. J. Virol. 87, 3324.

Maruyama, J., Miyamoto, H., Kajihara, M., Ogawa, H., Maeda, K., Sakoda, Y., Yoshida, R., Takada, A., 2014. Characterization of the envelope glycoprotein of a novel filovirus, Lloviu virus. J. Virol. 88, 99.

Marzi, A., Reinheckel, T., Feldmann, H., 2012. Cathepsin B & L are not required for ebola virus replication. PLoS Negl. Trop. Dis. 6, e1923.

Mateo, M., Carbonnelle, C., Martinez, M.J., Reynard, O., Page, A., Volchkova, V.A., Volchkov, V.E., 2011. Knockdown of Ebola virus VP24 impairs viral nucleocapsid assembly and prevents virus replication. J. Infect. Dis. 204, S892.

Mehedi, M., Falzarano, D., Seebach, J., Hu, X., Carpenter, M.S., Schnittler, H.-J., Feldmann, H., 2011. A new Ebola virus nonstructural glycoprotein expressed through RNA editing. J. Virol. 85, 5406.

Mehedi, M., Hoenen, T., Robertson, S., Ricklefs, S., Dolan, M.A., Taylor, T., Falzarano, D., Ebihara, H., Porcella, S.F., Feldmann, H., 2013. Ebola virus RNA editing depends on the primary editing site sequence and an upstream secondary structure. PLoS Pathog. 9, e1003677.

Miranda, M.E.G., Miranda, N.L.J., 2011. Reston ebolavirus in humans and animals in the Philippines: a review. J. Infect. Dis. 204, S757.

Modrof, J., Becker, S., Mühlberger, E., 2003. Ebola virus transcription activator VP30 is a zinc-binding protein. J. Virol. 77, 3334.

Mohan, G.S., Li, W., Ye, L., Compans, R.W., Yang, C., 2012. Antigenic subversion: a novel mechanism of host immune evasion by Ebola virus. PLoS Pathog. 8, e1003065.

Mühlberger, E., Sanchez, A., Randolf, A., Will, C., Kiley, M.P., Klenk, H.-D., Feldmann, H., 1992. The nucleotide sequence of the L gene of Marburg virus, a filovirus: homologies with paramyxoviruses and rhabdoviruses. Virology 187, 534.

Mühlberger, E., Lötfering, B., Klenk, H.-D., Becker, S., 1998. Three of the four nucleocapsid proteins of Marburg virus, NP, VP35, and L, are sufficient to mediate replication and transcription of Marburg virus-specific monocistronic minigenomes. J. Virol. 72, 8756.

Mühlberger, E., Weik, M., Volchkov, V.E., Klenk, H.-D., Becker, S., 1999. Comparison of the transcription and replication strategies of Marburg virus and Ebola virus by using artificial replication systems. J. Virol. 73, 2333.

Muyembe-Tamfum, J.-J., Mulangu, S., Masumu, J., Kayembe, J., Kemp, A., Paweska, J.T., 2012. Ebola virus outbreaks in Africa: past and present. Onderstepoort J. Vet. Res. 79, 451.

Nanbo, A., Imai, M., Watanabe, S., Noda, T., Takahashi, K., Neumann, G., Halfmann, P., Kawaoka, Y., 2010. Ebolavirus is internalized into host cells via macropinocytosis in a viral glycoprotein-dependent manner. PLoS Pathog. 6, e1001121.

Nanbo, A., Watanabe, S., Halfmann, P., Kawaoka, Y., 2013. The spatio-temporal distribution dynamics of Ebola virus proteins and RNA in infected cells. Sci. Rep. 3, 1206.

Negredo, A., Palacios, G., Vázquez-Morón, S., González, F., Dopazo, H., Molero, F., Juste, J., Quetglas, J., Savji, N., de la Cruz Martínez, M., 2011. Discovery of an ebolavirus-like filovirus in Europe. PLoS Pathog. 7, e1002304.

Neumann, G., Feldmann, H., Watanabe, S., Lukashevich, I., Kawaoka, Y., 2002. Reverse genetics demonstrates that proteolytic processing of the Ebola virus glycoprotein is not essential for replication in cell culture. J. Virol. 76, 406.

Ng, M., Ndungo, E., Kaczmarek, M.E., Herbert, A.S., Binger, T., Kuehne, A.I., Jangra, R.K., Hawkins, J.A., Gifford, R.J., Biswas, R., 2015. Filovirus receptor NPC1 contributes to species-specific patterns of ebolavirus susceptibility in bats. eLife 4, e11785.

Nidom, C.A., Nakayama, E., Nidom, R.V., Alamudi, M.Y., Daulay, S., Dharmayanti, I.N., Dachlan, Y.P., Amin, M., Igarashi, M., Miyamoto, H., 2012. Serological evidence of Ebola virus infection in Indonesian orangutans. PLoS One 7, e40740.

Noda, T., Sagara, H., Suzuki, E., Takada, A., Kida, H., Kawaoka, Y., 2002. Ebola virus VP40 drives the formation of virus-like filamentous particles along with GP. J. Virol. 76, 4855.

Noda, T., Hagiwara, K., Sagara, H., Kawaoka, Y., 2010. Characterization of the Ebola virus nucleoprotein–RNA complex. J. Gen. Virol. 91, 1478.

Ogawa, H., Miyamoto, H., Nakayama, E., Yoshida, R., Nakamura, I., Sawa, H., Ishii, A., Thomas, Y., Nakagawa, E., Matsuno, K., 2015. Seroepidemiological prevalence of multiple species of filoviruses in fruit bats (Eidolon helvum) migrating in Africa. J. Infect. Dis. 212, S101.

Olabode, A.S., Jiang, X., Robertson, D.L., Lovell, S.C., 2015. Ebolavirus is evolving but not changing: no evidence for functional change in EBOV from 1976 to the 2014 outbreak. Virology 482, 202.

Olival, K.J., Islam, A., Yu, M., Anthony, S.J., Epstein, J.H., Khan, S.A., Khan, S.U., Crameri, G., Wang, L.-F., Lipkin, W.I., 2013. Ebola virus antibodies in fruit bats, Bangladesh. Emerg. Infect. Dis. 19, 270.

Pan, Y., Zhang, W., Cui, L., Hua, X., Wang, M., Zeng, Q., 2014. Reston virus in domestic pigs in China. Arch. Virol. 159, 1129–1132.

Patel, M.R., Emerman, M., Malik, H.S., 2011. Paleovirology—ghosts and gifts of viruses past. Curr. Opin. Virol. 1, 304.

Pourrut, X., Souris, M., Towner, J.S., Rollin, P.E., Nichol, S.T., Gonzalez, J.-P., Leroy, E., 2009. Large serological survey showing cocirculation of Ebola and Marburg viruses in Gabonese bat populations, and a high seroprevalence of both viruses in Rousettus aegyptiacus. BMC Infect. Dis. 9, 159.

Prins, K.C., Cárdenas, W.B., Basler, C.F., 2009. Ebola virus protein VP35 impairs the function of interferon regulatory factor-activating kinases IKKε and TBK-1. J. Virol. 83, 3069.

Radoshitzky, S.R., Warfield, K.L., Chi, X., Dong, L., Kota, K., Bradfute, S.B., Gearhart, J.D., Retterer, C., Kranzusch, P.J., Misasi, J.N., 2011. Ebolavirus Δ-peptide immunoadhesins inhibit Marburgvirus and Ebolavirus cell entry. J. Virol. 85, 8502.

Reynard, O., Borowiak, M., Volchkova, V.A., Delpeut, S., Mateo, M., Volchkov, V.E., 2009. Ebolavirus glycoprotein GP masks both its own epitopes and the presence of cellular surface proteins. J. Virol. 83, 9596.

Richman, D.D., Cleveland, P.H., McCormick, J.B., Johnson, K.M., 1983. Antigenic analysis of strains of Ebola virus: identification of two Ebola virus serotypes. J. Infect. Dis. 147, 268.

Rodriguez, L., De Roo, A., Guimard, Y., Trappier, S., Sanchez, A., Bressler, D., Williams, A., Rowe, A., Bertolli, J., Khan, A., 1999. Persistence and genetic stability of Ebola virus during the outbreak in Kikwit, Democratic Republic of the Congo, 1995. J. Infect. Dis. 179, S170.

Rouquet, P., Froment, J.-M., Bermejo, M., Kilbourn, A., Karesh, W., Reed, P., Kumulungui, B., Yaba, P., Délicat, A., Rollin, P.E., 2005. Wild animal mortality monitoring and human Ebola outbreaks, Gabon and Republic of Congo, 2001–2003. Emerg. Infect. Dis. 11, 283.

Ruigrok, R.W., Schoehn, G., Dessen, A., Forest, E., Volchkov, V., Dolnik, O., Klenk, H.-D., Weissenhorn, W., 2000. Structural characterization and membrane binding properties of the matrix protein VP40 of Ebola virus. J. Mol. Biol. 300, 103.

Saeed, M.F., Kolokoltsov, A.A., Albrecht, T., Davey, R.A., 2010. Cellular entry of ebola virus involves uptake by a macropinocytosis-like mechanism and subsequent trafficking through early and late endosomes. PLoS Pathog. 6, e1001110.

Sanchez, A., 2007. Analysis of filovirus entry into vero e6 cells, using inhibitors of endocytosis, endosomal acidification, structural integrity, and cathepsin (B and L) activity. J. Infect. Dis. 196, S251.

Sanchez, A., Rollin, P.E., 2005. Complete genome sequence of an Ebola virus (Sudan species) responsible for a 2000 outbreak of human disease in Uganda. Virus Res. 113, 16.

Sanchez, A., Kiley, M.P., Holloway, B.P., Auperin, D.D., 1993. Sequence analysis of the Ebola virus genome: organization, genetic elements, and comparison with the genome of Marburg virus. Virus Res. 29, 215.

Sanchez, A., Trappier, S.G., Mahy, B., Peters, C.J., Nichol, S.T., 1996. The virion glycoproteins of Ebola viruses are encoded in two reading frames and are expressed through transcriptional editing. Proc. Natl. Acad. Sci. U.S.A. 93, 3602.

Sanchez, A., Ksiazek, T.G., Rollin, P.E., Miranda, M.E., Trappier, S.G., Khan, A.S., Peters, C.J., Nichol, S.T., 1999. Detection and molecular characterization of Ebola viruses causing disease in human and nonhuman primates. J. Infect. Dis. 179, S164.

Schlereth, J., Grünweller, A., Biedenkopf, N., Becker, S., Hartmann, R.K., 2016. RNA binding specificity of Ebola virus transcription factor VP30. RNA Biol. 13, 783.

Schudt, G., Dolnik, O., Kolesnikova, L., Biedenkopf, N., Herwig, A., Becker, S., 2015. Transport of Ebolavirus nucleocapsids is dependent on actin polymerization: live-cell imaging analysis of Ebolavirus-infected cells. J. Infect. Dis. 212, S160.

Scianimanico, S., Schoehn, G., Timmins, J., Ruigrok, R.H., Klenk, H.D., Weissenhorn, W., 2000. Membrane association induces a conformational change in the Ebola virus matrix protein. EMBO J. 19, 6732.

Sharp, P.M., Simmonds, P., 2011. Evaluating the evidence for virus/host co-evolution. Curr. Opin. Virol. 1, 436.

Siegert, R., Shu, H.-L., Slenczka, W., Peters, D., Müller, G., 1967. Zur Ätiologie einer unbekannten, von Affen ausgegangenen menschlichen Infektionskrankheit. Deutsch. Med. Wschr. 92, 2341.

Simmons, G., Reeves, J.D., Grogan, C.C., Vandenberghe, L.H., Baribaud, F., Whitbeck, J.C., Burke, E., Buchmeier, M.J., Soilleux, E.J., Riley, J.L., 2003. DC-SIGN and DC-SIGNR bind ebola glycoproteins and enhance infection of macrophages and endothelial cells. Virology 305, 115.

Slenczka, W., 1999. The Marburg virus outbreak of 1967 and subsequent episodes. Curr. Top. Microbiol. Immunol. 235, 49.

Soni, S.P., Stahelin, R.V., 2014. The Ebola virus matrix protein VP40 selectively induces vesiculation from phosphatidylserine-enriched membranes. J. Biol. Chem. 289, 33590.

Soni, S.P., Adu-Gyamfi, E., Yong, S.S., Jee, C.S., Stahelin, R.V., 2013. The Ebola virus matrix protein deeply penetrates the plasma membrane: an important step in viral egress. Biophys. J. 104, 1940.

Suzuki, Y., Gojobori, T., 1997. The origin and evolution of Ebola and Marburg viruses. Mol. Biol. Evol. 14, 800.

Swanepoel, R., Smit, S.B., Rollin, P.E., Formenty, P., Leman, P.A., Kemp, A., Burt, F.J., Grobbelaar, A.A., Croft, J., Bausch, D.G., 2007. Studies of reservoir hosts for Marburg virus. Emerg. Infect. Dis. 13, 1847.

Taniguchi, S., Watanabe, S., Masangkay, J.S., Omatsu, T., Ikegami, T., Alviola, P., Ueda, N., Iha, K., Fujii, H., Ishii, Y., Mizutani, T., Fukushi, S., Saijo, M., Kurane, I., Kyuwa, S., Akashi, H., Yoshikawa, Y., Morikawa, S., 2011. Reston ebolavirus antibodies in bats, the Philippines. Emerg. Infect. Dis. 17 (8), 1559–1560.

Taylor, D.J., Leach, R.W., Bruenn, J., 2010. Filoviruses are ancient and integrated into mammalian genomes. BMC Evol. Biol. 10, 193.

Taylor, D.J., Dittmar, K., Ballinger, M.J., Bruenn, J.A., 2011. Evolutionary maintenance of filovirus-like genes in bat genomes. BMC Evol. Biol. 11, 336.

Taylor, D.J., Ballinger, M.J., Zhan, J.J., Hanzly, L.E., Bruenn, J.A., 2014. Evidence that ebolaviruses and cuevaviruses have been diverging from marburgviruses since the Miocene. PeerJ 2, e556.

Timmins, J., Schoehn, G., Kohlhaas, C., Klenk, H.-D., Ruigrok, R.W., Weissenhorn, W., 2003. Oligomerization and polymerization of the filovirus matrix protein VP40. Virology 312, 359.

Towner, J.S., Rollin, P.E., Bausch, D.G., Sanchez, A., Crary, S.M., Vincent, M., Lee, W.F., Spiropoulou, C.F., Ksiazek, T.G., Lukwiya, M., 2004. Rapid diagnosis of Ebola hemorrhagic fever by reverse transcription-PCR in an outbreak setting and assessment of patient viral load as a predictor of outcome. J. Virol. 78, 4330.

Towner, J.S., Khristova, M.L., Sealy, T.K., Vincent, M.J., Erickson, B.R., Bawiec, D.A., Hartman, A.L., Comer, J.A., Zaki, S.R., Ströher, U., 2006. Marburgvirus genomics and association with a large hemorrhagic fever outbreak in Angola. J. Virol. 80, 6497.

Towner, J.S., Sealy, T.K., Khristova, M.L., Albariño, C.G., Conlan, S., Reeder, S.A., Quan, P.-L., Lipkin, W.I., Downing, R., Tappero, J.W., 2008. Newly discovered ebola virus associated with hemorrhagic fever outbreak in Uganda. PLoS Pathog. 4, e1000212.

Towner, J.S., Amman, B.R., Sealy, T.K., Carroll, S.A.R., Comer, J.A., Kemp, A., Swanepoel, R., Paddock, C.D., Balinandi, S., Khristova, M.L., 2009. Isolation of genetically diverse Marburg viruses from Egyptian fruit bats. PLoS Pathog. 5, e1000536.

Urbanowicz, R.A., McClure, C.P., Sakuntabhai, A., Sall, A.A., Kobinger, G., Müller, M.A., Holmes, E.C., Rey, F.A., Simon-Loriere, E., Ball, J.K., 2016. Human adaptation of Ebola virus during the West African outbreak. Cell 167, 1079.

Valmas, C., Grosch, M.N., Schümann, M., Olejnik, J., Martinez, O., Best, S.M., Krähling, V., Basler, C.F., Mühlberger, E., 2010. Marburg virus evades interferon responses by a mechanism distinct from ebola virus. PLoS Pathog. 6, e1000721.

Volchkov, V.E., Blinov, V.M., Netesov, S.V., 1992. The envelope glycoprotein of Ebola virus contains an immunosuppressive-like domain similar to oncogenic retroviruses. FEBS Lett. 305, 181.

Volchkov, V.E., Becker, S., Volchkova, V.A., Ternovoj, V.A., Kotov, A.N., Netesov, S.V., Klenk, H.-D., 1995. GP mRNA of Ebola virus is edited by the Ebola virus polymerase and by T7 and vaccinia virus polymerases. Virology 214, 421.

Volchkov, V.E., Volchkova, V.A., Slenczka, W., Klenk, H.-D., Feldmann, H., 1998a. Release of viral glycoproteins during Ebola virus infection. Virology 245, 110.

Volchkov, V.E., Feldmann, H., Volchkova, V.A., Klenk, H.-D., 1998b. Processing of the Ebola virus glycoprotein by the proprotein convertase furin. Proc. Natl. Acad. Sci. U.S.A. 95, 5762.

Volchkov, V.E., Volchkova, V.A., Chepurnov, A.A., Blinov, V.M., Dolnik, O., Netesov, S.V., Feldmann, H., 1999. Characterization of the L gene and 5' trailer region of Ebola virus. J. Gen. Virol. 80, 355.

Volchkova, V.A., Klenk, H.-D., Volchkov, V.E., 1999. Delta-peptide is the carboxy-terminal cleavage fragment of the nonstructural small glycoprotein sGP of Ebola virus. Virology 265, 164.

Wahl-Jensen, V.M., Afanasieva, T.A., Seebach, J., Ströher, U., Feldmann, H., Schnittler, H.-J., 2005. Effects of Ebola virus glycoproteins on endothelial cell activation and barrier function. J. Virol. 79, 10442.

Wamala, J.F., Lukwago, L., Malimbo, M., Nguku, P., Yoti, Z., Musenero, M., Amone, J., Mbabazi, W., Nanyunja, M., Zaramba, S., 2010. Ebola hemorrhagic fever associated with novel virus strain, Uganda, 2007–2008. Emerg. Infect. Dis. 16, 1087.

Wang, L.-F., Harcourt, B.H., Yu, M., Tamin, A., Rota, P.A., Bellini, W.J., Eaton, B.T., 2001. Molecular biology of Hendra and Nipah viruses. Microbes Infect. 3, 279.

Wang, H., Shi, Y., Song, J., Qi, J., Lu, G., Yan, J., Gao, G.F., 2016. Ebola viral glycoprotein bound to its endosomal receptor Niemann-Pick C1. Cell 164, 258.

Watanabe, S., Noda, T., Kawaoka, Y., 2006. Functional mapping of the nucleoprotein of Ebola virus. J. Virol. 80, 3743.

Watanabe, S., Noda, T., Halfmann, P., Jasenosky, L., Kawaoka, Y., 2007. Ebola virus (EBOV) VP24 inhibits transcription and replication of the EBOV genome. J. Infect. Dis. 196, S284.

Watt, A., Moukambi, F., Banadyga, L., Groseth, A., Callison, J., Herwig, A., Ebihara, H., Feldmann, H., Hoenen, T., 2014. A novel life cycle modeling system for Ebola virus shows a genome length-dependent role of VP24 in virus infectivity. J. Virol. 88, 10511.

Weik, M., Modrof, J., Klenk, H.-D., Becker, S., Mühlberger, E., 2002. Ebola virus VP30-mediated transcription is regulated by RNA secondary structure formation. J. Virol. 76, 8532.

Weik, M., Enterlein, S., Schlenz, K., Mühlberger, E., 2005. The Ebola virus genomic replication promoter is bipartite and follows the rule of six. J. Virol. 79, 10660.

Weissenhorn, W., Calder, L.J., Wharton, S.A., Skehel, J.J., Wiley, D.C., 1998a. The central structural feature of the membrane fusion protein subunit from the Ebola virus glycoprotein is a long triple-stranded coiled coil. Proc. Natl. Acad. Sci. U.S.A. 95, 6032.

Weissenhorn, W., Carfi, A., Lee, K.-H., Skehel, J.J., Wiley, D.C., 1998b. Crystal structure of the Ebola virus membrane fusion subunit, GP2, from the envelope glycoprotein ectodomain. Mol. Cell 2, 605.

Wertheim, J.O., Kosakovsky Pond, S.L., 2011. Purifying selection can obscure the ancient age of viral lineages. Mol. Biol. Evol. 28, 3355.

Whelan, S., Barr, J., Wertz, G., 2004. Transcription and replication of nonsegmented negative-strand RNA viruses. In: Kawaoka, Y. (Ed.), Biology of Negative Strand RNA Viruses: The Power of Reverse Genetics. Springer, p. 61.

WHO, 1978a. Ebola haemorrhagic fever in Sudan, 1976. Bull. World Health Organ. 56, 247.

WHO, 1978b. Ebola haemorrhagic fever in Zaire, 1976. Bull. World Health Organ. 56, 271.

WHO, 2016. Ebola Situation Report—2 March. World Health Organisation, Geneva, Switzerland.

Wool-Lewis, R.J., Bates, P., 1999. Endoproteolytic processing of the Ebola virus envelope glycoprotein: cleavage is not required for function. J. Virol. 73, 1419.

Yaddanapudi, K., Palacios, G., Towner, J.S., Chen, I., Sariol, C.A., Nichol, S.T., Lipkin, W.I., 2006. Implication of a retrovirus-like glycoprotein peptide in the immunopathogenesis of Ebola and Marburg viruses. FASEB J. 20, 2519.

Yuan, J., Zhang, Y., Li, J., Zhang, Y., Wang, L.-F., Shi, Z., 2012. Serological evidence of ebolavirus infection in bats, China. Virol. J. 9, 236.

CHAPTER TEN

An Orchestra of Reovirus Receptors: Still Searching for the Conductor

Danica M. Sutherland*,2, Pavithra Aravamudhan†,2, Terence S. Dermody†,1

*Vanderbilt University School of Medicine, Nashville, TN, United States
†University of Pittsburgh School of Medicine, Pittsburgh, PA, United States
1Corresponding author: e-mail address: terence.dermody@chp.edu

Contents

Abstract

Viruses are constantly engaged in a molecular arms race with the host, where efficient and tactical use of cellular receptors benefits critical steps in infection. Receptor use dictates initiation, establishment, and spread of viral infection to new tissues and hosts. Mammalian orthoreoviruses (reoviruses) are pervasive pathogens that use multiple receptors to overcome protective host barriers to disseminate from sites of initial infection and cause disease in young mammals. In particular, reovirus invades the central nervous system (CNS) with serotype-dependent tropism and disease. A single viral gene, encoding the attachment protein σ1, segregates with distinct patterns of CNS injury. Despite the identification and characterization of several reovirus receptors, host factors that dictate tropism via interaction with σ1 remain undefined. Here, we summarize the state of the reovirus receptor field and discuss open questions toward understanding how the reovirus attachment protein dictates CNS tropism.

---

2 Cofirst authors; contributed equally.

Advances in Virus Research, Volume 100
ISSN 0065-3527
https://doi.org/10.1016/bs.aivir.2017.10.005

1. INTRODUCTION

As obligate intracellular parasites, viruses must overcome an initial, critical barrier to succeed in infection: the cell membrane. Viral surface proteins engage host molecules, broadly termed as receptors, on target cell surfaces or within endocytic compartments to facilitate passage across membranes and access the cytosol. These receptors encompass a diverse array of molecules, including proteins, lipids, carbohydrates, or combinations of each. Viruses often bind several receptors to gain cell entry, as opposed to a simple interaction of a single virus protein with a host factor in a "lock-and-key" fashion. Multiple distinct receptors may be used on the same cell in a coordinated binding event or on different cell types within the host to mediate dissemination from sites of primary replication. Receptor engagement also can trigger signaling cascades to remodel host membranes, rearrange the cytoskeleton, or activate or suppress host immune responses (Danthi, 2011; Luisoni et al., 2015; Ong et al., 2016; Taylor et al., 2011). As the first, often multifunctional, step in the viral life cycle, receptors serve as attractive targets for prophylactic and therapeutic interventions.

Virus–receptor interactions vary greatly in stoichiometry and complexity, which can pose challenges in their study. Many viruses initially bind an "attachment factor" to dock onto the host cell for adhesion strengthening (Jolly and Sattentau, 2013). This mechanism narrows the search for high-affinity receptors to a two-dimensional membrane surface and aids the virus in locating receptors with specialized cellular distributions (e.g., receptors present in low abundance or localized to specific microdomains such as tight junctions). For example, to infect intestinal epithelial cells, group B coxsackieviruses bind to an apically localized, highly abundant protein called CD55/decay-accelerating factor (DAF) (Coyne and Bergelson, 2006). DAF binding triggers actin reorganization for translocation of the virus to tight junctions, where it can engage coxsackievirus and adenovirus receptor to undergo endocytosis (Coyne and Bergelson, 2006). In cases like hepatitis C virus, receptor-mediated entry is exceptionally complex, requiring interaction with more than four different cell-surface factors (Li et al., 2016; Lindenbach and Rice, 2013). While some viruses enter the cytosol at the plasma membrane, those internalized via endocytic routes must escape endosomal compartments. For many viruses, endosomal acidification, either directly or through proteolytic processing, triggers conformational changes in viral surface proteins to promote fusion with or penetration of endosomal membranes (White and Whittaker, 2016). However, for viruses like Ebola virus (Carette et al., 2011; Cote et al., 2011) and Lassa virus (Jae et al., 2014), engagement of an additional endosomal receptor is necessary for cytoplasmic entry. Despite these complexities in receptor use, many viruses employ similar strategies, and in some cases, even converge to use the same receptor families, to traverse host membrane barriers.

Virus interactions with receptors that exhibit tissue-specific expression in the host can dictate tropism and disease. For example, most human influenza virus strains engage $\alpha2,6$-linked sialic acid (SA) in the upper respiratory tract, but mutations in the receptor-binding domain of the viral attachment protein can alter binding specificity to target the more abundantly expressed $\alpha2,3$-linked SA in the lower respiratory tract, leading to more virulent disease (de Graaf and Fouchier, 2014). Receptor use also alters the capacity of a virus to transmit between species (Imai et al., 2012; Longdon et al., 2014) and receptor polymorphisms can limit virus infection to one or just a few species. For example, hepatitis B virus infection is restricted to humans, chimpanzees, and tree shrews. While the murine homolog of the hepatitis B receptor does not support virus entry, a chimeric murine receptor with a four amino acid replacement from the human receptor is sufficient to allow virus entry and replication (Yan et al., 2013). In addition, transgenic mice expressing the human receptor are susceptible to infection (Guidotti et al., 1995). In contrast, viruses that infect diverse host species commonly bind highly conserved receptor interfaces, thus promoting cross-species infection (Bhella, 2015; Woolhouse et al., 2012).

Mammalian orthoreoviruses (which will be referred to as reoviruses here) exhibit many of these complexities of virus–receptor interactions. Reoviruses engage multiple receptors to infect and spread systemically in young mammals and exhibit serotype-specific tropism and patterns of disease. There are three distinct serotypes of reovirus, with type 1 (T1) and type 3 (T3) being the best characterized. T1 and T3 reoviruses display comparable infection at sites of primary replication in the intestine and lungs but diverge in dissemination routes, central nervous system (CNS) tropism, and subsequent pathology. Reovirus research has led to the discovery of important, conserved mechanisms in virus cell biology and disease pathogenesis (Dermody et al., 2013). With ease of culture, efficient reverse genetics (Kanai et al., 2017; Kobayashi et al., 2010), and comparable disease across many well-established small animal models (Margolis and Kilham, 1969; Milhorat and Kotzen, 1994), questions about reovirus biology are attractive, addressable, and applicable to other systems. This review will describe what is known about reovirus–receptor interactions and their functions in serotype-specific tropism and disease, with a focus on the CNS, and discuss open questions in the field for further exploration.

2. REOVIRUS BACKGROUND

Reovirus displays a broad species tropism, causing age-restricted disease in many mammalian species, including mice, ferrets, rabbits, and pigs. While reovirus clinical manifestations in humans are rarely severe (Hermann et al., 2004; Johansson et al., 1996; Stanley et al., 1953; Tyler et al., 2004; Van Tongeren, 1957), strains isolated from human stools during a gastroenteritis outbreak induce lethal disease in animals (Sabin, 1959). Related *Reoviridae* members also cause severe disease. For example, rotavirus is a leading cause of gastroenteritis worldwide in young children, with over 215,000 estimated deaths in 2013 (Tate et al., 2016), and baboon reovirus initiates a fulminant meningoencephalitis in primates (Leland et al., 2000). Reovirus infection in animal models induces manifestations such as biliary inflammation, pneumonia, hydrocephalus, myocarditis, meningitis, and encephalitis (Dermody et al., 2013). Additionally, reovirus induces loss of oral tolerance in mice to food antigens such as gluten, making it a potential trigger for human disorders like celiac disease (Bouziat et al., 2017). Finally, reovirus exhibits preferential cytotoxicity in cancer cells and is being assessed in clinical trials as an oncolytic agent (Chakrabarty et al., 2015). Therefore, understanding mechanisms of reovirus pathogenesis and specific molecular interactions that dictate reovirus tropism could inform a diverse number of fields.

Reovirus particles are nonenveloped with two concentric capsid layers that encase 10 segments of double-stranded RNA. The viral genome encodes eight structural and three nonstructural proteins. The outer capsid is composed of repeating hexameric arrangements of σ3 in complex with μ1, interrupted at the 12 icosahedral vertices by pentameric arrangements of λ2 (Fig. 1A). The viral attachment protein, σ1, embeds in a turret formed by λ2 pentamers. σ1 is a long, filamentous trimer that can extend ~40 nm away from the capsid, doubling the virion diameter (Fig. 1A and B). Three σ1 monomers interweave to form tail, body, and head domains (Fig. 1B). The σ1 trimer structure has an α-helical coiled-coil tail domain that is anchored to the virion (Nagata et al., 1987; Nibert et al., 1990), followed by the body domain composed of β-spiral repeats interrupted by a short

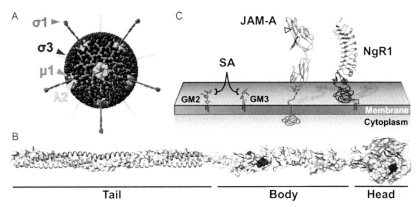

Fig. 1 The reovirus attachment protein σ1 engages multiple receptors. (A) The reovirus virion (2CSE) (Zhang et al., 2005) is modeled to scale with an extended conformer of σ1 (*gray*). Outer-capsid proteins σ3 (*blue*), μ1 (*green*), and λ2 (*yellow*) are indicated. (B) A model of reovirus attachment protein σ1 is shown in a ribbon diagram (*gray*), with one monomer of the trimer surface-shaded. Receptor-binding sites are colored for T1 SA (*red*), T3 SA (*blue*), and JAM-A (*green*). The tail, body, and head domains are indicated. The model was generated by linking the crystal structure of the T3 σ1 body and head (3S6X) with a predicted coiled-coil tail (Reiter et al., 2011). (C) Known reovirus receptors are shown to scale with the σ1 model displayed in (B). Representative sialylated glycans that bind T1 (GM2, *red*) and T3 (GM3, *blue*) σ1 are displayed as glycolipids but are also found linked to cellular proteins. The terminal SA moiety is indicated. JAM-A (1NBQ, *green*) (Kirchner et al., 2008; Prota et al., 2003) residues important for both JAM-A homodimerization and σ1 ligation are shown in *gray* and indicated with an *arrowhead*. Region of NgR1 (1OZN, *purple*) (He et al., 2003) that engages reovirus is unknown.

α-helix (Reiter et al., 2011), and terminates in a head domain composed of three β-barrel motifs (Reiss et al., 2012; Reiter et al., 2011).

Originally identified as the viral hemagglutinin for its capacity to agglutinate red blood cells (Weiner et al., 1978), σ1 is the primary target of the neutralizing antibody response and thus dictates the serotype (Weiner and Fields, 1977). The σ1 protein binds multiple receptors and is required for entry into all cells tested thus far. However, other capsid components also contribute to engagement of host factors for efficient cell entry (Konopka-Anstadt et al., 2014; Maginnis et al., 2006; Thete et al., 2016). Following σ1-mediated binding to cells, reovirus is internalized primarily through clathrin-mediated endocytosis (Maginnis et al., 2008). After internalization, outer-capsid proteins σ3 and μ1 undergo acid-dependent proteolytic processing to generate infectious subvirion particles (ISVPs), which lack σ3, contain cleaved μ1 fragments (Coombs, 1998; Sturzenbecker et al., 1987), and are hypothesized to display a more extended conformer of σ1 (Dietrich et al., 2017; Dryden et al., 1993). Further μ1 processing and loss of σ1 enables endosomal membrane penetration and release of the transcriptionally active viral core into the cytoplasm (Chandran and Nibert, 2003; Coombs, 1998; Silverstein et al., 1972). Fragments of µ1 entering the cytosol trigger apoptotic signaling (Danthi et al., 2008). Following genome replication and new particle assembly, reovirus progeny use both lytic and nonlytic pathways to exit infected cells (Excoffon et al., 2008; Lai et al., 2013).

Reovirus transmission occurs primarily through fecal-oral routes (Keroack and Fields, 1986). Following oral inoculation of newborn mice, reovirus establishes primary infection in intestinal epithelium and lymphoid tissue (Antar et al., 2009; Bass et al., 1988; Wolf et al., 1981), spreading systemically to several sites of secondary replication, including the CNS (Fig. 2A–C). The means of spread and sites of CNS infection depend on the viral serotype. T1 viruses spread hematogenously to infect ependymal cells and cause hydrocephalus, whereas T3 viruses spread by both hematogenous and neural routes to infect neurons, inducing apoptosis and lethal encephalitis (Oberhaus et al., 1997; Pruijssers et al., 2013) (Fig. 2A–C). Differences in spread, tropism, and disease caused by the two serotypes segregate genetically with the viral attachment protein, σ1. T1 σ1 preferentially binds ependymal cells (Tardieu and Weiner, 1982), and T3 σ1 preferentially binds neurons (Dichter and Weiner, 1984), suggesting that the σ1 protein mediates these disparate disease manifestations by binding distinct receptors on these cells. Despite identification and characterization of several cellular receptors for reovirus, host determinants of the serotype-dependent, σ1-mediated differences in tropism are not fully understood.

3. SIALIC ACID IS A SEROTYPE-SPECIFIC REOVIRUS ATTACHMENT FACTOR

Many viruses use cell-surface carbohydrates as attachment factors to enhance infectivity. While carbohydrates terminating in SA are commonly bound, neutrally charged glycans and glycosaminoglycans promote adhesion strengthening for different viruses (Haywood, 1994; Matrosovich et al., 2015; Stroh and Stehle, 2014). SAs are a heterogeneous family of more than 50 monosaccharides that share a nine carbon core (Varki and Schauer, 2009). The complexity of the SA family stems not just from varied glycosidic linkages and chemical modifications, but also from the glycans and structures to which they are linked. As the most common terminal glycan on oligosaccharides anchored to proteins or lipids, SA is expressed by all vertebrate cell

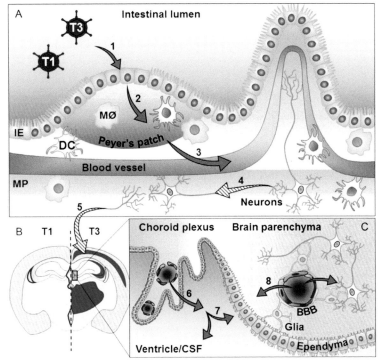

Fig. 2 Hematogenous and neural spread of reovirus to the CNS. (A) Reovirus bypasses harsh stomach conditions, intestinal bacteria, and mucus layers to translocate across the intestinal epithelial barrier (1) and access the bloodstream. In the intestine, reovirus infects cells in the intestinal epithelium (IE), lamina propria, and Peyer's patches (DC, dendritic cell; Mφ, macrophage) (2). When JAM-A is present, both T1 and T3 reovirus can invade the bloodstream efficiently to establish viremia (3). T3 reovirus also can access, infect, and traffic through neurons innervating the intestine, particularly in the myenteric plexus (MP) (4), and travel along the vagus nerve to invade the CNS (5). (B) Regions infected by T1 (*left*) and T3 (*right*) are shaded in the two halves of a coronally sectioned mouse brain. (C) Virus in the bloodstream may enter the CNS by crossing the blood–brain barrier (BBB) or exploiting gaps in the BBB, such as in the fenestrated blood capillaries of the choroid plexus (6). For T1, choroid plexus infection would provide direct access to ependymal cells throughout the ventricles (7). For T3, hematogenous spread into the CNS could be promoted by infection of glial cells (*yellow*) or neurons (*gray*) proximal to vasculature (8).

types and mediates many important physiological processes such as cell–cell adhesion and protein stability (Varki and Schauer, 2009). The broad distribution and abundance of SA is likely why many different viruses, including reoviruses, have converged to interact with SA as a receptor. Most reovirus field-isolate strains engage SA as an attachment factor at the cell surface to mediate adhesion strengthening. The low-affinity interaction of reovirus with SA allows rapid on–off kinetics (Barton et al., 2001a) and affords an opportunity for reovirus to sample nearby SAs and other cell-surface moieties to eventually engage in higher-affinity contacts with a receptor capable of mediating entry. Engagement of SA alone is not thought to yield a productive infection for reovirus. However, virus binding to SA could fortuitously allow its uptake by an internalization event already underway.

Despite similarities in sequence and structure, T1 and T3 σ1 use different domains to engage distinct sialylated glycans. For both serotypes, each σ1 monomer has an independent SA-binding site (Reiss et al., 2012; Reiter et al., 2011). T1 reoviruses specifically bind the terminal α2,3-linked N-acetyl-SA on GM2 glycan (displayed on glycoproteins or GM2 ganglioside) in a shallow groove located on the σ1 head domain (Reiss et al., 2012; Stencel-Baerenwald et al., 2015) (Fig. 1B and C). In contrast, T3 strains demonstrate more promiscuous glycan engagement and bind terminal α2,3-, α2,6-, or α2,8-linked SA using a deeper, larger groove located in the σ1 body domain (Reiter et al., 2011) (Fig. 1B and C). Point mutations engineered in these binding grooves specifically abrogate glycan engagement and convert SA-binding strains (referred to as SA$^+$) to non-SA-binding strains (referred to as SA$^-$). For example, two point mutations in the SA-binding groove of a prototype T1 strain, T1L, convert a T1 SA$^+$ virus to a T1 SA$^-$ virus (Stencel-Baerenwald et al., 2015). Multiple single amino acid polymorphisms in T3 σ1 generate T3 SA$^-$ viruses in different genetic backgrounds (Barton et al., 2003; Reiter et al., 2011; Weiner et al., 1980). These non-SA-binding strains are colloquially referred to as "glycan-blind" and have been instrumental in defining the contribution of SA engagement to reovirus infection of specific cell types.

SA binding is required for efficient reovirus attachment and infection of many cell types in vitro. Most commonly, cellular glycan requirements for binding and infection are demonstrated genetically using glycan-blind viruses or cell lines deficient in glycan expression, or chemically using neuraminidase to remove terminal SAs or lectins to block virus access to SA. Reovirus demonstrates little to no SA requirement for infection of some cell types, such as L929 fibroblasts. Diminishing reovirus access to SA on these cells using the methods mentioned above has a negligible effect on binding or infectivity, and different serotypes replicate comparably (Connolly et al., 2001; Reiss et al., 2012; Reiter et al., 2011). However, infection of other cell types, such as primary murine embryonic fibroblasts, is efficient only with T1 or T3 strains that exhibit intact glycan-binding capacity

(Connolly et al., 2001; Reiss et al., 2012). SA engagement also can permit reovirus infection in a serotype-specific manner. For example, murine erythroleukemia T3cl.2 cells are susceptible only to T3 glycan-binding strains (Reiter et al., 2011). These cell type-specific differences in glycan-requirement for infection are likely attributable to the relative abundance of other reovirus receptors present (Reiss et al., 2012). Interestingly, most cell lines that demonstrate glycan-dependent reovirus infection are more efficiently bound and infected by T3 strains, and, to our knowledge, no cell line has been identified that is exclusively susceptible to infection by T1 strains, likely demonstrating a significant consequence of the more promiscuous SA-binding capacity of T3 reovirus.

The function of SA engagement in reovirus-mediated cell signaling is unclear. Compared to T3 SA^-, T3 SA^+ virus induces more robust apoptosis in L929 fibroblasts, despite the two strains replicating comparably (Connolly et al., 2001). Preincubation of T3 SA^+ virus with sialylated glycans or pre-treatment of cells with neuraminidase abrogates apoptosis induction to the level of T3 SA^-, under the conditions tested (Connolly et al., 2001). It is not clear whether SA binding activates proapoptotic signaling pathways or alters other steps in viral infection like membrane lipid clustering, internalization, or virus disassembly, as has been observed for other viruses. For example, multivalent engagement of SA by influenza virus leads to clustering of lipid rafts (Eierhoff et al., 2010). Such ligand-induced clustering activates the epidermal growth factor receptor and leads to influenza virus internalization (Eierhoff et al., 2010; Hofman et al., 2010). While σ1 is capable of ligating multiple SA glycans simultaneously (Reiss et al., 2012; Reiter et al., 2011), it is unclear whether this occurs on the cell surface or whether SA ligation can mediate signaling processes in the absence of other receptors.

SA engagement contributes to reovirus pathogenesis and disease outcome (Barton et al., 2003). T1 and T3 glycan-blind viruses induce less severe disease in the CNS, compared to the cognate glycan-binding viruses. Following intracranial inoculation, T1 SA^- induces significantly less severe hydrocephalus than T1 SA^+, but reaches similar peak titers in the brain (Stencel-Baerenwald et al., 2015). Interestingly, ependymal infection is more localized to the inoculation site for T1 SA^-, suggesting that this virus may not efficiently disseminate through the ventricles (Stencel-Baerenwald et al., 2015). Reduced infectivity of T1 SA^- compared to T1 SA^+ also is observed in a human ependymoma xenograft model (Stencel-Baerenwald et al., 2015). A similar trend is true for T3 viruses. Following peroral inoculation of newborn mice, both T3 SA^+ and SA^- viruses establish efficient replication in the intestine, but T3 SA$^+$ is detected sooner at distant sites like the spleen, liver, and brain, suggesting an advantage in dissemination efficiency (Barton et al., 2003). However, T3 SA$^-$ reaches similar peak titers at later time points (Barton et al., 2003). In the CNS, T3 SA$^+$ often replicates to higher titers, induces more apoptosis, and is more neurovirulent than T3 SA$^-$ (Barton et al., 2003; Frierson et al., 2012). Cultured primary murine cortical neurons also are more susceptible to T3 SA$^+$ than T3 SA$^-$ infection (Frierson et al., 2012). However, while T3 SA$^+$ is more neurovirulent, both T3 SA$^+$ and SA$^-$ exhibit comparable CNS tropism. (Frierson et al., 2012). Therefore, although diminished SA-binding capacity alters the virulence of T1 and T3 reovirus, the tropism remains unaltered, suggesting that SA functions as an attachment factor and not as a tropism determinant in reovirus CNS infection.

4. JUNCTIONAL ADHESION MOLECULE A IS REQUIRED FOR HEMATOGENOUS DISSEMINATION OF REOVIRUS

Expression-cloning techniques have been used in the discovery of many viral receptors, including those for HIV (Deng et al., 1997), HCV (Evans et al., 2007), and measles virus (Tatsuo et al., 2000). This strategy involves transfection of cDNAs from susceptible cells into normally non-susceptible cells to identify cDNA constructs that confer virus binding capacity (Aruffo and Seed, 1987). To screen for a reovirus receptor, the cDNA library from a neuroblastoma cell line was transfected into non-susceptible COS-7 cells. These cells were screened for reovirus binding using T3 SA$^-$ as the affinity ligand to eliminate the potential confounding variable of SA binding. Using this strategy, junctional adhesion molecule A (JAM-A) was identified as a receptor for reovirus (Barton et al., 2001b).

JAM-A is an immunoglobulin superfamily glycoprotein that is grouped in the functional class of cell adhesion molecules (CAMs) (Martin-Padura et al., 1998; Williams et al., 1999). JAM-A is expressed by hematopoietic, endothelial, and epithelial cells, as well as some types of glial cells (Hwang et al., 2013; Stelzer et al., 2010). It serves critical functions in the maintenance of tight junction integrity and immune cell migration across epithelial and endothelial barriers (Del Maschio et al., 1999; Liu et al., 2000). Many tight junction proteins and immunoglobulin superfamily proteins, both CAMs and non-CAMs, serve as receptors for a variety of viruses (Bhella, 2015; Dermody et al., 2009). Distribution of these proteins to tight junctions would appear to impose a barrier to virus access. However, the repeated selection of tight junction proteins by widely different classes of viruses suggests a selective advantage in using these proteins for cell entry. This advantage could arise from the localization of these proteins, because viruses must cross barriers formed by epithelial and endothelial cells to gain access to sites of secondary replication. Infection of cells localized at junctions and subsequent release into the lumen provides a strategy for bloodstream access and systemic spread of virus.

JAM-A has two immunoglobulin-like extracellular domains, a transmembrane domain, and a short cytoplasmic tail that functions in intracellular signaling (Fig. 1C) (Kostrewa et al., 2001). The membrane-distal immunoglobulin domain engages in homotypic and heterotypic interactions at the cell surface (Kostrewa et al., 2001). Reovirus binds to JAM-A at this homodimerization surface via conserved residues within the head domain of $\sigma 1$ (Kirchner et al., 2008; Stettner et al., 2015). This interaction is serotype-independent; all prototype and field-isolate strains of the three reovirus serotypes tested to date use JAM-A as a receptor (Campbell et al., 2005; Stettner et al., 2015). The outer-capsid protein $\mu 1$ enhances reovirus binding to JAM-A-expressing cells by an unknown mechanism (Thete et al., 2016). This binding enhancement is serotype-dependent and displayed by T3 $\mu 1$ in a T1 background. $\sigma 1$ binds to JAM-A with a 1000-fold higher affinity than JAM-A for itself, which likely disrupts the homodimeric JAM-A interaction (Kirchner et al., 2008). Dimer disruption is a common mechanism to trigger CAM internalization and intracellular signaling (Salinas et al., 2014). Disruption of JAM-A dimers by $\sigma 1$ could function similarly to induce signaling and recruit additional interaction partners to internalize reovirus. There is evidence that JAM-A-mediated reovirus entry enhances apoptosis induction in cultured cells (Barton et al., 2001b). Interruption of JAM-A–reovirus interactions using a monoclonal antibody specific for JAM-A significantly decreases apoptosis without diminishing viral replication. However, JAM-A-independent, antibody-mediated uptake of reovirus into cells also efficiently induces apoptosis (Danthi et al., 2006), suggesting that reovirus triggers apoptotic signaling independent of the receptor mediating entry. Further work is required to define the function of JAM-A–reovirus interactions in apoptosis induction.

As a tight junction protein, the subcellular distribution of JAM-A is dynamically regulated to control junction plasticity. JAM-A is internalized into cells by multiple endocytic mechanisms, and both intra- and extracellular domains of JAM-A function in signaling and JAM-A internalization (Stamatovic et al., 2017). However, the intracellular domain of JAM-A is dispensable for internalization of reovirus (Maginnis et al., 2006), suggesting that other molecules coordinate signaling to internalize JAM-A–reovirus complexes. The extracellular domain of JAM-A interacts with integrins and integrin-associated proteins (Severson and Parkos, 2009), and expression of $\beta 1$ integrin is required for efficient reovirus entry in cultured cells (Maginnis et al., 2006, 2008). Integrins are transmembrane CAM proteins used by several viruses as attachment or internalization receptors (Guerrero et al., 2000; Schmidt et al., 2013; Wickham et al., 1993). For example, adenovirus binds an immunoglobulin superfamily receptor using a filamentous trimer that resembles reovirus $\sigma 1$ (Chappell et al., 2002) and subsequently undergoes integrin-dependent internalization (Wickham et al., 1993). Reovirus outer-capsid protein $\lambda 2$ contains conserved integrin-binding motifs that could mediate internalization via integrin interactions. Such interactions, however, are not required for reovirus binding to cells, suggesting that integrins function at a postbinding entry step (Maginnis et al., 2006). NPXY motifs in the cytoplasmic tail of $\beta 1$ integrin mediate sorting of cellular cargo, and mutations in this domain lead to mislocalization of internalized reovirus to lysosomes (Maginnis et al., 2008). These findings support an important role for $\beta 1$ integrin in reovirus infection, yet mechanisms of integrin-mediated internalization and sorting of reovirus remain to be defined.

JAM-A plays an essential role in hematogenous dissemination of both T1 and T3 reovirus from the intestine. Interestingly, primary replication of the virus in intestinal epithelium and other resident intestinal cells does not require JAM-A (Antar et al., 2009). To disseminate hematogenously, reovirus must first cross the endothelial barrier of the intestinal vasculature (Fig. 2A). JAM-A could facilitate this process through multiple potential mechanisms, including: (i) mediating virus binding to or infection of circulating leukocytes to penetrate the endothelial barrier, (ii) permitting virus to directly breach tight junctions, or (iii) enabling endothelial cell infection followed by apical release into the vascular lumen. Studies of reovirus infection using mice with tissue-specific knockdown of JAM-A revealed that hematopoietic expression of JAM-A is dispensable for the establishment of viremia, ruling out the first possibility (Lai et al., 2015). Additionally, disruption of endothelial cell tight junction integrity in vitro (Lai et al., 2013) or vasculature permeability in vivo (Lai et al., 2015) was not observed following reovirus infection. However, endothelial JAM-A is required for both reovirus entry and egress from the bloodstream, suggesting that JAM-A-dependent uptake, amplification, and apical release of reovirus by polarized endothelial cells promote viremia and systemic spread of reovirus (Fig. 2A) (Lai et al., 2013, 2015). Further work is required to establish the mechanism by which JAM-A promotes endothelium infection and bloodstream spread.

Although JAM-A is required for hematogenous spread of reovirus, it is dispensable for neural dissemination. Intracranial or intramuscular inoculation of virus provides direct access to neural routes to study the influence of receptors on neural spread of reovirus. Following intramuscular inoculation of wild-type mice, T3 reovirus infects sensory and motor neurons to travel the length of the spinal cord and reach the brain (Flamand et al., 1991). Following intramuscular inoculation of mice with genetic ablation of JAM-A (JAM-A$^{-/-}$), T3 viral titers increase in the spinal cord, suggesting that neural pathways of infection are intact (Antar et al., 2009). Furthermore, following intracranial inoculation, T3 virus tropism, replication, and virulence in the CNS are comparable in wild-type and JAM-A$^{-/-}$ mice. Infection of cortical neurons cultured from JAM-A$^{-/-}$ mice also demonstrates that JAM-A is dispensable for neuronal infection. Combined, these data suggest that additional receptors exist to mediate serotype-dependent neural spread and infection of T3 reovirus.

5. NOGO-66 RECEPTOR 1 IS A NEURAL RECEPTOR FOR REOVIRUS

Nogo-66 receptor 1 (NgR1) was discovered as a mediator of reovirus infectivity in an RNA interference screen to identify host genes required for reovirus-induced cytotoxicity (Konopka-Anstadt et al., 2014). NgR1 is expressed on the cell surface of neurons in a pattern overlapping with sites of T3 virus tropism in specific neural populations in the cortex, hippocampus, thalamus, and cerebellum (Fig. 2B) (Antar et al., 2009; Barrette et al., 2007). With the postnatal onset of myelination, NgR1 ligands are expressed on myelinating oligodendrocytes that encase neural axons. NgR1 engages these ligands (e.g., nogo-A, myelin-associated glycoprotein, and oligodendrocyte-myelin glycoprotein), recruits a signaling complex, and suppresses axonal outgrowth in the adult brain (Hunt et al., 2002). The timing of NgR1 occupation by oligodendrocyte ligands coincides with the onset of age restriction for reovirus infection (Llorens et al., 2011; Tardieu et al., 1983). Thus, it is possible that myelination may mechanically block reovirus access to neural receptors.

NgR1 has a curled shape (Fig. 1C) (He et al., 2003) characteristic of all leucine-rich repeat (LRR) superfamily proteins, many of which are involved in host detection of pathogens. For example, Toll-like receptors (Botos et al., 2011), NOD-like receptors (Motta et al., 2015), and the adaptive immune mediators in jawless vertebrates, variable lymphocyte receptors (Deng et al., 2013), all have the same LRR solenoid structure. NgR1 is composed of eight canonical LRR motifs capped on either end by noncanonical LRR motifs, and a C-terminal domain linked to glycosylphosphatidylinositol (GPI) that anchors the protein to the cell membrane (Fig. 1C). Like many LRR protein–ligand partners (Botos et al., 2011; Deng et al., 2013), NgR1 ligands appear to bind the highly conserved, concave face of NgR1 (Lauren et al., 2007). The binding surface of NgR1 that reovirus engages is not known, but preliminary evidence from our laboratory using mutant, chimeric, and deletion constructs of NgR1 suggests that similar sequences are used by reovirus (D.M. Sutherland and T.S. Dermody, unpublished data).

Ectopic expression of NgR1 allows infection of normally nonsusceptible Chinese hamster ovary (CHO) cells (Konopka-Anstadt et al., 2014). This infection is mediated by direct interaction of reovirus with NgR1, as evidenced by diminished infectivity following receptor blockade via either preincubation of cells with NgR1-specific antibodies or preincubation of virus with soluble NgR1 (Konopka-Anstadt et al., 2014). Importantly, these competition assays significantly diminish reovirus infectivity in primary cultures of cortical neurons, demonstrating a function for NgR1 as a neural receptor for reovirus. Reovirus virions but not ISVPs directly bind and use NgR1 as a receptor, suggesting that either $\sigma 3$, which is lost during ISVP formation, or a virion conformer of $\sigma 1$ interacts with NgR1 (Konopka-Anstadt et al., 2014).

Mechanisms of internalization, endocytic trafficking, and signaling initiated by reovirus binding to NgR1 are currently under investigation. NgR1 lacks a cytoplasmic domain and likely is incapable of intraneuronal signaling without cytoplasmic-domain-containing coreceptors. Under physiological conditions, NgR1 binds myelin-associated ligands and recruits two neural coreceptors to form a tripartite complex that initiates RhoA activation and actin reorganization to prevent axonal outgrowth (Nikolic, 2002). Many other viruses hijack the Rho pathway during entry (Taylor et al., 2011), but it is not known whether reovirus binding to NgR1 initiates signaling events or ligation of coreceptors.

The overlapping and specific expression of NgR1 in neural populations targeted by reovirus raises the possibility that NgR1 dictates T3-specific neurotropism (Antar et al., 2009; Oberhaus et al., 1997; Wang et al., 2002).

However, expression of NgR1 in CHO cells allows infection by both T1 and T3 strains (Konopka-Anstadt et al., 2014). Such promiscuous infection by both serotypes is not observed following inoculation of murine cortical neurons in culture (Antar et al., 2009). T3 infects these neurons in an NgR1-dependent manner, whereas T1 infects neurons poorly, independent of NgR1 expression (Konopka-Anstadt et al., 2014). The contrasting infectivity profile in different cell types could be due to cell-specific modifications of NgR1. Alternatively, an additional factor that promotes entry by specific serotypes, possibly glycans or coreceptors, may be differentially expressed in these cell types.

Our lab is currently investigating the function of NgR1 in reovirus spread and neural tropism. Preliminary results indicate that genetic ablation of NgR1 in mice has a protective effect on reovirus-induced encephalitis, supporting a role for NgR1 in reovirus neuropathogenesis (J.L. Konopka-Anstadt and T.S. Dermody, unpublished data). However, there is little difference in viral loads in the brains of infected NgR1-knockout and wild-type mice (J.L. Konopka-Anstadt and T.S. Dermody, unpublished data). This result suggests that additional cellular factors, perhaps receptors, mediate neural entry and serotype-dependent tropism of reovirus.

6. CONCLUDING THOUGHTS

Despite identification and characterization of three distinct reovirus receptors (sialylated glycans, JAM-A, and NgR1), mechanisms that mediate serotype-specific tropism in the CNS have not been uncovered. It is possible that currently known receptors coordinate unknown functions to orchestrate neural and ependymal tropism. Alternatively, we may be missing key receptors that dictate infection of discrete CNS cell types. Several approaches have been used to identify serotype-specific reovirus receptors. These include bioinformatic expression analyses, glycan microarrays, screens of cDNA libraries from NT2 cells and JAM-A$^{-/-}$ mouse brain, and genome-wide siRNA and CRISPR screens in cultured cells. A few potential reasons why these techniques have not been successful thus far are that the cell-surface receptor is displayed in low abundance or not expressed in the model system, tissue-specific posttranslational modifications in the receptor are required for binding, or ligation of multiple receptors is required for entry. Furthermore, cell lines may not recapitulate the complexities of primary neural and ependymal tissues, both of which are challenging to culture and scale for in vitro screens. The development and availability of better tools, including advanced microfluidic systems, iPS cells, coculture systems, and organoid models, should enable enhanced exploration of viral infection and transmission in systems that better recapitulate in vivo conditions.

Receptors are important not only for reovirus to infect neurons and ependyma, but also to cross cellular barriers to reach these protected replication sites. T1 reovirus in circulation must cross the blood–brain barrier (BBB) to access ependymal cells lining the ventricles. The BBB is weak or absent at certain sites, particularly in young animals, which are more susceptible to reovirus infection (Saunders et al., 2014). One such site is the fenestrated blood capillaries of the choroid plexus, which is particularly prone to viral targeting and composed of modified ependymal cells that secrete cerebrospinal fluid into ventricles (Fig. 2C) (Falangola et al., 1995; Feuer et al., 2003; Wolinsky et al., 1976). T1 reovirus is detected in endothelial cells lining blood capillaries (Kundin et al., 1966) and in epithelial cells of the choroid plexus (Margolis and Kilham, 1969). T1 virus may target these JAM-A-expressing cells to access the cerebrospinal fluid, which provides access to ependyma lining the ventricles (Fig. 2C).

T3 reovirus may use similar cell types as T1 to access neural tissue from blood (Fig. 2C). However, T3 reovirus also can enter the CNS directly through infection of neurons innervating peripheral tissue (Fig. 2A) (Flamand et al., 1991; Morrison et al., 1991; Tyler et al., 1986). Within the CNS, T3 reovirus infects specific neuronal subsets (Fig. 2B), which could result from cell-intrinsic factors such as receptor expression or innate immune regulators. Alternatively, virus could be transmitted and released directionally from polarized neurons, allowing virus to spread through specific neural tracts formed by synaptic connectivity. Such directional, nonlytic release of reovirus occurs in polarized epithelial and endothelial cells (Excoffon et al., 2008; Lai et al., 2013). The mechanism of nonlytic release and the form of released reovirus are not known. A variety of phylogenetically distinct nonenveloped viruses undergo nonlytic release in vesicles (Altan-Bonnet, 2016). These virus-containing vesicles are infectious and originate from different cellular pathways, including autophagy and exosome biogenesis. Mechanisms of vesicle docking, disassembly, and concomitant virus entry are under investigation. If nonlytic egress of reovirus occurs in membranous vesicles, this process may allow subsequent fusion-mediated entry into neighboring cells, potentially alleviating the dependence on viral receptors for entry beyond initial infection of a few neuronal cells.

Contributions of currently known receptors in reovirus spread to and preference for specific CNS sites require further exploration. For T1 reovirus, efficient SA binding dictates the magnitude of hydrocephalus (Stencel-Baerenwald et al., 2015). However, neither SA nor JAM-A is required for T1 reovirus replication in the brain, suggesting that other receptors exist that mediate ependymal infection. Further studies to evaluate tropism and replication of T1 SA$^-$ virus in JAM-A$^{-/-}$ mice will clarify whether an alternate receptor is targeted on ependyma and inform the mechanism by which T1 reovirus traffics from blood to this tissue. Similar to T1, T3 reovirus does not require SA or JAM-A interaction to infect CNS sites. Our preliminary studies suggest that NgR1 mediates infection in only a subset of neurons (J.L. Konopka-Anstadt and T.S. Dermody, unpublished data). It is possible that once T3 infects a few neurons in the brain, it bypasses receptors and spreads independently in membranous vesicles. For both T1 and T3 reovirus, the precise contributions of NgR1 in spread and disease require further investigation.

The cellular mediators of reovirus CNS tropism have been long hypothesized as cell-surface receptors expressed on ependyma and neurons. This idea primarily arose from the strong genetic segregation of σ1 with serotype-specific tropism. However, it is possible that σ1 mediates tropism via interaction with a noncell-surface factor. Cellular trafficking of reovirus requires functional microtubules (Mainou et al., 2013), which are especially critical for long-distance viral trafficking in axons (Tyler et al., 1986). T3 σ1, but not T1 σ1, may engage neuronal microtubule-based motors either directly or via endocytic adaptors for transport, which could explain serotype-specific infection of neurons. Serotype-specific virus interaction with an endosomal factor also may aid in efficient proteolytic processing of virions or act as a functional receptor to directly mediate cytosolic entry. Future studies will explore these alternate possibilities and identify host determinants of reovirus CNS tropism. Identification and exploration of reovirus tropism mediators will inform diverse fields of study and could lead to the design of improved reovirus oncolytics to target specific types of cancer.

ACKNOWLEDGMENTS

We acknowledge support from US Public Health Service awards R01 AI118887 (D.M.S. and T.S.D.), R01 AI038296 (P.A. and T.S.D.), and T32 AI007281 (D.M.S.). We thank Jonathan Knowlton, Anthony Lentscher, Laurie Silva, and Paula Zamora for critical review of the manuscript.

REFERENCES

Altan-Bonnet, N., 2016. Extracellular vesicles are the Trojan horses of viral infection. Curr. Opin. Microbiol. 32, 77–81.

Antar, A.A.R., Konopka, J.L., Campbell, J.A., Henry, R.A., Perdigoto, A.L., Carter, B.D., Pozzi, A., Abel, T.W., Dermody, T.S., 2009. Junctional adhesion molecule-A is required for hematogenous dissemination of reovirus. Cell Host Microbe 5, 59–71.

Aruffo, A., Seed, B., 1987. Molecular cloning of a CD28 cDNA by a high-efficiency COS cell expression system. Proc. Natl. Acad. Sci. U. S. A. 84, 8573–8577.

Barrette, B., Vallieres, N., Dube, M., Lacroix, S., 2007. Expression profile of receptors for myelin-associated inhibitors of axonal regeneration in the intact and injured mouse central nervous system. Mol. Cell. Neurosci. 34, 519–538.

Barton, E.S., Connolly, J.L., Forrest, J.C., Chappell, J.D., Dermody, T.S., 2001a. Utilization of sialic acid as a coreceptor enhances reovirus attachment by multistep adhesion strengthening. J. Biol. Chem. 276, 2200–2211.

Barton, E.S., Forrest, J.C., Connolly, J.L., Chappell, J.D., Liu, Y., Schnell, F.J., Nusrat, A., Parkos, C.A., Dermody, T.S., 2001b. Junction adhesion molecule is a receptor for reovirus. Cell 104, 441–451.

Barton, E.S., Youree, B.E., Ebert, D.H., Forrest, J.C., Connolly, J.L., Valyi-Nagy, T., Washington, K., Wetzel, J.D., Dermody, T.S., 2003. Utilization of sialic acid as a coreceptor is required for reovirus-induced biliary disease. J. Clin. Invest. 111, 1823–1833.

Bass, D.M., Trier, J.S., Dambrauskas, R., Wolf, J.L., 1988. Reovirus type I infection of small intestinal epithelium in suckling mice and its effect on M cells. Lab. Invest. 58, 226–235.

Bhella, D., 2015. The role of cellular adhesion molecules in virus attachment and entry. Philos. Trans. R. Soc. Lond. B Biol. Sci. 370, 20140035.

Botos, I., Segal, D.M., Davies, D.R., 2011. The structural biology of Toll-like receptors. Structure 19, 447–459.

Bouziat, R., Hinterleitner, R., Brown, J.J., Stencel-Baerenwald, J.E., Ikizler, M., Mayassi, T., Meisel, M., Kim, S.M., Discepolo, V., Pruijssers, A.J., Ernest, J.D., Iskarpatyoti, J.A., Costes, L.M., Lawrence, I., Palanski, B.A., Varma, M., Zurenski, M.A., Khomandiak, S., McAllister, N., Aravamudhan, P., Boehme, K.W., Hu, F., Samsom, J.N., Reinecker, H.C., Kupfer, S.S., Guandalini, S., Semrad, C.E., Abadie, V., Khosla, C., Barreiro, L.B., Xavier, R.J., Ng, A., Dermody, T.S., Jabri, B., 2017. Reovirus infection triggers inflammatory responses to dietary antigens and development of celiac disease. Science 356, 44–50.

Campbell, J.A., Schelling, P., Wetzel, J.D., Johnson, E.M., Forrest, J.C., Wilson, G.A.R., Aurrand-Lions, M., Imhof, B.A., Stehle, T., Dermody, T.S., 2005. Junctional adhesion molecule a serves as a receptor for prototype and field-isolate strains of mammalian reovirus. J. Virol. 79, 7967–7978.

Carette, J.E., Raaben, M., Wong, A.C., Herbert, A.S., Obernosterer, G., Mulherkar, N., Kuehne, A.I., Kranzusch, P.J., Griffin, A.M., Ruthel, G., Dal Cin, P., Dye, J.M., Whelan, S.P., Chandran, K., Brummelkamp, T.R., 2011. Ebola virus entry requires the cholesterol transporter Niemann-Pick C1. Nature 477, 340–343.

Chakrabarty, R., Tran, H., Selvaggi, G., Hagerman, A., Thompson, B., Coffey, M., 2015. The oncolytic virus, pelareorep, as a novel anticancer agent: a review. Invest. New Drugs 33, 761–774.

Chandran, K., Nibert, M.L., 2003. Animal cell invasion by a large nonenveloped virus: reovirus delivers the goods. Trends Microbiol. 11, 374–382.

Chappell, J.D., Prota, A., Dermody, T.S., Stehle, T., 2002. Crystal structure of reovirus attachment protein σ1 reveals evolutionary relationship to adenovirus fiber. EMBO J. 21, 1–11.

Connolly, J.L., Barton, E.S., Dermody, T.S., 2001. Reovirus binding to cell surface sialic acid potentiates virus-induced apoptosis. J. Virol. 75, 4029–4039.

Coombs, K.M., 1998. Stoichiometry of reovirus structural proteins in virus, ISVP, and core particles. Virology 243, 218–228.

Cote, M., Misasi, J., Ren, T., Bruchez, A., Lee, K., Filone, C.M., Hensley, L., Li, Q., Ory, D., Chandran, K., Cunningham, J., 2011. Small molecule inhibitors reveal Niemann-Pick C1 is essential for Ebola virus infection. Nature 477, 344–348.

Coyne, C.B., Bergelson, J.M., 2006. Virus-induced Abl and Fyn kinase signals permit cox-sackievirus entry through epithelial tight junctions. Cell 124, 119–131.

Danthi, P., 2011. Enter the kill zone: initiation of death signaling during virus entry. Virology 411, 316–324.

Danthi, P., Hansberger, M.W., Campbell, J.A., Forrest, J.C., Dermody, T.S., 2006. JAM-A-independent, antibody-mediated uptake of reovirus into cells leads to apoptosis. J. Virol. 80, 1261–1270.

Danthi, P., Coffey, C.M., Parker, J.S., Abel, T.W., Dermody, T.S., 2008. Independent regulation of reovirus membrane penetration and apoptosis by the mu1 phi domain. PLoS Pathog. 4, e1000248.

de Graaf, M., Fouchier, R.A., 2014. Role of receptor binding specificity in influenza A virus transmission and pathogenesis. EMBO J. 33, 823–841.

Del Maschio, A., De Luigi, A., Martin-Padura, I., Brockhaus, M., Bartfai, T., Fruscella, P., Adorini, L., Martino, G., Furlan, R., Desimoni, M.G., Dejana, E., 1999. Leukocyte recruitment in the cerebrospinal fluid of mice with experimental meningitis is inhabited by an antibody to junctional adhesion molecule (JAM). J. Exp. Med. 190, 1351–1356.

Deng, H.K., Unutmaz, D., Kewalramani, V.N., Littman, D.R., 1997. Expression cloning of new receptors used by simian and human immunodeficiency viruses. Nature 388, 296–300.

Deng, L., Luo, M., Velikovsky, A., Mariuzza, R.A., 2013. Structural insights into the evolution of the adaptive immune system. Annu. Rev. Biophys. 42, 191–215.

Dermody, T.S., Kirchner, E., Guglielmi, K.M., Stehle, T., 2009. Immunoglobulin superfamily virus receptors and the evolution of adaptive immunity. PLoS Pathog. 5, e1000481.

Dermody, T.S., Parker, J.S., Sherry, B., 2013. Orthoreoviruses. In: Knipe, D.M., Howley, P.M. (Eds.), Fields Virology, sixth ed. Lippincott Williams & Wilkins, Philadelphia.

Dichter, M.A., Weiner, H.L., 1984. Infection of neuronal cell cultures with reovirus mimics in vitro patterns of neurotropism. Ann. Neurol. 16, 603–610.

Dietrich, M.H., Ogden, K.M., Katen, S.P., Reiss, K., Sutherland, D.M., Carnahan, R.H., Goff, M., Cooper, T., Dermody, T.S., Stehle, T., 2017. Structural insights into reovirus sigma1 interactions with two neutralizing antibodies. J. Virol. 91, e01621-16.

Dryden, K.A., Wang, G., Yeager, M., Nibert, M.L., Coombs, K.M., Furlong, D.B., Fields, B.N., Baker, T.S., 1993. Early steps in reovirus infection are associated with dramatic changes in supramolecular structure and protein conformation: analysis of virions and subviral particles by cryoelectron microscopy and image reconstruction. J. Cell Biol. 122, 1023–1041.

Eierhoff, T., Hrincius, E.R., Rescher, U., Ludwig, S., Ehrhardt, C., 2010. The epidermal growth factor receptor (EGFR) promotes uptake of influenza A viruses (IAV) into host cells. PLoS Pathog. 6, e1001099.

Evans, M.J., von Hahn, T., Tscherne, D.M., Syder, A.J., Panis, M., Wolk, B., Hatziioannou, T., Mckeating, J.A., Bieniasz, P.D., Rice, C.M., 2007. Claudin-1 is a hepatitis C virus co-receptor required for a late step in entry. Nature 446, 801–805.

Excoffon, K.J.D.A., Guglielmi, K.M., Wetzel, J.D., Gansemer, N.D., Campbell, J.A., DermodY, T.S., Zabner, J., 2008. Reovirus preferentially infects the basolateral surface and is released from the apical surface of polarized human respiratory epithelial cells. J. Infect. Dis. 197, 1189–1197.

Falangola, M.F., Hanly, A., Galvao-Castro, B., Petito, C.K., 1995. HIV infection of human choroid plexus: a possible mechanism of viral entry into the CNS. J. Neuropathol. Exp. Neurol. 54, 497–503.

Feuer, R., Mena, I., Pagarigan, R.R., Harkins, S., Hassett, D.E., Whitton, J.L., 2003. Coxsackievirus B3 and the neonatal CNS: the roles of stem cells, developing neurons, and apoptosis in infection, viral dissemination, and disease. Am. J. Pathol. 163, 1379–1393.

Flamand, A., Gagner, J.P., Morrison, L.A., Fields, B.N., 1991. Penetration of the nervous systems of suckling mice by mammalian reoviruses. J. Virol. 65, 123–131.

Frierson, J.M., Pruijssers, A.J., Konopka, J.L., Reiter, D.M., Abel, T.W., Stehle, T., Dermod, T.S., 2012. Utilization of sialylated glycans as coreceptors enhances the neurovirulence of serotype 3 reovirus. J. Virol. 86, 13164–13173.

Guerrero, C.A., Mendez, E., Zarate, S., Isa, P., Lopez, S., Arias, C.F., 2000. Integrin alpha(v)beta(3) mediates rotavirus cell entry. Proc. Natl. Acad. Sci. U. S. A. 97, 14644–14649.

Guidotti, L.G., Matzke, B., Schaller, H., Chisari, F.V., 1995. High-level hepatitis B virus replication in transgenic mice. J. Virol. 69, 6158–6169.

Haywood, A.M., 1994. Virus receptors: binding, adhesion strengthening, and changes in viral structure. J. Virol. 68, 1–5.

He, X.L., Bazan, J.F., McDermott, G., Park, J.B., Wang, K., Tessier-Lavigne, M., He, Z., Garcia, K.C., 2003. Structure of the Nogo receptor ectodomain: a recognition module implicated in myelin inhibition. Neuron 38, 177–185.

Hermann, L., Embree, J., Hazelton, P., Wells, B., Coombs, R.T., 2004. Reovirus type 2 isolated from cerebrospinal fluid. Pediatr. Infect. Dis. J. 23, 373–375.

Hofman, E.G., Bader, A.N., Voortman, J., van den Heuvel, D.J., Sigismund, S., Verkleij, A.J., Gerritsen, H.C., van Bergen en Henegouwen, P.M., 2010. Ligand-induced EGF receptor oligomerization is kinase-dependent and enhances internalization. J. Biol. Chem. 285, 39481–39489.

Hunt, D., Coffin, R.S., Anderson, P.N., 2002. The Nogo receptor, its ligands and axonal regeneration in the spinal cord: a review. J. Neurocytol. 31, 93–120.

Hwang, I., An, B.S., Yang, H., Kang, H.S., Jung, E.M., Jeung, E.B., 2013. Tissue-specific expression of occludin, zona occludens-1, and junction adhesion molecule A in the duodenum, ileum, colon, kidney, liver, lung, brain, and skeletal muscle of C57BL mice. J. Physiol. Pharmacol. 64, 11–18.

Imai, M., Watanabe, T., Hatta, M., Das, S.C., Ozawa, M., Shinya, K., Zhong, G., Hanson, A., Katsura, H., Watanabe, S., Li, C., Kawakami, E., Yamada, S., Kiso, M., Suzuki, Y., Maher, E.A., Neumann, G., Kawaoka, Y., 2012. Experimental adaptation of an influenza H5 HA confers respiratory droplet transmission to a reassortant H5 HA/H1N1 virus in ferrets. Nature 486, 420–428.

Jae, L.T., Raaben, M., Herbert, A.S., Kuehne, A.I., Wirchnianski, A.S., Soh, T.K., Stubbs, S.H., Janssen, H., Damme, M., Saftig, P., Whelan, S.P., Dye, J.M., Brummelkamp, T.R., 2014. Virus entry. Lassa virus entry requires a trigger-induced receptor switch. Science 344, 1506–1510.

Johansson, P.J., Sveger, T., Ahlfors, K., Ekstrand, J., Svensson, L., 1996. Reovirus type 1 associated with meningitis. Scand. J. Infect. Dis. 28, 117–120.

Jolly, C.L., Sattentau, Q.J., 2013. Attachment factors. In: Poehlmann, S., Simmons, G. (Eds.), Viral Entry Into Host Cells. Springer Science + Business Media; Landes Bioscience, New York, NY.

Kanai, Y., Komoto, S., Kawagishi, T., Nouda, R., Nagasawa, N., Onishi, M., Matsuura, Y., Taniguchi, K., Kobayashi, T., 2017. Entirely plasmid-based reverse genetics system for rotaviruses. Proc. Natl. Acad. Sci. U. S. A. 114, 2349–2354.

Keroack, M., Fields, B.N., 1986. Viral shedding and transmission between hosts determined by reovirus L2-gene. Science 232, 1635–1638.

Kirchner, E., Guglielmi, K.M., Strauss, H.M., Dermody, T.S., Stehle, T., 2008. Structure of reovirus sigma1 in complex with its receptor junctional adhesion molecule-A. PLoS Pathog. 4, e1000235.

Kobayashi, T., Ooms, L.S., Ikizler, M., Chappell, J.D., Dermody, T.S., 2010. An improved reverse genetics system for mammalian orthoreoviruses. Virology 398, 194–200.

Konopka-Anstadt, J.L., Mainou, B.A., Sutherland, D.M., Sekine, Y., Strittmatter, S.M., Dermody, T.S., 2014. The Nogo receptor NgR1 mediates infection by mammalian reovirus. Cell Host Microbe 15, 681–691.

Kostrewa, D., Brockhaus, M., D'arcy, A., Dale, G.E., Nelboeck, P., Schmid, G., Mueller, F., Bazzoni, G., Dejana, E., Bartfai, T., Winkler, F.K., Hennig, M., 2001. X-ray structure of junctional adhesion molecule: structural basis for homophilic adhesion via a novel dimerization motif. EMBO J. 20, 4391–4398.

Kundin, W.D., Liu, C., Gigstad, J., 1966. Reovirus infection in suckling mice: immunofluorescent and infectivity studies. J. Immunol. 97, 393–401.

Lai, C.M., Mainou, B.A., Kim, K.S., Dermody, T.S., 2013. Directional release of reovirus from the apical surface of polarized endothelial cells. MBio 4, e00049-13.

Lai, C.M., Boehme, K.W., Pruijssers, A.J., Parekh, V.V., Van Kaer, L., Parkos, C.A., Dermody, T.S., 2015. Endothelial JAM-A promotes reovirus viremia and bloodstream dissemination. J. Infect. Dis. 211, 383–393.

Lauren, J., Hu, F., Chin, J., Liao, J., Airaksinen, M.S., Strittmatter, S.M., 2007. Characterization of myelin ligand complexes with neuronal Nogo-66 receptor family members. J. Biol. Chem. 282, 5715–5725.

Leland, M.M., Hubbard, G.B., Sentmore 3rd., H.T., Soike, K.F., Hilliard, J.K., 2000. Outbreak of Orthoreovirus-induced meningoencephalomyelitis in baboons. Comp. Med. 50, 199–205.

Li, Q., Sodroski, C., Lowey, B., Schweitzer, C.J., Cha, H., Zhang, F., Liang, T.J., 2016. Hepatitis C virus depends on E-cadherin as an entry factor and regulates its expression in epithelial-to-mesenchymal transition. Proc. Natl. Acad. Sci. U. S. A. 113, 7620–7625.

Lindenbach, B.D., Rice, C.M., 2013. The ins and outs of hepatitis C virus entry and assembly. Nat. Rev. Microbiol. 11, 688–700.

Liu, Y., Nusrat, A., Schnell, F.J., Reaves, T.A., Walsh, S., Pochet, M., Parkos, C.A., 2000. Human junction adhesion molecule regulates tight junction resealing in epithelia. J. Cell Sci. 113 (Pt. 13), 2363–2374.

Llorens, F., Gil, V., del Rio, J.A., 2011. Emerging functions of myelin-associated proteins during development, neuronal plasticity, and neurodegeneration. FASEB J. 25, 463–475.

Longdon, B., Brockhurst, M.A., Russell, C.A., Welch, J.J., Jiggins, F.M., 2014. The evolution and genetics of virus host shifts. PLoS Pathog. 10, e1004395.

Luisoni, S., Suomalainen, M., Boucke, K., Tanner, L.B., Wenk, M.R., Guan, X.L., Grzybek, M., Coskun, U., Greber, U.F., 2015. Co-option of membrane wounding enables virus penetration into cells. Cell Host Microbe 18, 75–85.

Maginnis, M.S., Forrest, J.C., Kopecky-Bromberg, S.A., Dickeson, S.K., Santoro, S.A., Zutter, M.M., Nemerow, G.R., Bergelson, J.M., Dermody, T.S., 2006. β1 integrin mediates internalization of mammalian reovirus. J. Virol. 80, 2760–2770.

Maginnis, M.S., Mainou, B.A., Derdowski, A.M., Johnson, E.M., Zent, R., Dermody, T.S., 2008. NPXY motifs in the β1 integrin cytoplasmic tail are required for functional reovirus entry. J. Virol. 82, 3181–3191.

Mainou, B.A., Zamora, P.F., Ashbrook, A.W., Dorset, D.C., Kim, K.S., Dermody, T.S., 2013. Reovirus cell entry requires functional microtubules. MBio 4, e00405-13.

Margolis, G., Kilham, L., 1969. Hydrocephalus in hamsters, ferrets, rats, and mice following inoculations with reovirus type I. II. Pathologic studies. Lab. Invest. 21, 189–198.

Martin-Padura, I., Lostaglio, S., Schneemann, M., Williams, L., Romano, M., Fruscella, P., Panzeri, C., Stoppacciaro, A., Ruco, L., Villa, A., Simmons, D., Dejana, E., 1998. Junctional adhesion molecule, a novel member of the immunoglobulin superfamily that distributes at intercellular junctions and modulates monocyte transmigration. J. Cell Biol. 142, 117–127.

Matrosovich, M., Herrler, G., Klenk, H.D., 2015. Sialic acid receptors of viruses. In: - Gerardy-Schahn, R., Delannoy, P., von Itzstein, M. (Eds.), SialoGlyco Chemistry and Biology II, 2013/07/23. Springer International Publishing, New York, NY.

Milhorat, T.H., Kotzen, R.M., 1994. Stenosis of the central canal of the spinal cord following inoculation of suckling hamsters with reovirus type I. J. Neurosurg. 81, 103–106.

Morrison, L.A., Sidman, R.L., Fields, B.N., 1991. Direct spread of reovirus from the intestinal lumen to the central nervous system through vagal autonomic nerve fibers. Proc. Natl. Acad. Sci. U. S. A. 88, 3852–3856.

Motta, V., Soares, F., Sun, T., Philpott, D.J., 2015. NOD-like receptors: versatile cytosolic sentinels. Physiol. Rev. 95, 149–178.

Nagata, L., Masri, S.A., Pon, R.T., Lee, P.W.K., 1987. Analysis of functional domains on reovirus cell attachment protein sigma 1 using cloned S1 gene deletion mutants. Virology 160, 162–168.

Nibert, M.L., Dermody, T.S., Fields, B.N., 1990. Structure of the reovirus cell-attachment protein: a model for the domain organization of σ1. J. Virol. 64, 2976–2989.

Nikolic, M., 2002. The role of Rho GTPases and associated kinases in regulating neurite outgrowth. Int. J. Biochem. Cell Biol. 34, 731–745.

Oberhaus, S.M., Smith, R.L., Clayton, G.H., Dermody, T.S., Tyler, K.L., 1997. Reovirus infection and tissue injury in the mouse central nervous system are associated with apoptosis. J. Virol. 71, 2100–2106.

Ong, E.Z., Chan, K.R., Ooi, E.E., 2016. Viral manipulation of host inhibitory receptor signaling for immune evasion. PLoS Pathog. 12, e1005776.

Prota, A.E., Campbell, J.A., Schelling, P., Forrest, J.C., Watson, M.J., Peters, T.R., Aurrand-Lions, M., Imhof, B.A., Dermody, T.S., Stehle, T., 2003. Crystal structure of human junctional adhesion molecule 1: implications for reovirus binding. Proc. Natl. Acad. Sci. U. S. A. 100, 5366–5371.

Pruijssers, A.J., Hengel, H., Abel, T.W., Dermody, T.S., 2013. Apoptosis induction influences reovirus replication and virulence in newborn mice. J. Virol. 87, 12980–12989.

Reiss, K., Stencel, J.E., Liu, Y., Blaum, B.S., Reiter, D.M., Feizi, T., Dermody, T.S., Stehle, T., 2012. The GM2 glycan serves as a functional co-receptor for serotype 1 reovirus. PLoS Pathog. 8, e1003078.

Reiter, D.M., Frierson, J.M., Halvorson, E.E., Kobayashi, T., Dermody, T.S., Stehle, T., 2011. Crystal structure of reovirus attachment protein sigma1 in complex with sialylated oligosaccharides. PLoS Pathog. 7, e1002166.

Sabin, A.B., 1959. Reoviruses: a new group of respiratory and enteric viruses formerly classified as ECHO type 10 is described. Science 130, 1387–1389.

Salinas, S., Zussy, C., Loustalot, F., Henaff, D., Menendez, G., Morton, P.E., Parsons, M., Schiavo, G., Kremer, E.J., 2014. Disruption of the coxsackievirus and adenovirus receptor-homodimeric interaction triggers lipid microdomain- and dynamin-dependent endocytosis and lysosomal targeting. J. Biol. Chem. 289, 680–695.

Saunders, N.R., Dreifuss, J.J., Dziegielewska, K.M., Johansson, P.A., Habgood, M.D., Mollgard, K., Bauer, H.C., 2014. The rights and wrongs of blood-brain barrier permeability studies: a walk through 100 years of history. Front. Neurosci. 8, 404.

Schmidt, K., Keller, M., Bader, B.L., Korytar, T., Finke, S., Ziegler, U., Groschup, M.H., 2013. Integrins modulate the infection efficiency of West Nile virus into cells. J. Gen. Virol. 94, 1723–1733.

Severson, E.A., Parkos, C.A., 2009. Structural determinants of Junctional Adhesion Molecule A (JAM-A) function and mechanisms of intracellular signaling. Curr. Opin. Cell Biol. 21, 701–707.

Silverstein, S.C., Astell, C., Levin, D.H., Schonberg, M., Acs, G., 1972. The mechanism of reovirus uncoating and gene activation in vivo. Virology 47, 797–806.

Stamatovic, S.M., Johnson, A.M., Sladojevic, N., Keep, R.F., Andjelkovic, A.V., 2017. Endocytosis of tight junction proteins and the regulation of degradation and recycling. Ann. N. Y. Acad. Sci. 1397, 54–65.

Stanley, N.F., Dorman, D.C., Ponsford, J., 1953. Studies on the pathogenesis of a hitherto undescribed virus (hepato-encephalomyelitis) producing unusual symptoms in suckling mice. Aust. J. Exp. Biol. Med. Sci. 31, 147–159.

Stelzer, S., Ebnet, K., Schwamborn, J.C., 2010. JAM-A is a novel surface marker for NG2-Glia in the adult mouse brain. BMC Neurosci. 11, 27.

Stencel-Baerenwald, J., Reiss, K., Blaum, B.S., Colvin, D., Li, X.N., Abel, T., Boyd, K., Stehle, T., Dermody, T.S., 2015. Glycan engagement dictates hydrocephalus induction by serotype 1 reovirus. MBio 6, e02356.

Stettner, E., Dietrich, M.H., Reiss, K., Dermody, T.S., Stehle, T., 2015. Structure of serotype 1 reovirus attachment protein sigma1 in complex with junctional adhesion molecule A reveals a conserved serotype-independent binding epitope. J. Virol. 89, 6136–6140.

Stroh, L.J., Stehle, T., 2014. Glycan engagement by viruses: receptor switches and specificity. Annu. Rev. Virol. 1, 285–306.

Sturzenbecker, L.J., Nibert, M.L., Furlong, D.B., Fields, B.N., 1987. Intracellular digestion of reovirus particles requires a low pH and is an essential step in the viral infectious cycle. J. Virol. 61, 2351–2361.

Tardieu, M., Weiner, H.L., 1982. Viral receptors on isolated murine and human ependymal cells. Science 215, 419–421.

Tardieu, M., Powers, M.L., Weiner, H.L., 1983. Age dependent susceptibility to Reovirus type 3 encephalitis: role of viral and host factors. Ann. Neurol. 13, 602–607.

Tate, J.E., Burton, A.H., Boschi-Pinto, C., Parashar, U.D., World Health Organization-Coordinated Global Rotavirus Surveillance, N, 2016. Global, regional, and national estimates of rotavirus mortality in children <5 years of age, 2000–2013. Clin. Infect. Dis. 62 (Suppl. 2), S96–S105.

Tatsuo, H., Ono, N., Tanaka, K., Yanagi, Y., 2000. SLAM (CDw150) is a cellular receptor for measles virus. Nature 406, 893–897.

Taylor, M.P., Koyuncu, O.O., Enquist, L.W., 2011. Subversion of the actin cytoskeleton during viral infection. Nat. Rev. Microbiol. 9, 427–439.

Thete, D., Snyder, A.J., Mainou, B.A., Danthi, P., 2016. Reovirus mu1 protein affects infectivity by altering virus-receptor interactions. J. Virol. 90, 10951–10962.

Tyler, K.L., McPhee, D.A., Fields, B.N., 1986. Distinct pathways of viral spread in the host determined by reovirus S1 gene segment. Science 233, 770–774.

Tyler, K.L., Barton, E.S., Ibach, M.L., Robinson, C., Campbell, J.A., O'Donnell, S.M., Valyi-Nagy, T., Clarke, P., Wetzel, J.D., Dermody, T.S., 2004. Isolation and molecular characterization of a novel type 3 reovirus from a child with meningitis. J. Infect. Dis. 189, 1664–1675.

van Tongeren, H.A.E., 1957. A familial infection with hepatoencephalomyelitis virus in the Netherlands: study on some properties of the infective agent. Arch. Gesamte Virusforsch. 7, 429–448.

Varki, A., Schauer, R., 2009. Sialic acids. In: Varki, A., Cummings, R.D., Esko, J.D., Freeze, H.H., Stanley, P., Bertozzi, C.R., Hart, G.W., Etzler, M.E. (Eds.), Essentials of Glycobiology, second ed. Cold Spring Harbor Laboratory Press, Cold Spring Harbor (NY).

Wang, X., Chun, S.J., Treloar, H., Vartanian, T., Greer, C.A., Strittmatter, S.M., 2002. Localization of Nogo-A and Nogo-66 receptor proteins at sites of axon-myelin and synaptic contact. J. Neurosci. 22, 5505–5515.

Weiner, H.L., Fields, B.N., 1977. Neutralization of reovirus: the gene responsible for the neutralization antigen. J. Exp. Med. 146, 1305–1310.

Weiner, H.L., Ramig, R.F., Mustoe, T.A., Fields, B.N., 1978. Identification of the gene coding for the hemagglutinin of reovirus. Virology 86, 581–584.

Weiner, H.L., Powers, M.L., Fields, B.N., 1980. Absolute linkage of virulence and central nervous system cell tropism of reoviruses to viral hemagglutinin. J. Infect. Dis. 141, 609–616.

White, J.M., Whittaker, G.R., 2016. Fusion of enveloped viruses in endosomes. Traffic 17, 593–614.

Wickham, T.J., Mathias, P., Cheresh, D.A., Nemerow, G.R., 1993. Integrins $\alpha_v\beta_3$ and $\alpha_v\beta_5$ promote adenovirus internalization but not virus attachment. Cell 73, 309–319.

Williams, L.A., Martin-Padura, I., Dejana, E., Hogg, N., Simmons, D.L., 1999. Identification and characterisation of human Junctional Adhesion Molecule (JAM). Mol. Immunol. 36, 1175–1188.

Wolf, J.L., Rubin, D.H., Finberg, R., Kaufman, R.S., Sharpe, A.H., Trier, J.S., Fields, B.N., 1981. Intestinal M cells: a pathway of entry for reovirus into the host. Science 212, 471–472.

Wolinsky, J.S., Klassen, T., Baringer, J.R., 1976. Persistence of neuroadapted mumps virus in brains of newborn hamsters after intraperitoneal inoculation. J. Infect. Dis. 133, 260–267.

Woolhouse, M., Scott, F., Hudson, Z., Howey, R., Chase-Topping, M., 2012. Human viruses: discovery and emergence. Philos. Trans. R. Soc. Lond. B Biol. Sci. 367, 2864–2871.

Yan, H., Peng, B., He, W., Zhong, G., Qi, Y., Ren, B., Gao, Z., Jing, Z., Song, M., Xu, G., Sui, J., Li, W., 2013. Molecular determinants of hepatitis B and D virus entry restriction in mouse sodium taurocholate cotransporting polypeptide. J. Virol. 87, 7977–7991.

Zhang, X., JI, Y., Zhang, L., Harrison, S.C., Marinescu, D.C., Nibert, M.L., Baker, T.S., 2005. Features of reovirus outer capsid protein mu1 revealed by electron cryomicroscopy and image reconstruction of the virion at 7.0 Angstrom resolution. Structure 13, 1545–1557.

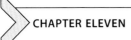

CHAPTER ELEVEN

Antiviral Immune Response and the Route of Infection in *Drosophila melanogaster*

Juan A. Mondotte, Maria-Carla Saleh[1]

Institut Pasteur, Viruses and RNA Interference Unit, CNRS Unité Mixte de Recherche 3569, Paris, France
[1]Corresponding author: e-mail address: carla.saleh@pasteur.fr

Contents

Abstract

The use of Drosophila as a model organism has made an important contribution to our understanding of the function and regulation of innate immunity in insects. Indeed, insects can discriminate between different types of pathogens and mount specific and effective responses. Strikingly, the same pathogen can trigger a different immune response in the same organism, depending solely on the route of infection by which the pathogen is delivered. In this review, we recapitulate what is known about antiviral responses in Drosophila, and how they are triggered depending on the route and the mode used for the virus to infect its host.

Advances in Virus Research, Volume 100
ISSN 0065-3527
https://doi.org/10.1016/bs.aivir.2017.10.006
247

1. INTRODUCTION

Insects are found in almost every environment on Earth. They are the largest and most diverse group of animals and are crucial components of many ecosystems where they participate in functions as diverse as plants pollinators or control of other insects and plant pests. Insects have economic importance: some produce useful substances, such as honey, wax, and silk (Foottit and Adler, 2009; Gullan and Cranston, 2010; Hill, 1997), but insects also cause severe economic losses by damaging crops and food production (Hill, 1997). In addition, some insects pose an increasing menace to human and animal health. Insects such as mosquitoes, lice, fleas, and bed bugs are able to transmit a number of disease-causing pathogens such as viruses, bacteria, protozoa, and nematodes (Baxter et al., 2017). Over one million people worldwide die from mosquito-borne diseases every year. Zika virus, West Nile virus, chikungunya virus, dengue virus, and *Plasmodium falciparum* (the causative agent of malaria) are examples of pathogens that are spread to people by mosquito bites (WHO, 2016).

Successful insect management requires intervening at some point during the insect's life cycle before they bite and infect a human or an animal. To achieve this, great efforts have been made in the recent years to understand the immune response in insects and how insects cope with a pathogen infection. To survive in a world full of microorganisms and parasites, insects developed potent defense mechanisms that depend on innate immunity. Most of our knowledge on insect innate immunity comes from studies performed on the fruit fly, *Drosophila melanogaster*. Fruit flies have a well-established genetic toolbox, are easy and inexpensive to culture in laboratory conditions, and have been the model insect of choice for the past 100 years (Jennings, 2011).

Studies of innate immunity in Drosophila initially focused on bacterial and fungal infection, and revealed that the production of antimicrobial peptides (AMPs) plays an important role in the host defense (Ganesan et al., 2011). Recently, several groups started to investigate the genetic basis of the antiviral resistance in Drosophila. It is now well established that RNA interference (RNAi) plays a central role in the control of viral infections in insects, while other inducible responses and restrictions factors contribute to resistance to viral infections (Mussabekova et al., 2017).

Most studies performed to understand host–virus interactions in Drosophila have been done by actively delivering the virus by injection into

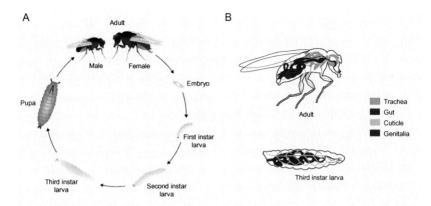

Fig. 1 Drosophila life cycle and routes of infection. (A) Drosophila exhibits complete metamorphism. The life cycle includes an embryo, larval forms, pupa, and finally emergence as an adult. (B) Potential routes of pathogen entry in Drosophila adult and larva. Each *color* depicts a physiological barrier breached by the pathogen during infection.

the flies. Although this approach has been shown to be relevant for identifying pathogen virulence factors and host defense mechanisms, injecting the virus bypasses the host's natural protection barriers. Several studies showed that the route used by pathogens to infect their hosts has an important impact on the outcome of an infection and can trigger differential immune responses (Behrens et al., 2014; Ferreira et al., 2014; Gupta et al., 2017b; Martins et al., 2013). In humans, for instance, pathogens infecting hosts through wounded skin results in significantly higher cases of fatality than if the pathogens are inhaled or ingested (Leggett et al., 2012).

In addition, Drosophila, as well as mosquito, is a holometabolous insect, undergoing metamorphosis between four life stages: embryo, larva, pupa, and imago or adult (Fig. 1A). Therefore, it could be postulated that depending on the route of infection of the pathogen and the developmental stage of the insect, the pathogen tropism and the infection outcome may be different.

This review is an attempt to cover the different elements of antiviral immunity in insects, with an emphasis on Drosophila and focusing in the different routes and modes of infection used to deliver the virus.

2. ROUTES OF INFECTION

To fight infections, insects rely on multiple innate defense responses, many of which are shared with higher organisms. They include the use of physical barriers together with local and systemic immune responses (Bergman et al., 2017).

Epithelia physically separate self from nonself and are the first line of defense against external pathogens. They fulfill the important task of preventing the penetration of pathogens that could cause systemic infections (Lemaitre and Hoffmann, 2007). The potential routes of pathogen entry in insects involve the penetration through the cuticle, the trachea, the gut, and the genital organ (Davis and Engstrom, 2012; Siva-Jothy et al., 2005) (Fig. 1B).

2.1 Through the Cuticle

The cuticle or exoskeleton is a protective integument over the external surface of insects. It is an extracellular matrix produced by the epidermis and consists mainly of proteins and the polysaccharide chitin (Tajiri, 2017). In addition to a physical barrier, the cuticle also provides an active biochemical barrier. When the epicuticle (outer layer of the cuticle) of a silkworm larva was abraded in the presence of live bacteria or bacterial cell wall components, the AMP cecropin was detected in the underlying epithelial cells, indicating a highly localized antibacterial response (Brey et al., 1993). Direct penetration of intact cuticle is the normal route of entry by most entomopathogenic fungi (Lu and St Leger, 2016). Insects in the wild are often wounded by predators (Kanbar and Engels, 2003) or during mating (Lange et al., 2013), increasing the risk for systemic infections through the cuticle. It was shown that bacteria entering the hemocoel through the site of cuticle injury trigger a systemic immune response, which results in the synthesis and secretion of a large set of humoral effector molecules. This reaction mainly consists of AMP production by the fat body, the stress response proteins, and factors required for phagocytosis and coagulation (Lemaitre and Hoffmann, 2007).

2.2 Through the Trachea

The respiratory tract of insects is another possible route of pathogen entry. The tracheae consist of an epithelium monolayer that wraps around the central, gas-transporting lumen. Air enters the respiratory systems of insects through a series of external openings called spiracles and passes through primary, secondary, and terminal branches, reaching all tissues in the body (Ghabrial et al., 2003).

The epithelial cells in the trachea not only constitute a physical barrier but also the first line of defense against airborne pathogens. Infection with the baculovirus *Autographa californica* multiple nucleopolyhedrovirus in Lepidoptera can be initiated on tracheae and is disseminated within the host via the trachea (Engelhard et al., 1994; Kirkpatrick et al., 1994).

In other insects such as Drosophila, the trachea is also a potential infection route, since the spiracles of larvae are in contact with potentially infectious organisms present in the food. Exposure of larva or adult flies to the Gram-negative bacteria results in the induction of the AMPs in the respiratory tract (Ferrandon et al., 1998; Tzou et al., 2000; Wagner et al., 2008).

2.3 Through the Gut

Many insect species mainly feed on decaying or contaminated food and are thus exposed to very large quantities of microorganisms. The gut is a tubular epithelium composed of a monolayer of cells surrounded by visceral muscles and tracheae. The tube structure of the digestive tract can be divided into the foregut, midgut, and hindgut. The midgut is the main site of digestion and food absorption and the one exposed to more pathogen threats. A semipermeable chitinous layer, the peritrophic matrix, protects the epithelium from physical damage and regulates the passage of particles between the lumen and the enterocytes (Linser and Dinglasan, 2014). A chitin-binding protein called Drosocrystallin (Dcy) has been identified as part of the peritrophic matrix in the adult Drosophila midgut. Dcy-deficient flies have a reduced peritrophic matrix and are more sensitive to pathogens (Kuraishi et al., 2011).

As a result of Gram-negative bacteria and Gram-positive bacilli infection in the gut, the immune deficiency (IMD) pathway is activated and AMPs produced (Buchon et al., 2009; Ryu et al., 2006; Tzou et al., 2000). Flies with deficiencies in this pathway are more sensitive to oral infections with bacteria (Liehl et al., 2006; Nehme et al., 2007).

The gut defense also comprises the production of reactive oxygen species (ROS) (Ha et al., 2005; Ryu et al., 2006). ROS are produced by the NADPH oxidase Duox. ROS act eliminating bacteria by damaging DNA, RNA, and proteins and also by producing the oxidative degradation of lipids in cell membranes (Vatansever et al., 2013). Duox-RNAi flies are more susceptible following infection with bacteria (Ha et al., 2005).

2.4 Through the Genital Organ

The genitalia are other organs potentially exposed to infectious organisms. Traumatic mating is widespread in the animal kingdom and copulation can involve the wounding of the mating partner (Lange et al., 2013). Drosophila females present wounds on their genitalia after copulation (Kamimura, 2007). This has been postulated as a significant cause of infection in the wild (Miest and Bloch-Qazi, 2008; Zhong et al., 2013). Highlighting the importance of this route of infection, many AMP genes are constitutively expressed in male and female genitalia of Drosophila (Tzou et al., 2000).

3. DROSOPHILA: MOST COMMON MODES OF INFECTION

Different modes of infection are used to study host–pathogens interactions in Drosophila (Fig. 2). Fruit flies can be infected by actively delivering the infective agent (bacteria, fungi, or virus) into the body cavity (abdomen or thorax) of the adult or the larva (Neyen et al., 2014). This is achieved by pricking the body cavity of the insect with a needle that has been immersed in the pathogen, or by microinjection of the pathogen directly into the body cavity, which might mimic the bite of the insect's parasites or a wound in the cuticle. For example, it was shown that mites serve as a vector to transmit bacteria from one *Drosophila* species to another (Jaenike et al., 2007), and wounds left by mites can become secondarily infected by bacteria in honey bees pupae (Kanbar and Engels, 2003). Alternatively, flies with the first pair of legs cut and removed can be exposed to medium contaminated with bacteria (Kari et al., 2013). This method mimics injuries that flies suffer in the natural habitat.

Although these approaches have been shown to be relevant for identifying pathogen virulence factors and host defense mechanisms, they bypass the entry of microbes through others routes of infection, such as the gut, trachea, or genitalia. Additionally, the injury produced by the inoculation could trigger immune mechanisms independent of the infection (Chambers et al., 2014).

Drosophila are naturally exposed to pathogens while foraging on decaying fruit, with the most common route of access of pathogens being oral infection in the digestive system and/or contact with the tracheal system. Different experimental methods for oral infection in Drosophila have been described: exposing larvae with virus particles from the beginning of the first instar (Gomariz-Zilber and Thomas-Orillard, 1993; Gomariz-Zilber et al., 1995, 1998; Jousset and Plus, 1975; Lautie-Harivel, 1992; Stevanovic and Johnson, 2015; Thomas-Orillard, 1984, 1988; Vale and Jardine, 2015) or by feeding adult flies with a mix of food and pathogen solution (Ferreira et al., 2014; Gomariz-Zilber et al., 1995; Gupta et al., 2017a; Jousset and Plus, 1975; Wong et al., 2016; Xu et al., 2013).

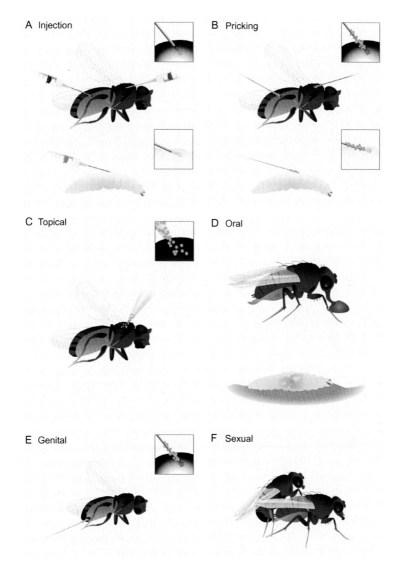

Fig. 2 Modes of infection used in Drosophila under laboratory conditions. Pathogens can be delivered by injection (A) or pricking (B) in the thorax or the abdomen. Alternatively, pathogens can be deposited over the cuticle (C) or orally ingested (D). Other possible modes of infection include the deposition of pathogens in the male genital plaque (E) or sexual transmission during mating (F).

Topical infection is another method of infection in which the pathogen is put directly in contact with the host cuticle. This infection mode has been used with the entomopathogenic fungi *Metarhizium anisopliae* that infects via direct penetration on the host cuticle during spore germination (Lu et al., 2015; Zhong et al., 2013).

The genital plate of Drosophila males is also a route of pathogen entry in males, and deposition of bacteria on genitalia is sufficient to trigger both systemic and local expression of AMPs (Gendrin et al., 2009). Furthermore, sexual transmission of bacteria and fungi from male to female during mating was observed under laboratory conditions (Miest and Bloch-Qazi, 2008; Zhong et al., 2013).

Interestingly, Martins et al. (2013) showed that host immune adaptation depends on the infection route taken by pathogens. They tested the evolution of resistance of *Drosophila melanogaster* against the *Pseudomonas entomophila* bacteria introduced through the cuticle (infection by pricking) or through the gut (upon oral infection). The host evolved resistance toward the bacteria for both routes of infection. However, adaptation to infection through one route does not protect from infection through the other. This route specificity indicates that the physiological mechanisms of resistance and the evolutionary trajectories of adaptation differ for each route of infection. An example comes from a transcription profile analysis of Drosophila larvae infected with bacteria by oral infection compared to injection; the analysis showed that during oral infection genes related to the chitinous peritrophic matrix and genes involved in general metabolism are the most induced. These may reflect modifications that the gut cells undergo due to the presence of bacteria in the food (Vodovar et al., 2005).

4. INFECTION OUTCOMES AND IMMUNE RESPONSES

A systemic infection is an infection in which the pathogen is distributed throughout the body rather than concentrated in one area. In contrast, a local infection is an infection that has not spread but remains contained near the entry site (Taber, 2017).

It is commonly accepted that bacterial systemic infections take place in the body cavity of the insect and produce a systemic immune response that concerns AMP production and release from the fat body into the hemolymph, and hemocyte activation. On the contrary, a local infection takes place in barrier epithelia such as the gut, the trachea, or the reproductive tract. In this case, AMPs are expressed in the epithelia and produce a local immune response (Lemaitre and Hoffmann, 2007). In Drosophila, AMP expression is detected in most tissues that are in contact with the external environment with a higher chance of encountering a pathogen (Ferrandon et al., 1998; Tzou et al., 2000). The secretion of AMPs locally helps to prevent the spreading of infections and provides a first line of defense, which does not require the triggering of a systemic response.

A septic injury in the body cavity of an insect is thought to start a systemic infection. However, it has been shown that oral infections with bacteria in Drosophila larvae (Basset et al., 2000; Vodovar et al., 2005) and adults (Nehme et al., 2007) are capable of also inducing systemic immune responses, even if bacteria only remain in the gut lumen (Liehl et al., 2006). These results indicate that an infection initiated at the epithelia could produce a systemic infection and trigger a systemic immune response. Similarly, in flies injected with Drosophila C virus (DCV), the virus is detected throughout the body. When flies are orally infected with DCV, the virus is found in other organs beyond the gut, even in hemocytes, showing a similar tropism to that of one after injection (Ferreira et al., 2014). Therefore, DCV is capable of generating a systemic infection independently of the infection mode.

Inducible responses such as the Janus kinase/signal transducer and activator of transcription (Jak–STAT), Toll, and IMD pathways (see Section 5.2) also contribute to the antiviral host defense in Drosophila, although they involve virus-specific mechanisms (in contrast to RNAi, which is a general antiviral response) that remain poorly characterized. For this reason, the production and release of AMPs from the fat body into the hemolymph following a viral infection is not a good parameter to differentiate local from systemic viral immune responses. One measurable parameter that reveals a systemic viral response is the spread of antiviral signals from infection sites to distant uninfected tissues (Saleh et al., 2009). For example, it was suggested that viral small RNAs act as an antiviral signal during systemic spread of RNAi-based immunity (Tassetto et al., 2017).

To simplify the interpretation of results in the bibliography, we distinguish the route of infection (through the cuticle, through the trachea, through the gut, through the genital organ), from the mode of infection (injection, pricking, topical infection, genitalia or trachea infection, sexual transmission, oral infection), and the infection outcome (systemic infection vs local infection) from the immune response triggered (systemic vs local immune response).

5. DROSOPHILA ANTIVIRAL IMMUNE RESPONSES UPON DIFFERENT ROUTES AND MODES OF INFECTION

Several natural viral pathogens have been described and used to investigate the genetic basis of antiviral resistance in Drosophila. The list includes the natural RNA viruses of Drosophila: DCV (Jousset and Plus, 1975), Nora virus (Habayeb et al., 2006), Drosophila A virus (DAV) (Brun, 1980), Drosophila X virus (DXV) (Teninges et al., 1979), Cricket Paralysis virus (CrPV) (Johnson and Christian, 1996), and Sigma virus (Berkaloff et al., 1965; Teissier, 1937). Also, nonnatural viruses of Drosophila have been actively used as infection models: the RNA viruses Flock House virus (FHV), Sindbis virus (SINV), Vesicular stomatitis virus (VSV), and the DNA virus Invertebrate Iridescent virus 6 (IIV6).

As mentioned earlier, the infection route plays an important role in the fate of the infection and the fate of the host. For instance, a DNA microarray analysis of flies injected with DCV revealed that 140 genes were induced after infection. Most AMP genes were not upregulated or were only weakly upregulated by the infection (Dostert et al., 2005). However, the genes *vir-1* (virus-induced RNA 1) and *Vago* (Deddouche et al., 2008; Dostert et al., 2005) that are host factors involved in DCV replication were upregulated. In another study the gene expression analysis was carried out in response to an oral infection with DCV (Roxstrom-Lindquist et al., 2004). Interestingly, only 80 genes showed upregulation in response to infection, and some of these were the genes for the AMPs Attacin A, Cecropin A1, Cecropin A2, Drosomycin, and Metchnikowin. Intriguingly, the genes *vir-1* and *Vago* were not upregulated. Even if the dramatic differences on gene expression reported in both studies could be due to the different routes of virus infection, one cannot exclude that changes might be due to differences in the experiment design and data analysis. Of note, a genome-wide transcriptome study by next-generation sequencing of DCV-injected wild-type flies reveled that just 31 genes were regulated by the infection (Merkling et al., 2015b). The number and the identity of the upregulated genes are very different than those in the DNA microarray analysis discussed earlier (Dostert et al., 2005).

With the current availability of next-generation sequencing techniques, it would be useful to perform gene expression studies in which flies of the same age, sex, genetic background, and reared in the same conditions are infected with different doses of DCV by injection or by oral infection. Only this kind of systematic and standardized comparative studies will shed light on the molecular mechanism underlying the effect of the route and mode of infection on the host immune response.

Below we will briefly describe the main responses involved in antiviral immunity in Drosophila and their differential regulation/expression depending on the infection route (Table 1). For more details in the different antiviral responses, see Merkling and Van Rij (2013) and Mussabekova et al. (2017).

Table 1 Antiviral Responses and Modes of Infection in Drosophila

Antiviral Response	Virus	Developmental Stage	Infection Mode	Evidence	References
RNA interference	DCV, FHV, SINV, CrPV, DXV, VSV, IIV6	Adult	Injection	– Viral accumulation and survival in mutant flies – vsiRNA accumulation – RNAi viral suppressors	Galiana-Arnoux et al. (2006), Van Rij et al. (2006), Wang et al. (2006), Zambon et al. (2006), Mueller et al. (2010), and Bronkhorst et al. (2012)
	DCV, CrPV	Adult	Intrathoracic injection	– Transcriptional induction – Viral accumulation and survival in *hopscotch* mutant flies	Dostert et al. (2005) and Kemp et al. (2013)
Jak–STAT	DCV	Adult	Intrathoracic injection	– Transcriptional induction – Survival in *G9a* mutant flies (negative regulator of JAK–STAT)	Merkling et al. (2015a)
	SINV	Adult	Intrathoracic injection, fly line expressing SINV replicon	– Transcriptional induction – Viral accumulation in *AttC* knockdown flies	Avadhanula et al. (2009) and Huang et al. (2013)
	SINV	Adult	Intrathoracic injection, fly line expressing SINV replicon	– Transcriptional induction – Viral accumulation in *Relish* and in *DptB* mutant flies	Avadhanula et al. (2009) and Huang et al. (2013)
IMD	SINV, VSV	Adult	Intrathoracic injection	– Transcriptional induction – Survival in *Diedel* mutant flies (negative regulator of IMD)	Lamiable et al. (2016b)

Continued

Table 1 Antiviral Responses and Modes of Infection in Drosophila—cont'd

Antiviral Response	Virus	Developmental Stage	Infection Mode	Evidence	References
IMD	CrPV	Adult	Abdominal injection	– Viral accumulation and survival in mutant flies	Costa et al. (2009)
	DCV, SINV	Adult	Oral	– Viral RNA accumulation in mutant fly intestines	Sansone et al. (2015)
	DXV	Adult	Injection	– Transcriptional induction – Viral accumulation and survival in *Dif* mutant flies	Zambon et al. (2005)
Toll	DCV, CrPV, FHV, Nora virus	Adult	Oral	– Viral RNA accumulation and survival in mutant flies	Ferreira et al. (2014)
	CrPV	Adult Larva	Abdominal injection	– Survival in phagocytosis-inhibited flies – Hemocytes depletion during infection	Costa et al. (2009)
Phagocytosis	CrPV, FHV, VSV	Adult	Intrathoracic injection	– Survival and viral RNA accumulation in phagocytosis-inhibited flies – Survival and viral RNA accumulation in *hemoless* mutant flies	Lamiable et al. (2016a)

	Virus	Stage	Method	Effect	Reference
	FHV	Adult	Intrathoracic injection	– Transcriptional and protein induction – Viral accumulation and survival in mutant flies	Liu et al. (2013)
Apoptosis					
	DCV	Adult	Abdominal injection	– Survival in phagocytosis-inhibited flies – Caspase activation in infected flies – Survival and viral accumulation in engulfment receptors mutant flies	Nainu et al. (2015)
	VSV, RVFV	Adult	Abdominal injection	– Survival and viral accumulation in mutant flies	Shelly et al. (2009) and Moy et al. (2014)
Autophagy					
	VSV	Adult	Intrathoracic injection	– Survival and viral accumulation in mutant flies	Lamiable et al. (2016a)
Vago	DCV	Adult	Intrathoracic injection	– Transcriptional induction – Viral accumulation in fat body of *Vago* mutant flies	Deddouche et al. (2008)
Heat shock	DCV, CrPV	Adult	Intrathoracic injection	– Transcriptional induction – Viral accumulation and survival in mutant flies	Merkling et al. (2015b)
pastrel Ubc-E2H	DCV, CrPV	Adult	Injection, intrathoracic pricking	– Knockdown of polymorphisms result in reduced fly survival	Magwire et al. (2012) and Martins et al. (2014)

Table 1 Antiviral Responses and Modes of Infection in Drosophila—cont'd

Antiviral Response	Virus	Developmental Stage	Infection Mode	Evidence	References
dFOXO	CrPV, FHV	Adult	Injection	– Survival in *dFOXO* null mutant flies	Spellberg and Marr (2015)
Gut microbiota	DCV, VSV	Adult	Oral	– Viral accumulation in intestines of axenic flies	Sansone et al. (2015)
	DCV, CrPV, FHV	Adult	Injection	– Survival in *Wolbachia*-free flies	Hedges et al. (2008)
	DCV, FHV, Nora virus	Adult	Intrathoracic injection	– Survival and viral accumulation in *Wolbachia*-free flies	Teixeira et al. (2008)
Wolbachia	DCV	Adult Larva	Oral	– Survival in *Wolbachia*-free flies	Ferreira et al. (2014) and Stevanovic et al. (2015)
	SINV	Adult	Intrathoracic injection	– *Wolbachia* increases the expression of the *Mt2* host gene – Viral and RNA accumulation in *Mt2* loss-of-function mutant flies and in flies over expressing *Mt2*	Bhattacharya et al. (2017)

5.1 RNA Interference

When challenged with any virus, the most robust insect response is the RNAi pathway. The most compelling results demonstrating the antiviral role of RNAi come, once again, from Drosophila: (i) flies with loss-of-function mutations for the three key genes of the small interfering RNA (siRNA) pathway, *Dicer-2* (*Dcr-2*), *Argonaute 2* (*Ago-2*), and *r2d2*, show increased sensitivity to infection by RNA and DNA viruses (Galiana-Arnoux et al., 2006; Van Rij et al., 2006; Wang et al., 2006; Zambon et al., 2006); (ii) Dicer-2-dependent 21-nucleotide siRNAs of viral origin accumulate in virus-infected flies (Galiana-Arnoux et al., 2006; Wang et al., 2006); (iii) several insect viruses express viral suppressors of RNAi (Li et al., 2002; Nayak et al., 2010; Van Rij et al., 2006).

The importance of the RNAi pathway in the control of viral infections has been confirmed in other insects, in particular, the disease vector mosquito genera *Aedes* and *Culex*, which transmit important human pathogens such as dengue virus, West Nile virus, and other arthropod-borne viruses (Brackney et al., 2009; Sanchez-Vargas et al., 2009).

Although the RNAi pathway has been proposed as the most important antiviral mechanism in insects, all the studies conducted in Drosophila were performed by injecting lethal doses of virus directly to the adult fly hemocel and producing viral systemic infections (Galiana-Arnoux et al., 2006; Van Rij et al., 2006; Wang et al., 2006; Zambon et al., 2006). The antiviral role of RNAi during oral infections (mimicking natural infections by feeding) remains to be confirmed.

5.2 Inducible Responses

Another component of the antiviral innate immune system are signal transduction pathways resulting in changes in cellular gene expression, such as the NF-κB pathways (Toll and IMD), which play essential roles in antibacterial and antifungal responses, and the cytokine-activated Jak–STAT pathway. Common downstream processes of these pathways include the production of humoral factors, such as AMPs secreted from the fat body, and phagocytosis, encapsulation, and melanization of the hemolymph (Lemaitre and Hoffmann, 2007). As already mentioned, their role during the antiviral response is secondary and involves virus-specific responses, which remain poorly characterized.

5.2.1 Jak–STAT Pathway

It was shown in Drosophila that injections with DCV and CrPV induce the expression of Jak–STAT-dependent genes (Dostert et al., 2005;

Kemp et al., 2013; Merkling et al., 2015a). Global transcription profiles of flies injected with DCV showed induction of *vir-1* dependent on Hopscotch, the sole Jak kinase of Drosophila. Deficient mutant flies in *hopscotch* showed increased viral load and sensitivity to DCV and CrPV injection (Dostert et al., 2005; Kemp et al., 2013). Thus, flies respond to DCV and CrPV injection by inducing a transcriptional response mediated in part by the Jak–STAT pathway. However, the overexpression of *vir-1* or the knockdown of *vir-1* in flies did not affect resistance to DCV infection. This suggests that *vir-1* does not have a direct role in the immune control of DCV infection (Dostert et al., 2005).

In another study, reduced expression of STAT resulted in increased production of SINV replicon, suggesting that the Jak–STAT pathway is involved in controlling SINV replication (Avadhanula et al., 2009). Of note, SINV replicon refers to a transgenic fly line that produces nonstructural SINV proteins and is capable of autonomous replication. In addition, several transcripts with STAT-binding sites are regulated by SINV infection, among them the AMP attacin C (AttC). The knockdown of AttC in flies resulted in an increase in virus titers after injection with SINV (Huang et al., 2013).

Interestingly, the histone methyltransferase G9a contributes to tolerance after viral infection by regulating the Jak–STAT pathway. In deficient mutant flies for *G9a*, the hyperactivation of the Jak–STAT pathway has been associated with an increase in lethality in DCV-injected flies (Merkling et al., 2015a).

It is important to note that the involvement of Jak–STAT pathway in the antiviral response in Drosophila has only been tested upon injection of viruses or replicon systems.

5.2.2 IMD Pathway

Different studies show that the IMD pathway is involved in antiviral immunity. Most of these studies were performed using viral replicons and viral injections. One study showed that intrathoracic injections of SINV into loss-of-function *relish* mutant flies produced higher viral loads and enhanced viral replication compared to wild-type flies. An induction of AMPs Diptericin and Metchnikowin was also detected using SINV replicon in flies (Avadhanula et al., 2009). Moreover, it was found that Diptericin B (DptB) was upregulated by the infection and flies with knockdown of DptB showed an increase in virus titers (Huang et al., 2013). More recently, it was shown that a protein encoded by Drosophila gene *diedel* (*die*) is induced after viral injection and also promotes host survival by modulating the activation of the IMD pathway (Lamiable et al., 2016b).

In others experiments CrPV was injected into mutants of the IMD pathway resulting in increased sensitivity to CrPV infection and higher viral load. The infection in wild-type flies did not induce AMP production, but hemocytes were depleted during the course of the infection (Costa et al., 2009). These results suggest that activation of the IMD pathway can be uncoupled from the induction of AMP genes and depends on cellular rather than humoral mechanisms during viral infections.

A recent study used oral infection of mutant flies for key players of the IMD pathway (Tak1, Relish, Imd). These flies displayed an increase in viral replication specifically in the intestine upon DCV or SINV oral challenge. Moreover, it was demonstrated that the microbiota in the fly gut activates the IMD signaling and boosts the antiviral defense (Sansone et al., 2015). See Section 6 for more information.

5.2.3 Toll Pathway

This pathway has been associated with resistance to the dsRNA DXV virus. Infection with DXV leads to a strong induction of AMPs and a loss-of-function mutant in *Dif* was more susceptible to viral challenge and allowed increased viral replication, but the role of the Toll pathway in resistance to DXV is not clear since other loss-of-function mutants from the pathway (*pelle*, *Toll*, *spätzle* and *tube*) were not found to be more susceptible to DXV infection. Constitutive activation of the pathway, in a *Toll* gain-of-function mutant, also leads to higher susceptibility to DXV but decreases in viral titer. This suggests that the constitutive activation of the Toll pathway is able to retard viral replication but not to affect the global result of the infection. It was proposed that DXV titer may be partially independent of the pathogenic effects of infection (Zambon et al., 2005) and that Dif regulates antiviral activity by a nonclassical mechanism (Mussabekova et al., 2017). Moreover, a direct antiviral activity of the induced AMPs could not be established since enhanced expression of single AMPs did not alter resistance to viral infection or viral titers (Zambon et al., 2005).

In recent work, the role of the Toll pathway in several RNA virus infections (DCV, CrPV, FHV, and Nora virus) was analyzed by comparing two different infections routes: through the gut (oral infection) vs the cuticle (pricking in the thorax). It was shown that several Toll pathway components are required to resist virus oral infections but not infection by pricking. The results showed that NF-κB-like transcription factors Dorsal, but not Dif, are required for viral resistance. Interestingly, DCV induced the translocation of Dorsal from the cytoplasm to the nucleus in fat body cells after both types of infections (oral and pricking). This indicates that the pathway is activated no matter the infection mode, but is only effective during an oral infection (Ferreira et al., 2014). These results confirm that the interaction of viruses with Drosophila change with the route of infection and that the antiviral action of the Toll pathway targets a step of the viral cycle specific to the infection route.

5.3 Cellular Responses

Phagocytosis, apoptosis, and autophagy are cellular processes that limit viral replication and dissemination in insects. Their involvement in antiviral response in Drosophila has also been investigated only in infections by injection.

5.3.1 Phagocytosis

It is a fundamental process in the immune response of animals, and it allows for rapid engulfment of pathogens and apoptotic cells.

It was observed that phagocytosis-inhibited flies succumbed to CrPV injection faster than controls flies indicating that phagocytosis is an important antiviral mechanism (Costa et al., 2009). In addition, by injecting a panel of different viruses in flies genetically depleted for hemocytes (blood cells), a decrease in survival upon intrathoracic injection with CrPV, FHV, and VSV, but not DCV, SINV, or IIV6 was observed (Lamiable et al., 2016a).

5.3.2 Apoptosis

The process of programmed cell death is considered a component of different cellular processes as cell turnover, development, and functioning of the immune system including the restriction of viral replication. Apoptosis limits the time and the cellular machinery available for the virus, decreasing viral dissemination in the viral host (Roulston et al., 1999). Evading or delaying apoptosis is an important mechanism for some viruses to establish infection. On the other hand, viruses may stimulate apoptosis at later stages of infection to induce the breakdown of infected cells to favor viral dissemination.

Studies in Drosophila flies injected with FHV showed induction of *reaper,* a proapoptotic gene, in a p53-dependent manner, indicating that apoptosis is capable of limiting viral replication. Moreover, *p53*-deficient mutant flies showed increased levels of FHV RNA and viral titers (Liu et al., 2013). In addition, a mechanism of apoptosis-dependent phagocytosis that removes virus-infected cells was induced in DCV-injected flies (Nainu et al., 2015).

5.3.3 Autophagy

It is a process by which cells degrade cytoplasmic components, including organelles, through the lysosomal degradation pathway. Several studies have implicated autophagy in restricting the replication and promoting the elimination of pathogens, including bacteria, protozoa, and viruses (Levine et al., 2009). It has been demonstrated that autophagy plays an important antiviral role against VSV and Rift Valley Fever virus (RVFV) in adult flies. Transgenic flies depleted for different autophagy genes and injected with VSV or RVFV became more sensitive to the virus and exhibited increased viral titers (Lamiable et al., 2016a; Moy et al., 2014; Shelly et al., 2009). SINV, DCV, CrPV, or IIV6 injected in *Atg7* (protein involved in autophagosome biogenesis)-deficient mutant flies did not show any difference in survival, suggesting that autophagy is not an important mechanism for the replication of these viruses (Lamiable et al., 2016a).

Of note, it was proposed that the Toll-7 receptor activates induced antiviral autophagy and restricts viral replication against VSV and RVFV in flies (Moy et al., 2014; Nakamoto et al., 2012). However, another study claims that Toll-7 does not participate in the autophagy against VSV (Lamiable et al., 2016a). All these results indicate that cellular antiviral responses in Drosophila involve virus-specific mechanisms, which need to be studied more thoroughly and should be verified using different infection routes.

5.4 Other Factors Involved in Antiviral Immunity

Other host factors have been identified as limiting or restricting viral replication in Drosophila.

5.4.1 Vago

Vago was identified as an upregulated RNA by microarray analysis of DCV-injected flies (Dostert et al., 2005). DCV replication is increased in the fat body of *Vago* loss-of-function mutant. However, these flies did not succumb to DCV infection more rapidly than wild-type flies. The DExD/H-box helicase domain of Dicer-2 was required for *Vago* induction, suggesting that in addition to its involvement in RNAi, Dicer-2 senses dsRNA and triggers an inducible antiviral response (Deddouche et al., 2008).

5.4.2 dFOXO

The Drosophila forkhead box O (FOXO) transcription factor binds to the promoters of *Ago-2* and *Dcr-2* activating their transcription. *dFOXO* null mutant flies are more sensitive to CrPV and FHV infection. This phenotype can be rescued by overexpressing Dcr-2, suggesting that the effect of *dFOXO* on viral immunity is likely due to RNAi expression defects (Spellberg and Marr, 2015).

5.4.3 Heat Shock Pathway
Analysis of global transcription upon DCV or CrPV injection in flies reveled a strong induction of the heat shock RNAs. Moreover, mutant flies deficient for the heat shock response are hypersensitive to the infection, and overexpression of the heat shock proteins induces resistance to infection. These results suggest that the heat shock response is important for the antiviral response (Merkling et al., 2015b).

5.4.4 Polymorphisms and Virus Sensitivity
pastrel (Magwire et al., 2012; Martins et al., 2014) and *Ubc-E2H* (Martins et al., 2014) are genes that are found as a cluster of polymorphisms that have been associated with resistance or susceptibility to DCV or CrPV viral injections, respectively. Importantly, the knockdown of *pastrel* or *Ubc-E2H* led to a reduced survival upon challenge with DCV or CrPV, but not FHV.

It remains to be demonstrated if Vago, dFOXO, the heat shock pathway, and the described polymorphisms are involved in the antiviral response after an oral challenge.

6. VIRUS–BACTERIA INTERACTIONS

Drosophila is associated with a microbiome that makes essential contributions to the host health and physiology, including nutrition, metabolic homeostasis, and mating preference (Mistry et al., 2016; Sharon et al., 2010). The midgut microbiota influences nutrition, development, behavior, and pathogen resistance (Buchon et al., 2013). The resident gut bacteria activate the IMD signaling in intestinal epithelial cells, but the pathway is negatively regulated to maintain the equilibrium and to prevent microbiota clearance from the gut (Ryu et al., 2008). Antibiotic-treated flies (axenic flies, without microbiota) showed higher viral replication levels in the intestine after an oral challenge with DCV or VSV (Sansone et al., 2015). These results suggest that the microbiota is required for the antiviral defense in the gut. Intriguingly, when the survival of DCV orally infected axenic flies was analyzed by Ferreira and coworkers, there was no difference when compared with nonaxenic-infected flies (Ferreira et al., 2014). This result suggests that microbiota could be important in controlling the local infection at the gut level, but other antiviral mechanisms could be relevant in determine the outcome of the infection.

Recently, it was shown that the nutrient responsive extracellular signal-regulated kinase (ERK) pathway is a regulator of intestinal immunity against different viruses. Using ERK pathway inhibitors and driving the reduction of ERK in the gut by genetic knockouts, it was found that this pathway restricts VSV, SINV, and DCV infection in the gut epithelia of orally infected adult flies (Xu et al., 2013). Moreover, the ligand Pvf2 is induced during a viral infection and activates the receptor tyrosine kinase (PVR), which activates the ERK pathway in enterocytes. Additionally, the induction of Pvf2 is also induced by the gut microbiota signaling through the NF-κB–IMD pathway, which primes the antiviral response (Sansone et al., 2015). Interestingly these findings provide a link between the gut as an active barrier against infection, the microbiota and the antiviral responses in the host.

Wolbachia pipientis are maternally transmitted, obligatory intracellular bacteria that infect a great number of species of arthropods and nematodes (Werren et al., 2008). *Wolbachia* mediates protection in adult flies following DCV, CrPV, FHV, or Nora virus injection (Hedges et al., 2008; Teixeira et al., 2008). Interestingly, the same *Drosophila–Wolbachia* associations have a protective effect against DCV following oral infection in adults (Ferreira et al., 2014; Stevanovic et al., 2015). The density of *Wolbachia* in adults and larvae orally infected and adults infected by injection correlates with protection against DCV (Osborne et al., 2012; Stevanovic et al., 2015); however, changing gut microbiota composition does not seem to be the way by which *Wolbachia* conveys antiviral protection to its host (Ye et al., 2017). Recently, new evidence indicates that *Wolbachia* acts by increasing the expression of the Drosophila methyltransferase gene *Mt2* to confer resistance to a SINV infection by injection (Bhattacharya et al., 2017).

7. THE MOST STUDIED DROSOPHILA VIRUS: DCV

DCV is the most studied Drosophila natural pathogen, a positive sense RNA virus that belongs to the *Dicistroviridae* family. Even though it is a widespread pathogenic enterovirus, most studies involving DCV have been performed by viral injections; while oral infection, probably the most frequent route of infection, has largely been unexplored. In general, DCV injected into flies causes complete mortality within 3–13 days postinfection, depending on the viral dose and the genetic background (Dostert et al., 2005; Galiana-Arnoux et al., 2006; Jousset et al., 1972; Merkling et al., 2015a; Van Rij et al., 2006). It is also possible to generate sublethal infections by injecting with low viral doses (Ferreira et al., 2014; Gupta et al., 2017a; Longdon et al., 2013). DCV-injected flies have a reduction in metabolic rate, an increase of fresh mass (Arnold et al., 2013) and a depression in loco-motor activity (Arnold et al., 2013; Gupta et al., 2017a). Also, DCV suble-thal injections were showen to increase fly fecundity (Gupta et al., 2017a).

From a cellular aspect, the clathrin-mediated endocytosis pathway is essen-tial for infection and pathogenesis of DCV (Cherry and Perrimon, 2004). Interestingly, midgut-specific genes are strongly repressed by infection. This repression is associated with nutritional stress and an intestinal obstruction pro-duced by a malfunctioning of the crop, a food storage organ (Chtarbanova et al., 2014). It would be interesting to determine if the midgut gene repression and the pathology affecting the crop are also observed upon an oral infection.

In different studies, when DCV was orally delivered in Drosophila larvae, a preadult mortality was observed (Gomariz-Zilber and Thomas-Orillard, 1993; Jousset and Plus, 1975; Stevanovic and Johnson, 2015; Thomas-Orillard, 1988). Despite this increased death rate, a selective advan-tage in the emerging DCV-infected adult flies was observed: (i) shorter development time, (ii) an increase in the number of ovarioles and in the fresh weight (Gomariz-Zilber and Thomas-Orillard, 1993; Thomas-Orillard, 1984), (iii) an increase in the egg production (Thomas-Orillard, 1990), (iv) an increase in fertility (Thomas-Orillard, 1988). This selective advantage could be due to a positive direct effect of DCV during the adult stage, but it could also be due to an indirect effect of the selection process produced by the infection. Maybe weaker larvae with lower fitness succumb to the infec-tion, and the remaining population with the described advantages is selected.

When adult flies were orally infected with DCV, the infection was sub-lethal (Gupta et al., 2017a), or lethal in just some flies (Ferreira et al., 2014; Jousset and Plus, 1975; Wong et al., 2016). In orally infected adult flies the benefits of DCV infections in fecundity were shown in only 2 of 10 genetic backgrounds tested, and the locomotor activity was not affected (Gupta et al., 2017a). However, in an ealier study in which flies were exposed to a higher viral concentration, female flies showed reduced locomotor activity (Vale and Jardine, 2015). The oral infection of adults was also associated with a general reduction in fecal excretion (Gupta et al., 2017a), in concordance with the phenotype of intestinal obstruction observed in DCV-injected flies (Chtarbanova et al., 2014).

8. DCV TROPISM AND THE INFECTION MODE

One of the most marked differences between a DCV infection initiated by injection or by an oral infection in flies is related to the fate of the infection. After a DCV injection, in most cases, all flies die. Nevertheless, in flies orally infected or coming from infected larvae, a mortality ranging from 10% to 25%, was observed, even when highly concentrated viral stock was used (Ferreira et al., 2014; Wong et al., 2016). This suggests once again that the viral tropism, the immune response, and the pathology associated with the infection could vary depending on the infection mode.

Several studies addressed the localization of DCV in tissues after injection in adult flies. The target organs were muscles surrounding the gut and trachea, tracheal cells, follicular cells, and Malpighi tubes (Cherry and Perrimon, 2004; Ferreira et al., 2014; Jousset et al., 1972; Lautie-Harivel, 1992; Lautie-Harivel and Thomas-Orillard, 1990). A more detailed analysis of the digestive tract showed that DCV can also be detected in the muscles surrounding the crop. Interestingly, this specific tropism was associated with a failed crop function, which ultimately induced starvation in infected flies (Chtarbanova et al., 2014). This result supports previous observations showing that DCV infection produces an increase in fresh mass and a decreased metabolic rate (Arnold et al., 2013).

In a comparative analysis of flies upon virus delivery by injection or by oral infection, it was found that, independent of the delivery route, DCV tropism remains the same (Ferreira et al., 2014). The virus was detected by immunofluorescence in the fat body, visceral muscles of the gut, gonads, and hemocytes. However, a closer look to these results revealed that only 2 out of 20 orally infected flies show this widespread virus distribution, with most of the infected flies showing virus at low intensity only in the gut and the fat body. Intriguingly, all orally infected flies showed viral presence when measuring DCV RNA levels of single flies by qRT-PCR. It is however remarkable that the relative DCV levels at 20 days postinfection are lower than at 5 days (Ferreira et al., 2014). It was also observed that flies from nature lose the virus through several passages in laboratory conditions after being collected in the field (Jousset and Plus, 1975; Thomas-Orillard, 1984). These observations suggested that a mechanism of control of the infection is involved, and that a viral clearance mechanism of DCV, so far unreported, could exist.

In another study DCV was detected in the intestinal visceral muscles in only 4% of the orally infected flies (Xu et al., 2013). This observation suggests that in most oral infections of DCV, the virus could localize and be controlled locally at the gut level. In some cases, the virus would be capable of breaching the midgut barrier, infecting the visceral muscles, reaching the hemolymph, spreading systemically, and eventually killing the fly. However, this hypothesis should be tested by performing a more exhaustive immune-staining analysis or by directly searching for the presence of DCV in fly hemolymph after an oral infection.

So far, only one study (Lautie-Harivel, 1992) analyzed the DCV tropism in Drosophila larvae infected orally and in the adults derived from these larvae. First instar larvae were exposed to DCV until the beginning of the third instar when they were collected and immunostained for DCV localization. The virus was principally detected in larvae that seemed unhealthy (those that move more slowly) in the lumen of the digestive tract and in the basal part of gut cells. Once again, two different scenarios could explain this observation: (i) DCV immunostaining is not sensitive enough to detect the virus when replication is weak and (ii) not all larvae became infected. In support of the first scenario, the viral infection was confirmed by a biological test, which consists of injecting a filtered crushing of the supposedly contaminated larvae into noninfected flies and scoring mortality. However, one can speculate that even if larvae were treated to eliminate the virus that was fixed on the exterior cuticle, the input virus could remain in the gut and does not reflect viral replication. Indeed, a study showed that DCV viral replication was only detected in only 10%–20% of larvae exposed to DCV (Stevanovic and Johnson, 2015). These differences in virus replication between larvae could explain the largely reported partial preadult mortality mentioned earlier.

Regarding the tissue tropism in adult flies derived from infected larvae, unexpectedly DCV was not detected by immunostaining in any of the tissues analyzed, even if the virus was detected by a biological test (Lautie-Harivel, 1992). Other study showed that in the emerging adults there was no virus actively replicating (Stevanovic and Johnson, 2015). These results suggest that adult flies coming from larvae infected with DCV are carrying the virus, but that the virus is not actively replicating. This observation negates a direct effect of viral replication in the adult stage on the selective advantage observed in the emerging DCV-infected adult flies (discussed earlier). Nevertheless, data produced in our own laboratory show that adult flies from infected larvae display a 15% mortality, and that the virus is actively replicating in adult emerged flies (Juan A. Mondotte et al., unpublished). These results highlight that variables, such as the DCV and fly strain used, viral concentration, time of infection, etc., are important to consider and could change the fate of the infection and the interpretation of the biological process.

9. CONCLUSIONS AND FUTURE PERSPECTIVES

The use of Drosophila as a model organism has made an important contribution to our understanding of the function and regulation of innate immunity in insects. Indeed, insects can discriminate between different types of pathogens and mount specific and effective responses. Strikingly, the same pathogen can trigger a different immune response in the same organism, depending solely on the route of infection by which the pathogen is delivered.

Different modes of infection have been used to study virus–host pathogens. Direct injection of the virus provides an efficient and reproducible mode of infection that has been widely used to understand the antiviral response of the host, to determine host factors involved in the control of the infection, and to identify suppressors encoded by viruses to avoid the antiviral response. Nevertheless, special attention should be paid to oral infections that are probably the most common route of infection during the natural insect life cycle. During an oral infection, viruses face specific antiviral pathways in the gut and trigger different immune responses compared to direct injection, and are probably subject to more layers of control. However, there are several limitations to the use of oral infections as a standard procedure in the laboratory, and the control of viral input and the developmental stage of the insect at the moment of infection represent a major challenge for this approach.

Analysis of immunity in the gut deserves special attention in light of its importance to restrict dissemination of viruses and the complexity imposed by the microbiota. Due to the current outbreaks of emerging and remerging mosquito-borne viral diseases, mosquitoes are being used more frequently as a model insect in laboratories. As the possibility of using genetically modified mosquitos become more accessible, it becomes of crucial importance to confirm findings of antiviral immunity discovered in Drosophila in mosquito using similar infection routes.

To conclude, one key message from this review is that the literature concerning the insect antiviral response is sparse, fragmentary, and sometimes inconsistent. The use of different insect and virus models, inoculation routes, and different experimental conditions makes it difficult to compare results on the mechanisms involved in response to virus infection. Systematic and standardized approaches are needed before any conclusions can be drawn on the antiviral activity of immune pathways in insects.

ACKNOWLEDGMENTS

We apologize to all of our colleagues whose work has not been cited due to space constraints. We thank Vanesa Mongelli and Elizabeth Jaworski for fruitful discussions and help with editing. Chloé Baron for artwork. This work was supported by the European Research Council (FP7/2013-2019 ERC CoG 615220) and the French Government's Investissement d'Avenir program, Laboratoire d'Excellence Integrative Biology of Emerging Infectious Diseases (Grant ANR-10-LABX-62-IBEID) to M.C.S. J.A.M. was supported by AXA Research fund.

REFERENCES

Arnold, P.A., Johnson, K.N., White, C.R., 2013. Physiological and metabolic consequences of viral infection in Drosophila melanogaster. J. Exp. Biol. 216, 3350–3357.

Avadhanula, V., Weasner, B.P., Hardy, G.G., Kumar, J.P., Hardy, R.W., 2009. A novel system for the launch of alphavirus RNA synthesis reveals a role for the Imd pathway in arthropod antiviral response. PLoS Pathog. 5, e1000582.

Basset, A., Khush, R.S., Braun, A., Gardan, L., Boccard, F., Hoffmann, J.A., Lemaitre, B., 2000. The phytopathogenic bacteria Erwinia carotovora infects Drosophila and activates an immune response. Proc. Natl. Acad. Sci. U.S.A. 97, 3376–3381.

Baxter, R.H., Contet, A., Krueger, K., 2017. Arthropod innate immune systems and vector-borne diseases. Biochemistry 56, 907–918.

Behrens, S., Peuss, R., Milutinovic, B., Eggert, H., Esser, D., Rosenstiel, P., Schulenburg, H., Bornberg-Bauer, E., Kurtz, J., 2014. Infection routes matter in population-specific responses of the red flour beetle to the entomopathogen Bacillus thuringiensis. BMC Genomics 15, 445.

Bergman, P., Seyedoleslami Esfahani, S., Engstrom, Y., 2017. Drosophila as a model for human diseases—focus on innate immunity in barrier epithelia. Curr. Top. Dev. Biol. 121, 29–81.

Berkaloff, A., Bregliano, J.C., Ohanessian, A., 1965. Demonstration of virions in Drosophila infected by the hereditary sigma virus. C. R. Acad. Sci. Hebd. Seances Acad. Sci. D. 260, 5956–5959.

Bhattacharya, T., Newton, I.L.G., Hardy, R.W., 2017. Wolbachia elevates host methyl-transferase expression to block an RNA virus early during infection. PLoS Pathog. 13, e1006427.

Brackney, D.E., Beane, J.E., Ebel, G.D., 2009. RNAi targeting of West Nile virus in mosquito midguts promotes virus diversification. PLoS Pathog. 5, e1000502.

Brey, P.T., Lee, W.J., Yamakawa, M., Koizumi, Y., Perrot, S., Francois, M., Ashida, M., 1993. Role of the integument in insect immunity: epicuticular abrasion and induction of cecropin synthesis in cuticular epithelial cells. Proc. Natl. Acad. Sci. U.S.A. 90, 6275–6279.

Bronkhorst, A.W., Van Cleef, K.W., Vodovar, N., Ince, I.A., Blanc, H., Vlak, J.M., Saleh, M.C., Van Rij, R.P., 2012. The DNA virus Invertebrate iridescent virus 6 is a target of the Drosophila RNAi machinery. Proc. Natl. Acad. Sci. U. S. A. 109, E3604–E3613.

Brun, G.P.N., 1980. The viruses of Drosophila. In: The Genetics and Biology of Drosophila. Academic Press, New York.

Buchon, N., Broderick, N.A., Poidevin, M., Pradervand, S., Lemaitre, B., 2009. Drosophila intestinal response to bacterial infection: activation of host defense and stem cell proliferation. Cell Host Microbe 5, 200–211.

Buchon, N., Broderick, N.A., Lemaitre, B., 2013. Gut homeostasis in a microbial world: insights from Drosophila melanogaster. Nat. Rev. Microbiol. 11, 615–626.

Chambers, M.C., Jacobson, E., Khalil, S., Lazzaro, B.P., 2014. Thorax injury lowers resistance to infection in Drosophila melanogaster. Infect. Immun. 82, 4380–4389.

Cherry, S., Perrimon, N., 2004. Entry is a rate-limiting step for viral infection in a Drosophila melanogaster model of pathogenesis. Nat. Immunol. 5, 81–87.

Chtarbanova, S., Lamiable, O., Lee, K.Z., Galiana, D., Troxler, L., Meignin, C., Hetru, C., Hoffmann, J.A., Daeffler, L., Imler, J.L., 2014. Drosophila C virus systemic infection leads to intestinal obstruction. J. Virol. 88, 14057–14069.

Costa, A., Jan, E., Sarnow, P., Schneider, D., 2009. The Imd pathway is involved in antiviral immune responses in Drosophila. PLoS One 4, e7436.

Davis, M.M., Engstrom, Y., 2012. Immune response in the barrier epithelia: lessons from the fruit fly Drosophila melanogaster. J. Innate Immun. 4, 273–283.

Deddouche, S., Matt, N., Budd, A., Mueller, S., Kemp, C., Galiana-Arnoux, D., Dostert, C., Antoniewski, C., Hoffmann, J.A., Imler, J.L., 2008. The DExD/H-box helicase Dicer-2 mediates the induction of antiviral activity in Drosophila. Nat. Immunol. 9, 1425–1432.

Dostert, C., Jouanguy, E., Irving, P., Troxler, L., Galiana-Arnoux, D., Hetru, C., Hoffmann, J.A., Imler, J.L., 2005. The Jak-STAT signaling pathway is required but not sufficient for the antiviral response of Drosophila. Nat. Immunol. 6, 946–953.

Engelhard, E.K., Kam-Morgan, L.N., Washburn, J.O., Volkman, L.E., 1994. The insect tracheal system: a conduit for the systemic spread of Autographa californica M nuclear polyhedrosis virus. Proc. Natl. Acad. Sci. U.S.A. 91, 3224–3227.

Ferrandon, D., Jung, A.C., Criqui, M., Lemaitre, B., Uttenweiler-Joseph, S., Michaut, L., Reichhart, J., Hoffmann, J.A., 1998. A drosomycin-GFP reporter transgene reveals a local immune response in Drosophila that is not dependent on the Toll pathway. EMBO J. 17, 1217–1227.

Ferreira, A.G., Naylor, H., Esteves, S.S., Pais, I.S., Martins, N.E., Teixeira, L., 2014. The Toll-dorsal pathway is required for resistance to viral oral infection in Drosophila. PLoS Pathog. 10, e1004507.

Foottit, R., Adler, P.H., 2009. Insect Biodiversity: Science and Society. Wiley-Blackwell, Chichester, UK; Hoboken, NJ.

Galiana-Arnoux, D., Dostert, C., Schneemann, A., Hoffmann, J.A., Imler, J.L., 2006. Essential function in vivo for Dicer-2 in host defense against RNA viruses in Drosophila. Nat. Immunol. 7, 590–597.

Ganesan, S., Aggarwal, K., Paquette, N., Silverman, N., 2011. NF-kappaB/Rel proteins and the humoral immune responses of Drosophila melanogaster. Curr. Top. Microbiol. Immunol. 349, 25–60.

Gendrin, M., Welchman, D.P., Poidevin, M., Herve, M., Lemaitre, B., 2009. Long-range activation of systemic immunity through peptidoglycan diffusion in Drosophila. PLoS Pathog. 5, e1000694.

Ghabrial, A., Luschnig, S., Metzstein, M.M., Krasnow, M.A., 2003. Branching morphogenesis of the Drosophila tracheal system. Annu. Rev. Cell Dev. Biol. 19, 623–647.

Gomariz-Zilber, E., Thomas-Orillard, M., 1993. Drosophila C virus and Drosophila hosts a good association in various environments. J. Evol. Biol. 6 (5), 677–689.

Gomariz-Zilber, E., Poras, M., Thomas-Orillard, M., 1995. Drosophila C virus: experimental study of infectious yields and underlying pathology in Drosophila melanogaster laboratory populations. J. Invertebr. Pathol. 65, 243–247.

Gomariz-Zilber, E., Jeune, B., Thomas-Orillard, M., 1998. Limiting conditions of the horizontal transmission of the Drosophila C virus in its host (D-melanogaster). Acta Oecol. 19, 125–137.

Gullan, P.J., Cranston, P.S., 2010. The Insects: An Outline of Entomology. Wiley-Blackwel, Chichester, West Sussex, UK; Hoboken, NJ.

Gupta, V., Stewart, C.O., Rund, S.S.C., Monteith, K., Vale, P.F., 2017a. Costs and benefits of sublethal Drosophila C virus infection. J. Evol. Biol. 30, 1325–1335.

Gupta, V., Vasanthakrishnan, R.B., Siva-Jothy, J., Monteith, K.M., Brown, S.P., Vale, P.F., 2017b. The route of infection determines Wolbachia antibacterial protection in Drosophila. Proc. Biol. Sci. 284.

Ha, E.M., Oh, C.T., Bae, Y.S., Lee, W.J., 2005. A direct role for dual oxidase in Drosophila gut immunity. Science 310, 847–850.

Habayeb, M.S., Ekengren, S.K., Hultmark, D., 2006. Nora virus, a persistent virus in Drosophila, defines a new picorna-like virus family. J. Gen. Virol. 87, 3045–3051.

Hedges, L.M., Brownlie, J.C., O'Neill, S.L., Johnson, K.N., 2008. Wolbachia and virus protection in insects. Science 322, 702.

Hill, D.S., 1997. The Economic Importance of Insects. Institute of Biology; Chapman & Hall, London; New York.

Huang, Z., Kingsolver, M.B., Avadhanula, V., Hardy, R.W., 2013. An antiviral role for antimicrobial peptides during the arthropod response to alphavirus replication. J. Virol. 87, 4272–4280.

Jaenike, J., Polak, M., Fiskin, A., Helou, M., Minhas, M., 2007. Interspecific transmission of endosymbiotic Spiroplasma by mites. Biol. Lett. 3, 23–25.

Jennings, B.H., 2011. Drosophila—a versatile model in biology and medicine. Mater. Today 14, 190–195.

Johnson, K.N., Christian, P.D., 1996. A molecular taxonomy for cricket paralysis virus including two new isolates from Australian populations of Drosophila (Diptera: Drosophilidae). Arch. Virol. 141, 1509–1522.

Jousset, F.X., Plus, N., 1975. Study of the vertical transmission and horizontal transmission of "Drosophila melanogaster" and "Drosophila immigrans" picornavirus (author's transl). Ann. Microbiol. (Paris) 126, 231–249.

Jousset, F.X., Plus, N., Croizier, G., Thomas, M., 1972. Existence in Drosophila of 2 groups of picornavirus with different biological and serological properties. C. R. Acad. Sci. Hebd. Seances Acad. Sci. D. 275, 3043–3046.

Kamimura, Y., 2007. Twin intromittent organs of Drosophila for traumatic insemination. Biol. Lett. 3, 401–404.

Kanbar, G., Engels, W., 2003. Ultrastructure and bacterial infection of wounds in honey bee (Apis mellifera) pupae punctured by Varroa mites. Parasitol. Res. 90, 349–354.

Kari, B., Zsamboki, J., Honti, V., Csordas, G., Markus, R., Ando, I., Kurucz, E., 2013. A novel method for the identification of factors involved in host-pathogen interactions in Drosophila melanogaster. J. Immunol. Methods 398-399, 76–82.

Kemp, C., Mueller, S., Goto, A., Barbier, V., Paro, S., Bonnay, F., Dostert, C., Troxler, L., Hetru, C., Meignin, C., Pfeffer, S., Hoffmann, J.A., Imler, J.L., 2013. Broad RNA interference-mediated antiviral immunity and virus-specific inducible responses in Drosophila. J. Immunol. 190, 650–658.

Kirkpatrick, B.A., Washburn, J.O., Engelhard, E.K., Volkman, L.E., 1994. Primary infection of insect tracheae by Autographa californica M nuclear polyhedrosis virus. Virology 203, 184–186.

Kuraishi, T., Binggeli, O., Opota, O., Buchon, N., Lemaitre, B., 2011. Genetic evidence for a protective role of the peritrophic matrix against intestinal bacterial infection in Drosophila melanogaster. Proc. Natl. Acad. Sci. U.S.A. 108, 15966–15971.

Lamiable, O., Arnold, J., de Faria, I.J., Olmo, R.P., Bergami, F., Meignin, C., Hoffmann, J.A., Marques, J.T., Imler, J.L., 2016a. Analysis of the contribution of Hemocytes and autophagy to Drosophila antiviral immunity. J. Virol. 90, 5415–5426.

Lamiable, O., Kellenberger, C., Kemp, C., Troxler, L., Pelte, N., Boutros, M., Marques, J.T., Daeffler, L., Hoffmann, J.A., Roussel, A., Imler, J.L., 2016b. Cytokine Diedel and a viral homologue suppress the IMD pathway in Drosophila. Proc. Natl. Acad. Sci. U.S.A. 113, 698–703.

Lange, R., Reinhardt, K., Michiels, N.K., Anthes, N., 2013. Functions, diversity, and evolution of traumatic mating. Biol. Rev. 88, 585–601.

Lautie-Harivel, N., 1992. Drosophila C virus cycle during the development of two Drosophila melanogaster strains (Charolles and Champetieres) after larval contamination by food. Biol. Cell 76, 151–157.

Lautie-Harivel, N., Thomas-Orillard, M., 1990. Location of Drosophila C virus target organs in Drosophila host population by an immunofluorescence technique. Biol. Cell 69, 35–39.

Leggett, H.C., Cornwallis, C.K., West, S.A., 2012. Mechanisms of pathogenesis, infective dose and virulence in human parasites. PLoS Pathog. 8, e1002512.

Lemaitre, B., Hoffmann, J., 2007. The host defense of Drosophila melanogaster. Annu. Rev. Immunol. 25, 697–743.

Levine, B., Yoshimori, T., Deretic, V., 2009. Autophagy in Infection and Immunity. Springer, Dordrecht; New York.

Li, H., Li, W.X., Ding, S.W., 2002. Induction and suppression of RNA silencing by an animal virus. Science 296, 1319–1321.

Liehl, P., Blight, M., Vodovar, N., Boccard, F., Lemaitre, B., 2006. Prevalence of local immune response against oral infection in a Drosophila/Pseudomonas infection model. PLoS Pathog. 2, e56.

Linser, P.J., Dinglasan, R.R., 2014. Insect gut structure, function, development and target of biological toxins. In: Dhadialla, T., Gill, S. (Eds.), Insect Midgut and Insecticidal Proteins, first ed. In: Advances in Insect Physiology, vol. 47. Academic Press, 436 pp.

Liu, B., Behura, S.K., Clem, R.J., Schneemann, A., Becnel, J., Severson, D.W., Zhou, L., 2013. P53-mediated rapid induction of apoptosis conveys resistance to viral infection in Drosophila melanogaster. PLoS Pathog. 9, e1003137.

Longdon, B., Cao, C., Martinez, J., Jiggins, F.M., 2013. Previous exposure to an RNA virus does not protect against subsequent infection in Drosophila melanogaster. PLoS One 8, e73833.

Lu, H.L., St Leger, R.J., 2016. Insect immunity to entomopathogenic fungi. In: Lovett, B., St. Leger, R.J. (Eds.), Genetics and Molecular Biology of Entomopathogenic Fungi. In: Advances in Genetics, vol. 94. Academic Press, pp. 1–489.

Lu, H.L., Wang, J.B., Brown, M.A., Euerle, C., St Leger, R.J., 2015. Identification of Drosophila mutants affecting defense to an entomopathogenic fungus. Sci. Rep. 5, 12350.

Magwire, M.M., Fabian, D.K., Schweyen, H., Cao, C., Longdon, B., Bayer, F., Jiggins, F.M., 2012. Genome-wide association studies reveal a simple genetic basis of resistance to naturally coevolving viruses in Drosophila melanogaster. PLoS Genet. 8, e1003057.

Martins, N.E., Faria, V.G., Teixeira, L., Magalhaes, S., Sucena, E., 2013. Host adaptation is contingent upon the infection route taken by pathogens. PLoS Pathog. 9, e1003601.

Martins, N.E., Faria, V.G., Nolte, V., Schlotterer, C., Teixeira, L., Sucena, E., Magalhaes, S., 2014. Host adaptation to viruses relies on few genes with different cross-resistance properties. Proc. Natl. Acad. Sci. U.S.A. 111, 5938–5943.

Merkling, S.H., Van Rij, R.P., 2013. Beyond RNAi: antiviral defense strategies in Drosophila and mosquito. J. Insect Physiol. 59, 159–170.

Merkling, S.H., Bronkhorst, A.W., Kramer, J.M., Overheul, G.J., Schenck, A., Van Rij, R.P., 2015a. The epigenetic regulator G9a mediates tolerance to RNA virus infection in Drosophila. PLoS Pathog. 11, e1004692.

Merkling, S.H., Overheul, G.J., van Mierlo, J.T., Arends, D., Gilissen, C., Van Rij, R.P., 2015b. The heat shock response restricts virus infection in Drosophila. Sci. Rep. 5, 12758.

Miest, T.S., Bloch-Qazi, M., 2008. Sick of mating: sexual transmission of a pathogenic bacterium in Drosophila melanogaster. Fly (Austin) 2, 215–219.

Mistry, R., Kounatidis, I., Ligoxygakis, P., 2016. Exploring interactions between pathogens and the Drosophila gut. Dev. Comp. Immunol. 64, 3–10.

Moy, R.H., Gold, B., Molleston, J.M., Schad, V., Yanger, K., Salzano, M.V., Yagi, Y., Fitzgerald, K.A., Stanger, B.Z., Soldan, S.S., Cherry, S., 2014. Antiviral autophagy restricts Rift Valley fever virus infection and is conserved from flies to mammals. Immunity 40, 51–65.

Mueller, S., Gausson, V., Vodovar, N., Deddouche, S., Troxler, L., Perot, J., Pfeffer, S., Hoffmann, J.A., Saleh, M.C., Imler, J.L., 2010. RNAi-mediated immunity provides strong protection against the negative-strand RNA vesicular stomatitis virus in Drosophila. Proc. Natl. Acad. Sci. U. S. A. 107, 19390–19395.

Mussabekova, A., Daeffler, L., Imler, J.L., 2017. Innate and intrinsic antiviral immunity in Drosophila. Cell. Mol. Life Sci. 74, 2039–2054.

Nainu, F., Tanaka, Y., Shiratsuchi, A., Nakanishi, Y., 2015. Protection of insects against viral infection by apoptosis-dependent phagocytosis. J. Immunol. 195, 5696–5706.

Nakamoto, M., Moy, R.H., Xu, J., Bambina, S., Yasunaga, A., Shelly, S.S., Gold, B., Cherry, S., 2012. Virus recognition by Toll-7 activates antiviral autophagy in Drosophila. Immunity 36, 658–667.

Nayak, A., Berry, B., Tassetto, M., Kunitomi, M., Acevedo, A., Deng, C.H., Krutchinsky, A., Gross, J., Antoniewski, C., Andino, R., 2010. Cricket paralysis virus antagonizes Argonaute 2 to modulate antiviral defense in Drosophila. Nat. Struct. Mol. Biol. 17547-U41.

Nehme, N.T., Liegeois, S., Kele, B., Giammarinaro, P., Pradel, E., Hoffmann, J.A., Ewbank, J.J., Ferrandon, D., 2007. A model of bacterial intestinal infections in Drosophila melanogaster. PLoS Pathog. 3, e173.

Neyen, C., Bretscher, A.J., Binggeli, O., Lemaitre, B., 2014. Methods to study Drosophila immunity. Methods 68, 116–128.

Osborne, S.E., Iturbe-Ormaetxe, I., Brownlie, J.C., O'Neill, S.L., Johnson, K.N., 2012. Antiviral protection and the importance of Wolbachia density and tissue tropism in Drosophila simulans. Appl. Environ. Microbiol. 78, 6922–6929.

Roulston, A., Marcellus, R.C., Branton, P.E., 1999. Viruses and apoptosis. Annu. Rev. Microbiol. 53, 577–628.

Roxstrom-Lindquist, K., Terenius, O., Faye, I., 2004. Parasite-specific immune response in adult Drosophila melanogaster: a genomic study. EMBO Rep. 5, 207–212.

Ryu, J.H., Ha, E.M., Oh, C.T., Seol, J.H., Brey, P.T., Jin, I., Lee, D.G., Kim, J., Lee, D., Lee, W.J., 2006. An essential complementary role of NF-kappaB pathway to microbicidal oxidants in Drosophila gut immunity. EMBO J. 25, 3693–3701.

Ryu, J.H., Kim, S.H., Lee, H.Y., Bai, J.Y., Nam, Y.D., Bae, J.W., Lee, D.G., Shin, S.C., Ha, E.M., Lee, W.J., 2008. Innate immune homeostasis by the homeobox gene caudal and commensal-gut mutualism in Drosophila. Science 319, 777–782.

Saleh, M.C., Tassetto, M., Van Rij, R.P., Goic, B., GAUSSON, V., Berry, B., Jacquier, C., Antoniewski, C., Andino, R., 2009. Antiviral immunity in Drosophila requires systemic RNA interference spread. Nature 458, 346–350.

Sanchez-Vargas, I., Scott, J.C., Poole-Smith, B.K., Franz, A.W., Barbosa-Solomieu, V., Wilusz, J., Olson, K.E., Blair, C.D., 2009. Dengue virus type 2 infections of Aedes aegypti are modulated by the mosquito's RNA interference pathway. PLoS Pathog. 5, e1000299.

Sansone, C.L., Cohen, J., Yasunaga, A., Xu, J., Osborn, G., Subramanian, H., Gold, B., Buchon, N., Cherry, S., 2015. Microbiota-dependent priming of antiviral intestinal immunity in Drosophila. Cell Host Microbe 18, 571–581.

Sharon, G., Segal, D., Ringo, J.M., Hefetz, A., Zilber-Rosenberg, I., Rosenberg, E., 2010. Commensal bacteria play a role in mating preference of Drosophila melanogaster. Proc. Natl. Acad. Sci. U.S.A. 107, 20051–20056.

Shelly, S., Lukinova, N., Bambina, S., Berman, A., Cherry, S., 2009. Autophagy is an essential component of Drosophila immunity against vesicular stomatitis virus. Immunity 30, 588–598.

Siva-Jothy, M.T., Moret, Y., Rolff, J., 2005. Insect immunity: an evolutionary ecology perspective. Adv. Insect Phys. 32, 1–48.

Spellberg, M.J., Marr 2nd., M.T., 2015. FOXO regulates RNA interference in Drosophila and protects from RNA virus infection. Proc. Natl. Acad. Sci. U.S.A. 112, 14587–14592.

Stevanovic, A.L., Johnson, K.N., 2015. Infectivity of Drosophila C virus following oral delivery in Drosophila larvae. J. Gen. Virol. 96, 1490–1496.

Stevanovic, A.L., Arnold, P.A., Johnson, K.N., 2015. Wolbachia-mediated antiviral protection in Drosophila larvae and adults following oral infection. Appl. Environ. Microbiol. 81, 8215–8223.

Taber, C.W., 2017. In: Donald Venes, M., MSJ, FACP (Eds.), Taber's Cyclopedic Medical Dictionary, 23 ed. Davis Company, Philadelphia, PA.

Tajiri, R., 2017. Cuticle itself as a central and dynamic player in shaping cuticle. Curr. Opin. Insect Sci. 19, 30–35.

Tassetto, M., Kunitomi, M., Andino, R., 2017. Circulating immune cells mediate a systemic RNAi-based adaptive antiviral response in Drosophila. Cell 169 (314–325). e13.

Teissier, L.H.E.G., 1937. Une anomalie physiologique héréditaire chez la Drosophile. C. R. Acad. Sci. Paris 231, 192–194.

Teixeira, L., Ferreira, A., Ashburner, M., 2008. The bacterial symbiont Wolbachia induces resistance to RNA viral infections in Drosophila melanogaster. PLoS Biol. 6, e2.

Teninges, D., Ohanessian, A., Richardmolard, C., Contamine, D., 1979. Isolation and biological properties of Drosophila X-virus. J. Gen. Virol. 42, 241–254.

Thomas-Orillard, M., 1984. Modifications of mean Ovariole number, fresh weight of adult females and developmental time in Drosophila melanogaster induced by Drosophila C virus. Genetics 107, 635–644.

Thomas-Orillard, M., 1988. Interaction between a picornavirus and a wild population of Drosophila melanogaster. Oecologia 75, 516–520.

Thomas-Orillard, M., 1990. Paradoxical influence of an RNA virus on Drosophila host population. Endocyt. Cell Res. 7, 97–104.

Tzou, P., Ohresser, S., Ferrandon, D., Capovilla, M., Reichhart, J.M., Lemaitre, B., Hoffmann, J.A., Imler, J.L., 2000. Tissue-specific inducible expression of antimicrobial peptide genes in Drosophila surface epithelia. Immunity 13, 737–748.

Vale, P.F., Jardine, M.D., 2015. Sex-specific behavioural symptoms of viral gut infection and Wolbachia in Drosophila melanogaster. J. Insect Physiol. 82, 28–32.

Van Rij, R.P., Saleh, M.C., Berry, B., Foo, C., Houk, A., Antoniewski, C., Andino, R., 2006. The RNA silencing endonuclease Argonaute 2 mediates specific antiviral immunity in Drosophila melanogaster. Genes Dev. 20, 2985–2995.

Vatansever, F., de Melo, W.C.M.A., Avci, P., Vecchio, D., Sadasivam, M., Gupta, A., Chandran, R., Karimi, M., Parizotto, N.A., Yin, R., Tegos, G.P., Hamblin, M.R.,

2013. Antimicrobial strategies centered around reactive oxygen species—bactericidal antibiotics, photodynamic therapy, and beyond. FEMS Microbiol. Rev. 37, 955–989.

Vodovar, N., Vinals, M., Liehl, P., Basset, A., Degrouard, J., Spellman, P., Boccard, F., Lemaitre, B., 2005. Drosophila host defense after oral infection by an entomopathogenic Pseudomonas species. Proc. Natl. Acad. Sci. U.S.A. 102, 11414–11419.

Wagner, C., Isermann, K., Fehrenbach, H., Roeder, T., 2008. Molecular architecture of the fruit fly's airway epithelial immune system. BMC Genomics 9, 446.

Wang, X.H., Aliyari, R., Li, W.X., Li, H.W., Kim, K., Carthew, R., Atkinson, P., Ding, S.W., 2006. RNA interference directs innate immunity against viruses in adult Drosophila. Science 312, 452–454.

Werren, J.H., Baldo, L., Clark, M.E., 2008. Wolbachia: master manipulators of invertebrate biology. Nat. Rev. Microbiol. 6, 741–751.

WHO, 2016. Vector-Borne Diseases. [Online]. Available:http://www.who.int/mediacentre/factsheets/fs387/en/.

Wong, Z.S., Brownlie, J.C., Johnson, K.N., 2016. Impact of ERK activation on fly survival and Wolbachia-mediated protection during virus infection. J. Gen. Virol. 97, 1446–1452.

Xu, J., Hopkins, K., Sabin, L., Yasunaga, A., Subramanian, H., Lamborn, I., Gordesky-Gold, B., Cherry, S., 2013. ERK signaling couples nutrient status to antiviral defense in the insect gut. Proc. Natl. Acad. Sci. U.S.A. 110, 15025–15030.

Ye, Y.H., Seleznev, A., Flores, H.A., Woolfit, M., McGraw, E.A., 2017. Gut microbiota in Drosophila melanogaster interacts with Wolbachia but does not contribute to Wolbachia-mediated antiviral protection. J. Invertebr. Pathol. 143, 18–25.

Zambon, R.A., Nandakumar, M., Vakharia, V.N., Wu, L.P., 2005. The Toll pathway is important for an antiviral response in Drosophila. Proc. Natl. Acad. Sci. U.S.A. 102, 7257–7262.

Zambon, R.A., Vakharia, V.N., Wu, L.P., 2006. RNAi is an antiviral immune response against a dsRNA virus in Drosophila melanogaster. Cell. Microbiol. 8, 880–889.

Zhong, W., McClure, C.D., Evans, C.R., Mlynski, D.T., Immonen, E., Ritchie, M.G., Priest, N.K., 2013. Immune anticipation of mating in Drosophila: Turandot M promotes immunity against sexually transmitted fungal infections. Proc Biol Sci 280. 20132018.

CHAPTER TWELVE

Changing Role of Wild Birds in the Epidemiology of Avian Influenza A Viruses

Rogier Bodewes*[,1], Thijs Kuiken[†]
*Utrecht University, Utrecht, The Netherlands
[†]ErasmusMC, Rotterdam, The Netherlands
[1]Corresponding author: e-mail address: r.bodewes@uu.nl

Contents

Abstract

Waterbirds are the main reservoir for low pathogenic avian influenza A viruses (LPAIV), from which occasional spillover to poultry occurs. When circulating among poultry, LPAIV may become highly pathogenic avian influenza A viruses (HPAIV). In recent years, the epidemiology of HPAIV viruses has changed drastically. HPAIV H5N1 are currently endemic among poultry in a number of countries. In addition, global spread of HPAIV H5Nx viruses has resulted in major outbreaks among wild birds and poultry worldwide. Using data collected during these outbreaks, the role of migratory birds as a vector became increasingly clear. Here we provide an overview of current data about various aspects of the changing role of wild birds in the epidemiology of avian influenza A viruses.

Advances in Virus Research, Volume 100
ISSN 0065-3527
https://doi.org/10.1016/bs.aivir.2017.10.007

1. INTRODUCTION

Influenza A viruses (IAV) are an important cause of mainly respiratory tract disease among humans and animals worldwide. IAV are single-stranded negative-sense RNA viruses with a genome consisting of eight segments. IAV have been detected in multiple species, including humans, birds, dogs, cats, seals, horses, and pigs (Fereidouni et al., 2016; Short et al., 2015; Webster et al., 1992). The eight segments of IAV encode for multiple proteins, with segments 4 and 6 encoding for the viral glycoproteins hemagglutinin (HA) and neuraminidase (NA), respectively. These glycoproteins are present on the surface of virus particles. HA binds to sialic acids present on host cells and is responsible for fusion of the viral membrane with the endosomal membrane after endocytosis, while the NA facilitates the release of virus particles from virus-infected host cells by cleaving sialic acids from the cell surface. Based on antigenic and genetic differences of the two viral glycoproteins, IAV are categorized into different subtypes, e.g., H5N1 or H3N2 (Webster et al., 1992). Currently, 18 different subtypes of HA and 11 subtypes of NA are known (Fouchier et al., 2005; Tong et al., 2012, 2013,; Verhagen et al., 2017; Webster et al., 1992). In addition to the classification based on antigenic and genetic differences, avian IAV are divided based on their pathogenicity in chickens, namely, low pathogenic avian influenza A virus (LPAIV) and highly pathogenic avian influenza A virus (HPAIV). Circulation of IAV of the H5 and H7 subtypes in poultry may result in these viruses becoming highly pathogenic by introduction of basic amino acids in the hemagglutinin cleavage site (HACS) (Capua et al., 2000; García et al., 1996; Horimoto and Kawaoka, 1994; Senne et al., 1996; Webster and Rott, 1987). Infections of chickens with LPAIV may be subclinical or cause mild clinical signs, while infection with HPAIV results in severe clinical signs and high mortality rates (Swayne and Pantin-Jackwood, 2006). By sequencing of the HACS motif of the virus, either a multibasic cleavage site or a monobasic cleavage site can be detected. Hemagglutinins with a monobasic cleavage site can be cleaved by trypsin-like proteases, which are mainly present in the respiratory and gastrointestinal tract of chickens. In contrast, HA with a multibasic cleavage site can be cleaved by proprotein convertases, such as furin, that are ubiquitously expressed throughout the body. Replication of viruses with a monobasic cleavage site is generally restricted to epithelial surfaces of the respiratory and gastrointestinal tracts and the kidneys, whereas viruses with a multibasic cleavage site will spread systemically (Brown et al., 1992; Swayne and Pantin-Jackwood, 2006).

2. CIRCULATION OF LPAIV AMONG WILD BIRDS

Wild waterbirds from the orders Anseriformes (mainly ducks, geese, and swans) and Charadriiformes (mainly gulls, terns, and waders) form the natural reservoir of IAV of subtypes H1–16 and N1–9. Within the orders in which LPAIV are most frequently detected, variation exists among species in the frequency in which LPAIV are detected. Although it cannot be completely excluded that sampling bias plays a role, LPAIV are frequently isolated from members of the subfamily Anatinae (dabbling and diving ducks), in particular dabbling ducks (Munster et al., 2007). Among dabbling ducks, most viruses have been isolated from the mallard (*Anas platyrhynchos*) (Munster et al., 2007; Nishiura et al., 2009; Wilcox et al., 2011). Especially LPAIV of the subtypes H1–H12 have been isolated from mallards in multiple combinations. Within the order of Charadriiformes, there are also family- and species-specific patterns present. LPAIV of various subtypes have been isolated from multiple species of the families Scolopacidae, Charadriidae, Laridae, and Alcidae, with members of the family of Laridae (gulls, terns, and skimmers) most often being positive for LPAIV. Gulls are most likely the reservoir of LPAIV of the subtypes H13 and H16 (Arnal et al., 2015; Munster et al., 2007; Verhagen et al., 2014a). The diversity of LPAIV subtypes also differs between years (Krauss et al., 2004; Sharp et al., 1993; Wilcox et al., 2011).

In addition to species of the order Anseriformes and Charadriiformes, IAV have been discovered in various other birds, although in relatively low frequencies. The presence of IAV in these additional hosts is most likely at least partially associated with spillover of viruses from birds of the orders Anseriformes and Charadriiformes (Stallknecht and Brown, 2017).

Besides species-specific variation in the prevalence of LPAIV among wild birds, there are also spatiotemporal differences in the prevalence of LPAIV. Typically, the virus prevalence in mallards in North America and Europe varies from very low in spring and summer to high in autumn (autumn migration) and winter (Hinshaw et al., 1985). This high prevalence during autumn migration is most likely due to aggregation of large numbers of juvenile birds before and during migration that have not yet been exposed to IAV. When birds migrate southward, the AIV prevalence decreases rapidly, as has been demonstrated during studies in the northern part of USA, Europe, and Asia, although in parts of northern Europe the period of high prevalence continues until the end of the autumn (Stallknecht and Shane,

1988; Wallensten et al., 2007). In addition to the peak during autumn migration, there is also a peak, although lower, during spring migration (Hanson et al., 2005; Wallensten et al., 2006). In other regions, such as Africa, Australia, and South America, the temporal patterns in LPAIV prevalence of ducks are less obvious (Gaidet, 2016; Gaidet et al., 2007, 2012; Mackenzie et al., 1984; Pereda et al., 2008). However, although there are no major changes in temperature between the different seasons, there is a strong seasonality of rainfall and surface areas of wetlands in Africa which in combination with extended and nonsynchronized breeding periods results in different patterns of the infection dynamics of LPAIV (Gaidet, 2016).

In several studies, it has been demonstrated that infection with an IAV induces, at least partial, immunity in wild birds (Costa et al., 2010; Jourdain et al., 2010; Latorre-Margalef et al., 2013; Tolf et al., 2013; Verhagen et al., 2015b). Infection of ducks with a LPAIV results in immunity against the same LPAIV, but also to a certain extent against IAV of other subtypes (heterosubtypic immunity) (Costa et al., 2010; Latorre-Margalef et al., 2013). These results were confirmed by another study in Canada geese (*Branta canadensis*) (Berhane et al., 2014). However, results of an experimental study with black-headed gulls (*Chroicocephalus ridibundus*) using H13N2 and H16N3 viruses indicated that infection after 1 year with the homologous virus resulted in less virus excretion, but infection with the heterologous virus did not have any impact on either duration or level of virus shedding. In another study focusing on the age structure of immune responses to avian IAV in a free-living mute swan (*Cygnus olor*) population (Abbotsbury, United Kingdom) before and after an outbreak of HPAIV H5N1 in 2008, it was demonstrated that the breadth of the immune response accumulated with age indicating that these swans can develop long-term immune memory, but it remained unclear whether this also resulted in reduced infections at an older age (Hill et al., 2016).

LPAIV primarily replicates in the intestinal tract of ducks and, thus, transmission of LPAIV among wild birds occurs mainly via the fecal–oral route. LPAIV are shed in high concentrations in feces, and it has been demonstrated that LPAIV are able to remain infectious for a long time in water, dependent on various aspects, such as temperature, pH, salinity, and the number of freeze–thaw cycles (Stallknecht and Brown, 2017). Therefore, it was suggested that transmission via water could play a key role in transmission of LPAIV among waterbirds. This was confirmed by mathematical modeling which showed that indirect transmission of LPAIV within an environmental virus reservoir could play an important role in the

epidemiology of LPAIV (Rohani et al., 2009). Since many of the host species of LPAIV fly long distances during migration, wild birds could carry
LPAIV over large distances and between different hosts, populations, and
continents. In addition, migrating birds could also act as local amplifiers if
immunologically naïve migrating birds arrive at a certain location where a
LPAIV is circulating among resident birds (Verhagen et al., 2014b).
Although migrating birds may carry LPAIV over long distances, there are
still two main phylogenetic lineages of LPAIV which are geographically separated: the Eurasian and the American lineage (Donis et al., 1989; Olsen
et al., 2006; Yoon et al., 2014). In addition, there is evidence for an additional southern South American lineage (Pereda et al., 2008). However,
despite the fact that a number of species of both ducks and shorebirds cross
the Bering Strait regularly and there is exchange of genes between Eurasian
and American LPAIV lineages, persistence of genes from LPAIV of one lineage within the other is limited. Crossover of genes has been described for
the Eurasian H6 gene that replaced the North American H6 (Bahl et al.,
2009), and the introduction and persistence of the H14 HA gene in North
America (Fries et al., 2013; Ramey et al., 2014). It was also demonstrated by
Pearce et al. (2009), who performed a phylogenetic and population genetic
analysis of LPAIV that were collected from the northern pintail (*Anas acuta*),
a species that is known to migrate between North America and Eurasia
(Miller, 2006; Nicolai et al., 2005), at both sides of the Pacific migratory flyway in North America. Analysis of genetic data of LPAIV revealed that
Asian lineage viruses are circulating among northern pintails in Alaska, adjacent to the Bering Strait, but there was limited evidence for Asian LPAIV in
wintering areas of northern pintails in California, further south (Pearce
et al., 2009).

An important question about the role of wild waterbirds as a reservoir of
LPAIV is whether infection causes clinical signs. Although it was originally
thought that LPAIV have adapted to waterbirds in such a way that they are
not pathogenic, in various studies it has been demonstrated that LPAIV
infection was negatively correlated with body weight (for review, see
Kuiken, 2013). In addition, results of a recent study by Hoye and colleagues
indicated that LPAIV infection of Bewick's swans (*Cygnus columbianus
bewickii*) may have resulted in indirect effects on individual performance
and recruitment (Hoye et al., 2016). However, a causal relationship between
infection and reduced migration has not been shown in any of these studies
(for review, see Kuiken, 2013). Besides the impact of LPAIV infection on
body weight and migration pattern, it was also hypothesized that body

condition and annual migration could have an impact on the susceptibility to LPAIV infection (Flint and Franson, 2009). However, in a study performed by Dannemiller and colleagues with secondary LPAIV infections in mallards, no relationship between body condition, infection, and immunocompetence was found (Dannemiller et al., 2017). Also in a study of Van Dijk and colleagues in wild mallards, only weak associations between infection and shedding of LPAIV and the body condition and immune status were found. Although the exact role of infection with LPAIV on migration patterns of wild birds has not been elucidated yet, current evidence supports the hypothesis that wild birds are primarily asymptomatic carriers of LPAIV.

The availability of novel techniques to sequence viral genomes has greatly enhanced the possibility to analyze LPAIV sequences in time and space, which has provided very interesting results. In various studies, it has been demonstrated that as a result of the circulation of multiple subtypes at the same time, location, and host population, reassortments between different LPAIV occur frequently (Dugan et al., 2008; Macken et al., 2006; Olsen et al., 2015). Therefore, it has been proposed that LPAIV in wild birds form transient genome constellations, which continuously reshuffle by reassortment (Dugan et al., 2008; Olsen et al., 2015). Despite the continuous exchange of gene segments of LPAIV among wild birds, it has been demonstrated for H4 and H6 viruses that their evolutionary rate is significantly slower than H5N1 viruses and a poultry-associated lineage of H6 influenza (Fourment and Holmes, 2015).

3. TRANSMISSION OF LPAIV FROM WILD BIRDS TO POULTRY

From wild birds, there is occasional spillover of LPAIV to domestic and aquatic poultry. Transmission of LPAIV from wild birds to poultry or waterfowl most likely results from either direct or indirect contact between wild birds and poultry (Alexander, 2007; Velkers et al., 2017). Data from the Dutch LPAIV surveillance program from 2007 to 2010 were analyzed to quantify the rate of introduction of LPAIV into different types of poultry farms. It was found that outdoor-layer, turkey, duck-breeder, and meat-duck farms had a higher rate of introduction of LPAIV than indoor farms (Gonzales et al., 2013). There is also a seasonal occurrence of LPAIV outbreaks among poultry (Halvorson et al., 1985; Verhagen et al., 2017). Transmission of LPAIV from wild birds to poultry occurs regularly, but for various reasons, most outbreaks of LPAIV remain limited in time and space. Recent exceptions are the widespread occurrence of the LPAIV H9N2 in poultry populations since the mid-1990s (Alexander, 2007), and the recent emergence of the LPAIV H7N9 in Southeast Asian poultry populations (Alexander, 2007; Bui et al., 2017; Gonzales et al., 2013).

4. THE EMERGENCE OF HPAIV H5N1 IN 1997, AND ITS SPILLOVER TO WILD BIRDS FROM 2002 TO 2005

Until a few decades ago, there has been only one major outbreak of HPAIV reported among wild birds, namely, HPAIV H5N3 in common terns (*Sterna hirundo*) in South Africa (Alexander, 2000; Becker, 1966), causing the death of at least 1300 birds. In addition, there were occasionally outbreaks of HPAIV among wild birds as a result of spillover from infected poultry (Lipkind et al., 1982; Morgan and Kelly, 1990; Philippa et al., 2005).

However, this situation changed drastically with the emergence of the HPAIV H5N1 in Southeast Asia. In 1996, the HPAIV A(H5N1) virus A/Goose/Guangdong/1/1996 was isolated from a domestic goose during an outbreak with 40% morbidity on a goose farm in Guangdong province, Southern China (Xu et al., 1999). In 1997, an outbreak of a HPAIV A(H5N1) in Hong Kong occurred in poultry, which also resulted in infection of 18 humans with 6 fatalities. Phylogenetic analysis of the virus that was isolated from a human case, A/Hong Kong/156/97, revealed that this virus was a reassortant with a HA similar to A/Goose/Guangdong/1/1996, and other gene segments from LPAIV from a quail and a teal (Duan et al., 2008). HPAIV H5N1 closely related to A/Goose/Guangdong/1/1996 (the Gs/Gd-lineage) continued to circulate among domestic geese from 1996 to 2000 and from 2000 in domestic ducks (Guan et al., 2002). In addition, several reassortments with LPAIV were detected, and genetic changes resulted in several novel genotypes (Chen et al., 2006a; Guan et al., 2002; Nguyen et al., 2005).

The first outbreaks among wild birds as a result of spillover of HPAIV H5N1 from poultry to wild birds were detected at the end of 2002. During two outbreaks at two waterfowl parks in Hong Kong, HPAIV H5N1 was detected in several species of waterbirds (Ellis et al., 2004). During follow-up surveillance studies, no influenza HPAIV H5N1 was detected, indicating that the outbreak was limited. From 2003, outbreaks of HPAIV H5N1 occurred among poultry in Indonesia, with the initial introduction originating either from wild migratory birds or poultry trade (Kilpatrick et al., 2006; Vijaykrishna et al., 2008; Wang et al., 2008).

In the winter of 2003/2004, several outbreaks of HPAIV H5N1 occurred in South Korea and Japan, with viruses closely related to viruses from Southern China. Since Japan and South Korea are frequently visited by migratory birds that fly along the East Asian/Australasian flyway, it was speculated that they played a major role in these outbreaks. However, HPAIV H5N1 was not detected in migratory waterfowl during active surveillance after the outbreaks (Lee et al., 2005; Mase et al., 2005; Yamane, 2006).

Before 2005, wild birds infected with HPAIV H5N1 were only found at limited locations, and these locations were mostly in close association with outbreaks among poultry. However, in April 2005 a large outbreak occurred among several wild bird species at Qinghai Lake, China (Chen et al., 2005; Liu et al., 2005). Qinghai Lake is used as a breeding site by a large number of migratory bird species of both the Central Asian and the East Asia/Australasian Flyway. The first telltale signs were bar-headed geese (*Anser indicus*) on an islet that had neurological symptoms, such as paralysis, unusual head tilt, staggering, tremor, opisthotonus, and neck thrill. Diarrhea also was reported (Liu et al., 2005). An increasing number of birds was found dead, with in total more than 6000 birds within 2 months (Chen et al., 2005, 2006a; Liu et al., 2005). The majority of the birds that were found dead were indeed bar-headed geese, but also brown-headed gulls (*Larus brunnicephalus*), great black-headed gulls (*Larus ichthyaetus*), ruddy shelducks (*Tadorna ferruginea*), great cormorants (*Phalacrocorax carbo*), whooper swans (*Cygnus cygnus*), black-headed cranes (*Grus nigricollis*), and pochards (*Aythya ferina*) were found dead during this outbreak (Chen et al., 2005, 2006a; Liu et al., 2005). The exact origin of this outbreak remained unclear; it could have occurred via migratory birds, but also via captive-bred bar-headed geese that were housed in close vicinity of the lake (Butler, 2006; Feare, 2007). Sequencing of viruses isolated from samples collected from the birds revealed that this virus was a reassortment between clade 2.2 (genotype V) and clade 1 (genotype Z) (Chen et al., 2005; Vijaykrishna et al., 2008). Also in Poyang Lake, about 1700 km southeast of Qinghai Lake, HPAIV H5N1 was found in healthy migratory ducks in early 2005 (Chen et al., 2006b).

The Qinghai outbreak was the first step in the rapid westward spread of HPAIV H5N1 across Eurasia and into Africa. After the outbreak of HPAIV H5N1 in Qinghai, viruses from this lineage were found in Mongolia, Russia, and Northeast China in wild and domestic birds (Chen et al., 2006a; Lipatov et al., 2007; Prosser et al., 2011;

Shestopalov et al., 2006). Subsequently, the HPAIV H5N1 spread to Europe, India, the Middle East, and northern and central Africa in late 2005 and in 2006. This spread overlapped in time and space with wild bird migration via the flyways in Europe and Asia. HPAIV H5N1 were found in samples collected from multiple migratory bird species, including various species of swan, duck, goose, and grebe (Feare, 2007). The exact role of wild birds in the spread of HPAIV H5N1 from Asia to Europe and Africa in 2005 and 2006 has been a matter of debate (Feare, 2007; Normile, 2006; Olsen et al., 2006).

5. CONTINUED DETECTION OF HPAIV H5N1 IN WILD BIRDS, 2006–11

While HPAIV H5N1 of the Qinghai lineage spread from Asia to Europe, the Middle East and Africa in 2005–06, HPAIV H5N1 of clade 2.3.4 continued to expand within China and to other parts of Asia, including South Korea, Mongolia, and Japan (Smith et al., 2006; Sonnberg et al., 2013). These data highlight the complexity of the spread of HPAIV H5N1 with a possible, but not clearly defined, role of wild birds on several occasions.

In China, more than 14,000 samples were collected between April 2004 until August 2007 from 56 different species of wild birds in 14 provinces to monitor the prevalence of HPAIV H5N1 (Kou et al., 2009). A total of 149 samples tested positive, and sequence analysis of the obtained isolates revealed that these strains could be differentiated into five different clades, highlighting the genetic diversity of HPAIV H5N1 among wild birds in China in these years. The highest prevalence was found in mallards and most frequently in Qinghai province, where all virus isolates belonged to clade 2.2. In another study in the same period, birds from mostly forested sites of the southern part of China were sampled and tested for the presence of HPAIV H5N1 (Peterson et al., 2008). In this study, 939 samples were collected from 153 species of which 24 samples tested positive, with the relatively highest proportion from migratory birds. A novel reassortant of HPAIV H5N1 was detected in tree sparrows (*Passer montanus*) in 2004 in China (Kou et al., 2005), suggesting a minor role for terrestrial birds in HPAIV H5N1 epidemiology because of spill-over from poultry or wild waterbirds. Smith and colleagues sampled wild birds in Hong Kong from 2004 to 2008 for influenza (Smith et al., 2009).

While no HPAIV H5N1 was detected on farms and markets in Hong Kong during this period, HPAIV H5N1 from clades 2.3.2 and 2.3.4 was detected in various species of wild birds. These results indicated that viruses from these clades also were circulating extensively in wild birds (Smith et al., 2009).

In South Korea, there were several outbreaks of HPAIV H5N1 among poultry in winter 2006–07 with viruses of the Qinghai lineage closely related to viruses detected in Russia and Mongolia (Lee et al., 2008). Closely related HPAIV H5N1 were also detected in migratory birds at the time of these outbreaks (Lee et al., 2008). Subsequently, in April 2008, HPAIV H5N1 broke out again in South Korea with 19 duck and chicken farms affected in 7 different provinces. Remarkably, this outbreak occurred in April–May, while previous outbreaks had occurred in the winter season. While trade of unheated poultry products had not occurred between South Korea and China or between South Korea and Vietnam since 2003 (Kim et al., 2010), it was shown that several species of wild ducks migrated from Southeast Asia and China to South Korea in April and May 2008 (U.S. Geological Survey (USGS), 2009). Also, viruses isolated from this outbreak were closely related to viruses isolated from dead and moribund whooper swans in Japan in April–May 2008 and viruses isolated from chickens in Russia in April 2008 (Uchida et al., 2008; Usui et al., 2009). Therefore, it was suggested that wild birds may have introduced the HPAIV H5N1 virus to South Korea. Two years later, in November and December 2010, HPAIV H5N1 (clade 2.3.2.1) was again detected in both wild birds (mallard; Baikal teal, *Anas formosa*; Mandarin duck, *Aix galericulata*; whooper swan; and Eurasian eagle-owl, Bubo bubo) and poultry in South Korea (Kim et al., 2012; Kwon et al., 2011).

In Mongolia, HPAIV H5N1 were isolated at multiple locations and at multiple time points from carcasses of various species of waterbirds. In 2005 and 2006 isolates (bar-headed goose; whooper swan, common goldeneye; *Bucephala clangula*) belonged to clade 2.2, while isolates from 2009 and 2010 (whooper swan, bar-headed goose, ruddy shelduck, common goldeneye) belonged to clade 2.3.2.1 (Kang et al., 2011; Sakoda et al., 2010). In June 2009 an outbreak of HPAIV H5N1 occurred among wild birds (great crested grebe, *Podiceps cristatus*; little grebe, *Tachybaptus ruficollis*; black-headed gull, *Chroicocephalus ridibundus*; and common spoonbill, *Platalea leucorodia*) at Uvs-Nuur Lake, Russia. Phylogenetic analysis of the viruses isolated from a black-headed gull and a great crested grebe revealed that also these viruses belonged to clade 2.3.2.1 (Sharshov et al., 2010). Since there were no reports of HPAIV outbreaks in Russia since 2008 and poultry are not present in the Uvs-Nuur Lake, it was suggested that the virus was introduced by migratory birds from Southeast Asia (Sharshov et al., 2010).

After the detection of HPAIV H5N1 at Uvs-Nuur Lake, Russia, HPAIV H5N1 of clade 2.3.2.1 was detected both further west and further east. In October 2009, a virus from clade 2.3.2.1 was isolated from a feral pigeon (*Columbia livia*) and in February 2010 from poultry during outbreaks in Nepal. Viruses from this clade were subsequently found even further west in March 2010: in poultry in Romania, and in a dead common buzzard (*Buteo buteo*) from the Black Sea coast of Bulgaria. The latter location is a bottleneck bird migration site of global importance (Marinova-Petkova et al., 2012; Reid et al., 2011), suggesting that migratory birds played a role in the spread of this virus. Viruses of clade 2.3.2.1 were also detected further eastward: in the fall of 2010, feces collected from apparently healthy southward migrating ducks in Hokkaido, Japan (Kajihara et al., 2011) tested positive, and appeared later to be the start of an outbreak among wild and domestic birds that lasted until March 2011 (Sakoda et al., 2012).

6. GLOBAL SPREAD OF HPAIV CLADE 2.3.4.4 H5N8, 2014–16

In 2014 and 2016, HPAIV H5N8 spread from Asia to other geographical regions. These global outbreaks differed in several aspects from the global outbreak of HPAIV H5N1 in 2005–06 and possibly suggested increased adaptation of HPAIV to wild waterbird populations.

In January 2014, clinical signs of infection with a HPAIV were detected in domestic ducks on a breeder duck farm near Donglim reservoir, South Korea, an important resting site for migratory Baikal teal and other waterbirds. The next day, another farmer reported clinical signs in breeder ducks and 100 dead Baikal teals were found in the reservoir. From samples collected from these birds, a HPAIV of the H5N8 subtype was isolated that was a reassortant between a H5N8 virus detected in China in 2010 and other avian IAV circulating in China (Lee et al., 2014). These detections marked the start of a major outbreak of HPAIV H5N8, subsequently categorized as clade 2.3.4.4, among poultry and wild birds in South Korea. Indeed it was confirmed in another study that the HPAIV H5N8 isolated in South Korea were closely related to viruses detected in domestic ducks on live poultry markets in eastern China in 2013 (Wu et al., 2014). In-depth phylogenetic analysis revealed that two distinct groups of HPAIV H5N8 were introduced into the Donglim reservoir at the same time. Jeong and colleagues demonstrated that viruses of one of these groups spread subsequently among migratory bird habitats in the western part of South Korea and the nearby poultry farms (Jeong et al., 2014). Besides in South Korea and China, closely related HPAIV H5N8 also were detected from a chicken farm in Japan in April 2014 (Kanehira et al., 2015).

Like HPAIV H5N1 in 2005, HPAIV H5N8 clade 2.3.4.4 subsequently made a far jump to Europe. First, it was detected in a Eurasian wigeon (*Anas penelope*) in Russia in September 2014 (Marchenko et al., 2015). Subsequently, from November 2014 until February 2015, HPAIV H5N8 clade 2.3.4.4 spread widely across Europe, with detections in 11 poultry farms and in small number of waterfowl in a total of six countries (Germany, Hungary, Italy, the Netherlands, Sweden, and United Kingdom) (Global Consortium for H5N8 and Related Influenza Viruses, 2016).

At the same time as HPAIV H5N8 clade 2.3.4.4 reached Europe, it was detected in wild birds and poultry farms in North America. This was different from the HPAIV H5N1 2005–06 outbreak, which did not reach North America. The HPAIV H5N8 reassorted with locally circulating LPAIV, which resulted in HPAIV H5N2 containing five gene segments of the H5N8 virus and three from North American LPAIV and HPAIV H5N1 (Pasick et al., 2015; Torchetti et al., 2015). This HPAIV H5N2 subsequently spread among poultry farms in the mid-western region of the United States in 2015. Hill and colleagues also reported the occurrence of LPAIV H5N2 and H1N1 in mallards sampled in Alaska during September 2014 and April 2015. Phylogenetic analysis of these viruses indicated that they had the same ancestor as reassortant HPAIV H5N1 and H5N2 viruses and molecular clock analysis revealed that reassortment of these viruses occurred soon after crossing the Bering Strait from Asia to North America of HPAIV H5N8 (Hill et al., 2017). The widespread presence of HPAIV clade 2.3.4.4 viruses in wild birds of the United States was further demonstrated by collection of oral and cloacal swabs from wild birds along the Pacific flyway from December 2014 until February 2015, including many apparently healthy wild birds (Bevins et al., 2016). It was concluded that HPAIV likely disappeared from wild birds after February 2015, possibly because of stamping out and quarantine policies for poultry and because this HPAIV apparently could not be maintained in wild bird populations. It was speculated that wild birds played a major role in the global spread of this virus from Southeast Asia to Europe and North America.

After HPAIV clade 2.3.4.4 H5N8 disappeared in Europe and North-America in mid-2015, it continued to circulate in Asia. A reassortment event in China also resulted in a HPAIV clade 2.3.4.4 H5N6 that subsequently spread to Lao and Vietnam and also resulted in human infections (Claes et al., 2016; Shen et al., 2015, 2016). In 2016, HPAIV clade 2.3.4.4 again spread to Europe. The first signs of this were an outbreak of mortality among wild birds (mainly bar-headed geese) at Qinghai Lake, China, that were found positive for HPAIV H5N8 (Li et al., 2017) from the beginning of May to June 2016. Also at Uvs-Nuur Lake, Russia, HPAIV H5N8 clade 2.3.4.4 was isolated from live and dead wild birds found in late May (Marchenko et al., 2017). Subsequently the virus spread to Europe and Africa causing the death of thousands of wild birds and hundreds of thousands of domestic birds (More et al., 2017; Pohlmann et al., 2017).

7. ROUTES OF SPREAD OF HPAIV FROM POULTRY TO WILD BIRDS

While transmission of HPAIV from wild birds to poultry has been the focus of a number of studies, the opposite route has received only little attention. Given that wild waterbirds normally are not infected with HPAIV and that the transition from LPAIV to HPAIV only is known to occur in poultry, the detection of HPAIV in wild waterbirds suggests that transmission of HPAIV from poultry to wild birds must occur.

There are several case studies that support such transmission. During several HPAIV outbreaks in poultry, the virus also was detected in wild birds such as house sparrows (*Passer domesticus*), European starlings (*Sturnus vulgaris*), and waterbirds living in close proximity to poultry farms (Lipkind et al., 1982; Morgan and Kelly, 1990; Philippa et al., 2005). The outbreak of HPAIV H5N1 at Qinghai Lake in 2005 has been suggested to be related to the presence of domestic bar-headed geese in the vicinity, which could have transmitted the virus to wild birds of the same species living in the lake (Butler, 2006; Feare, 2007).

The specific route of spread from poultry to wild birds may differ. Possibilities are via direct contact, via air, or via vectors. Direct contact between wild waterbirds and poultry infected with HPAIV could occur at farms with a low level of biosecurity. Especially farming of domestic ducks in rice fields, common in Southeast Asia, could facilitate the transfer of HPAIV to wild waterbirds (Gilbert et al., 2006). In addition, other types of free-range poultry, as well as live animal markets, may be suitable locations for the spread of HPAIV from poultry to wild birds via direct contact.

Another possibility for spread of HPAIV from poultry to wild birds is via air. Influenza A viral RNA was detected in the air of a chicken and duck pen in a live poultry market in Taipei, Taiwan, and in chicken houses in China (Chen et al., 2009; Lv et al., 2011). Furthermore, influenza A viral RNA has been detected in the air up to 60 m downwind from barns during outbreaks of LPAIV at commercial indoor farms in the Netherlands (Jonges et al., 2015).

Finally, spread from poultry to wild birds could also occur via vector species, such as rats, mice, or flies, which have been suggested for virus spread in the opposite direction (Velkers et al., 2017). However, this is unlikely to be an important route of spread except in particular farms where such species occur in dense populations.

8. WILD WATERBIRDS AS A LONG-DISTANCE VECTOR OF HPAIV

Wild waterbirds could play a role in the local transmission of HPAIV between farms, but birds that migrate over longer distances can also play a role in the spread of HPAIV between regions, countries, or even continents (Verhagen et al., 2015a,b). It was hypothesized that suitable wild waterbird species are those that migrate over long distances directly after infection, do not develop disease, and shed high amounts of virus in the feces for a relatively long time. By use of experimental infections, it was demonstrated that several wild duck species were potentially suitable as long-distance vectors of HPAIV H5N1, because they shed virus for an average of 5 days without showing clinical signs (Brown et al., 2006; Keawcharoen et al., 2008).

Further evidence for wild waterbirds as long-distance vectors of HPAIV came from a recent in-depth study of the 2014–15 global HPAIV H5N8 outbreak, in which analysis of HPAIV H5N8 sequences, epidemiological investigations, migratory patterns of wild birds in which HPAIV H5N8 was detected and poultry trade data were combined. This study showed that long distance migratory wild waterbirds played a major role in the global spread of this virus. Most likely, they carried the virus in two steps: first, during spring migration from East Asia to their breeding grounds in Siberia and Beringia; second, during autumn migration from these breeding grounds along different flyways to Europe, North America, or back to East Asia (Global Consortium for H5N8 and Related Influenza Viruses, 2016; Lee et al., 2015) (Fig. 1).

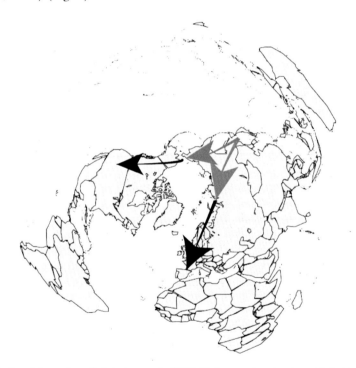

Fig. 1 Possible routes of global spread of HPAIV viruses via migratory birds. Upon spill-over from poultry in Southeast Asia, wild bird populations can become infected and spread the virus to their northern breeding grounds during spring migration (*gray arrows*). After being maintained in wild bird populations during the summer breeding season, HPAIV can spread to their southern wintering grounds during autumn migration (*black arrows*).

9. WILD BIRDS AS A MAINTENANCE RESERVOIR OF HPAIV?

While the role of wild birds as a vector of HPAIV became clear during recent outbreaks, an important remaining question is whether wild birds are able to serve as a maintenance reservoir of HPAIV in the absence of its circulation in poultry. The outbreak of HPAIV H5N1 among wild and domestic birds in Europe from 2005 to 2007 appeared to have a limited duration based on extensive monitoring, but still a few isolated cases were detected in 2008 in various European countries (Globig et al., 2009). Therefore, it could not be excluded that the virus remained present in the population, although at a low prevalence and in limited populations. Of interest, Reperant and colleagues determined that the occurrence of HPAI H5N1 outbreaks in waterbirds in the winter of 2005–06 in Europe was associated with temperatures close to 0°C. This was related to the high density of waterbirds along cold fronts close to the 0°C during winter (Reperant et al., 2010). Since in many European and North American studies it was demonstrated that HPAIV clade 2.3.4.4 were widespread among wild birds from Autumn 2014 until mid-2015, it was surprising that no HPAIV H5Nx were detected in the United States after June 11, 2015, despite intensive sampling (Krauss et al., 2016a). However, the exact implications of the lack of detection in the samples have been a matter of debate, and additional studies are necessary to elucidate if wild birds can indeed become a maintenance reservoir of HPAIV H5N8 or if regular spillover from poultry to wild birds is necessary (Krauss et al., 2016a,b; Ramey et al., 2016). Of interest, also after the HPAIV H5Nx outbreak in Europe in 2014/2015, there was no serological or virological evidence that these viruses continued to circulate among wild birds in the Netherlands (Poen et al., 2016). However, after the very recent outbreak of HPAIV H5Nx in Europe in autumn and winter of 2016/2017, HPAIV H5N5 was found in two dead greylag goose (*Anser anser*) in the Netherlands in the end of May, a few months after the last cases had been detected (OiE, 2017).

10. DISCUSSION

Avian IAV continue to circulate among wild birds and poultry. The increase in the global human population, together with a per capita increase in demand for meat, has resulted in an enormous increase in production of chickens and domestic ducks, especially in Asia (Food and Agriculture

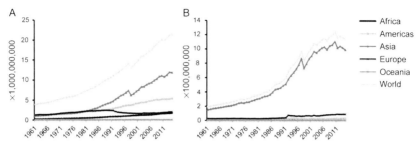

Fig. 2 Number of live chickens (A) and domestic ducks (B) in various continents from 1961 to 2014, according to data from the FAO (Food and Agriculture Organization of the United Nations, n.d.).

Organization of the United Nations, n.d.) (Fig. 2). In the past, LPAIV circulated mainly among wild birds with occasional transmission to poultry. Circulation of LPAIV of the H5 and H7 subtype in poultry did in certain cases result in mutation of the virus into a HPAIV, but only limited outbreaks were reported. However, this situation changed drastically in the past decades. Nowadays, LPAIV H9N2 and HPAIV H5N1 are endemic among poultry in a number of countries, with an increasing number of genetic variants and an increasing number of reassortments that coexist (Alexander, 2007; Perez and Sjaak de Wit, 2016). The continuous presence of HPAIV among poultry has resulted in occasional spillover to wild birds. Various characteristics of wild birds and their populations have allowed HPAIV to continue to circulate among these birds, at least for a certain period of time. This has resulted in an unexpected spread of HPAIV in recent years that is worrying for the future. Evidence that wild birds could play a role in the global spread of HPAIV came from the outbreak in 2005/2006 that started with a die-off among wild birds at Qinghai Lake (Feare, 2007; Normile, 2006; Olsen et al., 2006). More convincing evidence was collected during outbreaks in Europe and North America in 2014–15 (Global Consortium for H5N8 and Related Influenza Viruses, 2016). However, the detailed epidemiology of HPAIV among wild birds is still unclear. Therefore, additional studies are necessary to elucidate the exact routes of spread of HPAIV among different populations of wild birds and to determine whether wild bird species in which viruses are found are indeed the long-distance vectors. Furthermore, it is crucial to find out whether wild birds only remain occasional vectors for HPAIV spreading among poultry, or whether wild birds can become maintenance reservoirs of HPAIV (Fig. 3). In the latter case, the global epidemiology of avian influenza would definitely enter a new era.

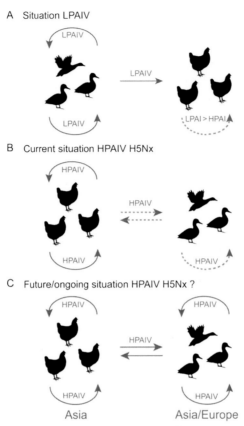

Fig. 3 Schematic overview of the current and putative future situation of the circulation of LPAIV and HPAIV among wild and domestic birds worldwide and on specific continents. *Curved solid arrows*: continuous circulation among wild waterbirds or poultry. *Curved dotted arrows*: temporary circulation among wild waterbirds or poultry. *Straight solid arrows*: regular transmission from poultry to wild waterbirds or vice versa. *Straight dotted arrows*: occasional transmission from poultry to wild waterbirds or vice versa.

REFERENCES

Alexander, D.J., 2000. A review of avian influenza in different bird species. Vet. Microbiol. 74, 3–13.

Alexander, D.J., 2007. An overview of the epidemiology of avian influenza. Vaccine 25, 5637–5644. https://doi.org/10.1016/j.vaccine.2006.10.051.

Arnal, A., Vittecoq, M., Pearce-Duvet, J., Gauthier-Clerc, M., Boulinier, T., Jourdain, E., 2015. Laridae: a neglected reservoir that could play a major role in avian influenza virus epidemiological dynamics. Crit. Rev. Microbiol. 41, 508–519. https://doi.org/10.3109/1040841X.2013.870967.

Bahl, J., Vijaykrishna, D., Holmes, E.C., Smith, G.J.D., Guan, Y., 2009. Gene flow and competitive exclusion of avian influenza a virus in natural reservoir hosts. Virology 390, 289–297. https://doi.org/10.1016/j.virol.2009.05.002.

Becker, W.B., 1966. The isolation and classification of Tern virus: influenza A-Tern South Africa—1961. J. Hyg. (Lond.) 64, 309–320.

Berhane, Y., Embury-Hyatt, C., Leith, M., Kehler, H., Suderman, M., Pasick, J., 2014. Pre-exposing Canada geese (*Branta canadensis*) to a low-pathogenic H1N1 avian influenza virus protects them against H5N1 HPAI virus challenge. J. Wildl. Dis. 50, 84–97. https://doi.org/10.7589/2012-09-237.

Bevins, S.N., Dusek, R.J., White, C.L., Gidlewski, T., Bodenstein, B., Mansfield, K.G., DeBruyn, P., Kraege, D., Rowan, E., Gillin, C., Thomas, B., Chandler, S., Baroch, J., Schmit, B., Grady, M.J., Miller, R.S., Drew, M.L., Stopak, S., Zscheile, B., Bennett, J., Sengl, J., Brady, C., Ip, H.S., Spackman, E., Killian, M.L., Torchetti, M.K., Sleeman, J.M., Deliberto, T.J., 2016. Widespread detection of highly pathogenic H5 influenza viruses in wild birds from the Pacific flyway of the United States. Sci. Rep. 6, 28980. https://doi.org/10.1038/srep28980.

Brown, C.C., Olander, H.J., Senne, D.A., 1992. A pathogenesis study of highly pathogenic avian influenza virus H5N2 in chickens, using immunohistochemistry. J. Comp. Pathol. 107, 341–348.

Brown, J., Stallknecht, D., Beck, J., Suarez, D., Swayne, D., 2006. Susceptibility of north American ducks and gulls to H5N1 highly pathogenic avian influenza viruses. Emerg. Infect. Dis. 12, 1663–1670. https://doi.org/10.3201/eid1211.060652.

Bui, C., Rahman, B., Heywood, A.E., MacIntyre, C.R., 2017. A meta-analysis of the prevalence of influenza a H5N1 and H7N9 infection in birds. Transbound. Emerg. Dis. 64, 967–977. https://doi.org/10.1111/tbed.12466.

Butler, D., 2006. Doubts hang over source of bird flu spread. Nature 439, 772. https://doi.org/10.1038/439772a.

Capua, I., Mutinelli, F., Marangon, S., Alexander, D.J., 2000. H7N1 avian influenza in Italy (1999 to 2000) in intensively reared chickens and turkeys. Avian Pathol. 29, 537–543. https://doi.org/10.1080/03079450020016779.

Chen, H., Smith, G.J.D., Zhang, S.Y., Qin, K., Wang, J., Li, K.S., Webster, R.G., Peiris, J.S.M., Guan, Y., 2005. Avian flu: H5N1 virus outbreak in migratory waterfowl. Nature 436, 191–192. https://doi.org/10.1038/nature03974.

Chen, H., Li, Y., Li, Z., Shi, J., Shinya, K., Deng, G., Qi, Q., Tian, G., Fan, S., Zhao, H., Sun, Y., Kawaoka, Y., 2006a. Properties and dissemination of H5N1 viruses isolated during an influenza outbreak in migratory waterfowl in Western China. J. Virol. 80, 5976–5983. https://doi.org/10.1128/JVI.00110-06.

Chen, H., Smith, G.J.D., Li, K.S., Wang, J., Fan, X.H., Rayner, J.M., Vijaykrishna, D., Zhang, J.X., Zhang, L.J., Guo, C.T., Cheung, C.L., Xu, K.M., Duan, L., Huang, K., Qin, K., Leung, Y.H.C., Wu, W.L., Lu, H.R., Chen, Y., Xia, N.S., Naipospos, T.S.P., Yuen, K.Y., Hassan, S.S., Bahri, S., Nguyen, T.D., Webster, R.G., Peiris, J.S.M., Guan, Y., 2006b. Establishment of multiple sublineages of H5N1 influenza virus in Asia: implications for pandemic control. Proc. Natl. Acad. Sci. U.S.A. 103, 2845–2850. https://doi.org/10.1073/pnas.0511120103.

Chen, P.-S., Kun Lin, C., Ta Tsai, F., Yang, C.-Y., Lee, C.-H., Liao, Y.-S., Yeh, C.-Y., King, C.-C., Wu, J.-L., Wang, Y.-C., Lin, K.-H., 2009. Quantification of airborne influenza and avian influenza virus in a wet poultry market using a filter/real-time qPCR method. Aerosol Sci. Technol. 43 (4), 290–297. https://doi.org/10.1080/02786820802621232.

Claes, F., Morzaria, S.P., Donis, R.O., 2016. Emergence and dissemination of clade 2.3.4.4 H5Nx influenza viruses—how is the Asian HPAI H5 lineage maintained. Curr. Opin. Virol. 16, 158–163. https://doi.org/10.1016/j.coviro.2016.02.005.

Costa, T.P., Brown, J.D., Howerth, E.W., Stallknecht, D.E., 2010. The effect of age on avian influenza viral shedding in mallards (Anas platyrhynchos). Avian Dis. 54, 581–585. https://doi.org/10.1637/8692-031309-ResNote.1.

Dannemiller, N.G., Webb, C.T., Wilson, K.R., Bentler, K.T., Mooers, N.L., Ellis, J.W., Root, J.J., Franklin, A.B., Shriner, S.A., 2017. Impact of body condition on influenza A virus infection dynamics in mallards following a secondary exposure. PLoS One 12, e0175757. https://doi.org/10.1371/journal.pone.0175757.

Donis, R.O., Bean, W.J., Kawaoka, Y., Webster, R.G., 1989. Distinct lineages of influenza virus H4 hemagglutinin genes in different regions of the world. Virology 169, 408–417.

Duan, L., Bahl, J., Smith, G.J.D., Wang, J., Vijaykrishna, D., Zhang, L.J., Zhang, J.X., Li, K.S., Fan, X.H., Cheung, C.L., Huang, K., Poon, L.L.M., Shortridge, K.F., Webster, R.G., Peiris, J.S.M., Chen, H., Guan, Y., 2008. The development and genetic diversity of H5N1 influenza virus in China, 1996–2006. Virology 380, 243–254. https://doi.org/10.1016/j.virol.2008.07.038.

Dugan, V.G., Chen, R., Spiro, D.J., Sengamalay, N., Zaborsky, J., Ghedin, E., Nolting, J., Swayne, D.E., Runstadler, J.A., Happ, G.M., Senne, D.A., Wang, R., Slemons, R.D., Holmes, E.C., Taubenberger, J.K., 2008. The evolutionary genetics and emergence of avian influenza viruses in wild birds. PLoS Pathog. 4, e1000076. https://doi.org/10.1371/journal.ppat.1000076.

Ellis, T.M., Barry Bousfield, R., Bissett, L.A., Dyrting, K.C., Luk, G.S.M., Tsim, S.T., Sturm-ramirez, K., Webster, R.G., Guan, Y., Peiris, J.S.M., 2004. Investigation of outbreaks of highly pathogenic H5N1 avian influenza in waterfowl and wild birds in Hong Kong in late 2002. Avian Pathol. 33, 492–505. https://doi.org/10.1080/03079450400003601.

Feare, C.J., 2007. The role of wild birds in the spread of HPAI H5N1. Avian Dis. 51, 440–447. https://doi.org/10.1637/7575-040106R1.1.

Fereidouni, S., Munoz, O., Von Dobschuetz, S., De Nardi, M., 2016. Influenza virus infection of marine mammals. Ecohealth 13, 161–170. https://doi.org/10.1007/s10393-014-0968-1.

Flint, P.L., Franson, J.C., 2009. Does influenza A affect body condition of wild mallard ducks, or vice versa? Proc. Biol. Sci 276 (1666), 2345–2346 (discussion 2347–2349). https://doi.org/10.1098/rspb.2008.1962. (Epub 2009 Apr 1).

Food and Agriculture Organization of the United Nations, n.d. FAOSTAT [WWW Document]. URL http://www.fao.org/faostat/en/#data/QA (accessed 1.25.17).

Fouchier, R.A.M., Munster, V., Wallensten, A., Bestebroer, T.M., Herfst, S., Smith, D., Rimmelzwaan, G.F., Olsen, B., Osterhaus, A.D.M.E., 2005. Characterization of a novel Influenza A virus Hemagglutinin subtype (H16) obtained from black-headed gulls. J. Virol. 79, 2814–2822. https://doi.org/10.1128/JVI.79.5.2814-2822.2005.

Fourment, M., Holmes, E.C., 2015. Avian influenza virus exhibits distinct evolutionary dynamics in wild birds and poultry. BMC Evol. Biol. 15, 120. https://doi.org/10.1186/s12862-015-0410-5.

Fries, A.C., Nolting, J.M., Danner, A., Webster, R.G., Bowman, A.S., Krauss, S., Slemons, R.D., 2013. Evidence for the circulation and inter-hemispheric movement of the H14 subtype influenza A virus. PLoS One 8, e59216. https://doi.org/10.1371/journal.pone.0059216.

Gaidet, N., 2016. Ecology of avian influenza virus in wild birds in tropical Africa. Avian Dis. 60, 296–301. https://doi.org/10.1637/11149-051115-Review.

Gaidet, N., Dodman, T., Caron, A., Balança, G., Desvaux, S., Goutard, F., Cattoli, G., Lamarque, F., Hagemeijer, W., Monicat, F., 2007. Avian influenza viruses in water birds, Africa. Emerg. Infect. Dis. 13, 626–629. https://doi.org/10.3201/eid1304.061011.

Gaidet, N., Caron, A., Cappelle, J., Cumming, G.S., Balança, G., Hammoumi, S., Cattoli, G., Abolnik, C., de Almeida, R.S., Gil, P., Fereidouni, S.R., Grosbois, V., Tran, A., Mundava, J., Fofana, B., El Mamy, A.B.O., Ndlovu, M., Mondain-Monval, J.Y., Triplet, P., Hagemeijer, W., Karesh, W.B., Newman, S.H., Dodman, T., 2012. Understanding the ecological drivers of avian influenza virus infection in wildfowl: a continental-scale study across Africa. Proc. Biol. Sci. 279, 1131–1141. https://doi.org/10.1098/rspb.2011.1417.

García, M., Crawford, J.M., Latimer, J.W., Rivera-Cruz, E., Perdue, M.L., 1996. Heterogeneity in the haemagglutinin gene and emergence of the highly pathogenic phenotype among recent H5N2 avian influenza viruses from Mexico. J. Gen. Virol. 77 (Pt. 7), 1493–1504. https://doi.org/10.1099/0022-1317-77-7-1493.

Gilbert, M., Chaitaweesub, P., Parakamawongsa, T., Premashthira, S., Tiensin, T., Kalpravidh, W., Wagner, H., Slingenbergh, J., 2006. Free-grazing ducks and highly pathogenic avian influenza, Thailand. Emerg. Infect. Dis. 12, 227–234. https://doi.org/10.3201/eid1202.050640.

Global Consortium for H5N8 and Related Influenza Viruses, 2016. Role for migratory wild birds in the global spread of avian influenza H5N8. Science 354, 213–217. https://doi.org/10.1126/science.aaf8852.

Globig, A., Staubach, C., Beer, M., Köppen, U., Fiedler, W., Nieburg, M., Wilking, H., Starick, E., Teifke, J.P., Werner, O., Unger, F., Grund, C., Wolf, C., Roost, H., Feldhusen, F., Conraths, F.J., Mettenleiter, T.C., Harder, T.C., 2009. Epidemiological and ornithological aspects of outbreaks of highly pathogenic avian influenza virus H5N1 of Asian lineage in wild birds in Germany, 2006 and 2007. Transbound. Emerg. Dis. 56, 57–72. https://doi.org/10.1111/j.1865-1682.2008.01061.x.

Gonzales, J.L., Stegeman, J.A., Koch, G., de Wit, S.J., Elbers, A.R.W., 2013. Rate of introduction of a low pathogenic avian influenza virus infection in different poultry production sectors in the Netherlands. Influenza Other Respir. Viruses 7, 6–10. https://doi.org/10.1111/j.1750-2659.2012.00348.x.

Guan, Y., Peiris, M., Kong, K.F., Dyrting, K.C., Ellis, T.M., Sit, T., Zhang, L.J., Shortridge, K.F., 2002. H5N1 influenza viruses isolated from geese in Southeastern China: evidence for genetic reassortment and interspecies transmission to ducks. Virology 292, 16–23. https://doi.org/10.1006/viro.2001.1207.

Halvorson, D.A., Kelleher, C.J., Senne, D.A., 1985. Epizootiology of avian influenza: effect of season on incidence in sentinel ducks and domestic turkeys in Minnesota. Appl. Environ. Microbiol. 49, 914–919.

Hanson, B.A., Swayne, D.E., Senne, D.A., Lobpries, D.S., Hurst, J., Stallknecht, D.E., 2005. Avian influenza viruses and paramyxoviruses in wintering and resident ducks in Texas. J. Wildl. Dis. 41, 624–628. https://doi.org/10.7589/0090-3558-41.3.624.

Hill, S.C., Manvell, R.J., Schulenburg, B., Shell, W., Wikramaratna, P.S., Perrins, C., Sheldon, B.C., Brown, I.H., Pybus, O.G., 2016. Antibody responses to avian influenza viruses in wild birds broaden with age. Proc. Biol. Sci. 283. https://doi.org/10.1098/rspb.2016.2159.

Hill, N.J., Hussein, I.T.M., Davis, K.R., Ma, E.J., Spivey, T.J., Ramey, A.M., Puryear, W.B., Das, S.R., Halpin, R.A., Lin, X., Fedorova, N.B., Suarez, D.L., Boyce, W.M., Runstadler, J.A., 2017. Reassortment of Influenza A viruses in wild birds in Alaska before H5 clade 2.3.4.4 outbreaks. Emerg. Infect. Dis. 23, 654–657. https://doi.org/10.3201/eid2304.161668.

Hinshaw, V.S., Wood, J.M., Webster, R.G., Deibel, R., Turner, B., 1985. Circulation of influenza viruses and paramyxoviruses in waterfowl originating from two different areas of North America. Bull. World Health Organ. 63, 711–719.

Horimoto, T., Kawaoka, Y., 1994. Reverse genetics provides direct evidence for a correlation of hemagglutinin cleavability and virulence of an avian influenza A virus. J. Virol. 68, 3120–3128.

Hoye, B.J., Munster, V.J., Huig, N., de Vries, P., Oosterbeek, K., Tijsen, W., Klaassen, M., Fouchier, R.A.M., van Gils, J.A., 2016. Hampered performance of migratory swans: intra- and inter-seasonal effects of avian influenza virus. Integr. Comp. Biol. 56, 317–329. https://doi.org/10.1093/icb/icw038.

Jeong, J., Kang, H.-M., Lee, E.-K., Song, B.-M., Kwon, Y.-K., Kim, H.-R., Choi, K.-S., Kim, J.-Y., Lee, H.-J., Moon, O.-K., Jeong, W., Choi, J., Baek, J.-H., Joo, Y.-S., Park, Y.H., Lee, H.-S., Lee, Y.-J., 2014. Highly pathogenic avian influenza virus (H5N8) in domestic poultry and its relationship with migratory birds in South Korea during 2014. Vet. Microbiol. 173, 249–257. https://doi.org/10.1016/j.vetmic.2014.08.002.

Jonges, M., van Leuken, J., Wouters, I., Koch, G., Meijer, A., Koopmans, M., 2015. Wind-mediated spread of low-pathogenic avian influenza virus into the environment during outbreaks at commercial poultry farms. PLoS One 10, e0125401. https://doi.org/10.1371/journal.pone.0125401.

Jourdain, E., Gunnarsson, G., Wahlgren, J., Latorre-Margalef, N., Bröjer, C., Sahlin, S., Svensson, L., Waldenström, J., Lundkvist, Å., Olsen, B., 2010. Influenza virus in a natural host, the mallard: experimental infection data. PLoS One 5, e8935. https://doi.org/10.1371/journal.pone.0008935.

Kajihara, M., Matsuno, K., Simulundu, E., Muramatsu, M., Noyori, O., Manzoor, R., Nakayama, E., Igarashi, M., Tomabechi, D., Yoshida, R., Okamatsu, M., Sakoda, Y., Ito, K., Kida, H., Takada, A., 2011. An H5N1 highly pathogenic avian influenza virus that invaded Japan through waterfowl migration. Jpn. J. Vet. Res. 59, 89–100.

Kanehira, K., Uchida, Y., Takemae, N., Hikono, H., Tsunekuni, R., Saito, T., 2015. Characterization of an H5N8 influenza A virus isolated from chickens during an outbreak of severe avian influenza in Japan in April 2014. Arch. Virol. 160, 1629–1643. https://doi.org/10.1007/s00705-015-2428-9.

Kang, H.-M., Batchuluun, D., Kim, M.-C., Choi, J.-G., Erdene-Ochir, T.-O., Paek, M.-R., Sugir, T., Sodnomdarjaa, R., Kwon, J.-H., Lee, Y.-J., 2011. Genetic analyses of H5N1 avian influenza virus in Mongolia, 2009 and its relationship with those of Eastern Asia. Vet. Microbiol. 147, 170–175. https://doi.org/10.1016/j.vetmic.2010.05.045.

Keawcharoen, J., van Riel, D., van Amerongen, G., Bestebroer, T., Beyer, W.E., van Lavieren, R., Osterhaus, A.D.M.E., Fouchier, R.A.M., Kuiken, T., 2008. Wild ducks as long-distance vectors of highly pathogenic avian influenza virus (H5N1). Emerg. Infect. Dis. 14, 600–607. https://doi.org/10.3201/eid1404.071016.

Kilpatrick, A.M., Chmura, A.A., Gibbons, D.W., Fleischer, R.C., Marra, P.P., Daszak, P., 2006. Predicting the global spread of H5N1 avian influenza. Proc. Natl. Acad. Sci. U.S.A. 103, 19368–19373. https://doi.org/10.1073/pnas.0609227103.

Kim, H.-R., Park, C.-K., Lee, Y.-J., Woo, G.-H., Lee, K.-K., Oem, J.-K., Kim, S.-H., Jean, Y.-H., Bae, Y.-C., Yoon, S.-S., Roh, I.-S., Jeong, O.-M., Kim, H.-Y., Choi, J.-S., Byun, J.-W., Song, Y.-K., Kwon, J.-H., Joo, Y.-S., 2010. An outbreak of highly pathogenic H5N1 avian influenza in Korea, 2008. Vet. Microbiol. 141, 362–366. https://doi.org/10.1016/j.vetmic.2009.09.011.

Kim, H.-R., Lee, Y.-J., Park, C.-K., Oem, J.-K., Lee, O.-S., Kang, H.-M., Choi, J.-G., Bae, Y.-C., 2012. Highly pathogenic avian influenza (H5N1) outbreaks in wild birds and poultry, South Korea. Emerg. Infect. Dis. 18, 480–483. https://doi.org/10.3201/eid1803.111490.

Kou, Z., Lei, F.M., Yu, J., Fan, Z.J., Yin, Z.H., Jia, C.X., Xiong, K.J., Sun, Y.H., Zhang, X.W., Wu, X.M., Gao, X.B., Li, T.X., 2005. New genotype of avian influenza H5N1 viruses isolated from tree sparrows in China. J. Virol. 79, 15460–15466. https://doi.org/10.1128/JVI.79.24.15460-15466.2005.

Kou, Z., Li, Y., Yin, Z., Guo, S., Wang, M., Gao, X., Li, P., Tang, L., Jiang, P., Luo, Z., Xin, Z., Ding, C., He, Y., Ren, Z., Cui, P., Zhao, H., Zhang, Z., Tang, S., Yan, B., Lei, F., Li, T., 2009. The survey of H5N1 flu virus in wild birds in 14 provinces of China from 2004 to 2007. PLoS One 4, e6926. https://doi.org/10.1371/journal.pone.0006926.

Krauss, S., Walker, D., Pryor, S.P., Niles, L., Chenghong, L., Hinshaw, V.S., Webster, R.G., 2004. Influenza A viruses of migrating wild aquatic birds in North America. Vector Borne Zoonotic Dis. 4, 177–189. https://doi.org/10.1089/vbz.2004.4.177.

Krauss, S., Stallknecht, D.E., Slemons, R.D., Bowman, A.S., Poulson, R.L., Nolting, J.M., Knowles, J.P., Webster, R.G., 2016a. The enigma of the apparent disappearance of Eurasian highly pathogenic H5 clade 2.3.4.4 influenza A viruses in North American waterfowl. Proc. Natl. Acad. Sci. U.S.A. 113, 9033–9038. https://doi.org/10.1073/pnas.1608853113.

Krauss, S., Stallknecht, D.E., Slemons, R.D., Bowman, A.S., Poulson, R.L., Nolting, J.M., Knowles, J.P., Webster, R.G., 2016b. Reply to Ramey et al.: let time be the arbiter. Proc. Natl. Acad. Sci. U.S.A. 113, E6553–E6554. https://doi.org/10.1073/pnas.1614678113.

Kuiken, T., 2013. Is low pathogenic avian influenza virus virulent for wild waterbirds? Proc. Biol. Sci. 280, 20130990. https://doi.org/10.1098/rspb.2013.0990.

Kwon, H., Song, M.-S., Pascua, P.N.Q., Baek, Y.H., Lee, J.H., Hong, S.-P., Rho, J.-B., Kim, J.-K., Poo, H., Kim, C.-J., Choi, Y.K., 2011. Genetic characterization and pathogenicity assessment of highly pathogenic H5N1 avian influenza viruses isolated from migratory wild birds in 2011, South Korea. Virus Res. 160, 305–315. https://doi.org/10.1016/j.virusres.2011.07.003.

Latorre-Margalef, N., Grosbois, V., Wahlgren, J., Munster, V.J., Tolf, C., Fouchier, R.A.M., Osterhaus, A.D.M.E., Olsen, B., Waldenström, J., 2013. Heterosubtypic immunity to influenza A virus infections in mallards may explain existence of multiple virus subtypes. PLoS Pathog. 9, e1003443. https://doi.org/10.1371/journal.ppat.1003443.

Lee, C.-W., Suarez, D.L., Tumpey, T.M., Sung, H.-W., Kwon, Y.-K., Lee, Y.-J., Choi, J.-G., Joh, S.-J., Kim, M.-C., Lee, E.-K., Park, J.-M., Lu, X., Katz, J.M., Spackman, E., Swayne, D.E., Kim, J.-H., 2005. Characterization of highly pathogenic H5N1 avian influenza A viruses isolated from South Korea. J. Virol. 79, 3692–3702. https://doi.org/10.1128/JVI.79.6.3692-3702.2005.

Lee, Y.-J., Choi, Y.-K., Kim, Y.-J., Song, M.-S., Jeong, O.-M., Lee, E.-K., Jeon, W.-J., Jeong, W., Joh, S.-J., Choi, K., Her, M., Kim, M.-C., Kim, A., Kim, M.-J., ho Lee, E., Oh, T.-G., Moon, H.-J., Yoo, D.-W., Kim, J.-H., Sung, M.-H., Poo, H., Kwon, J.-H., Kim, C.-J., 2008. Highly pathogenic avian influenza virus (H5N1) in domestic poultry and relationship with migratory birds, South Korea. Emerg. Infect. Dis. 14, 487–490. https://doi.org/10.3201/eid1403.070767.

Lee, Y.-J., Kang, H.-M., Lee, E.-K., Song, B.-M., Jeong, J., Kwon, Y.-K., Kim, H.-R., Lee, K.-J., Hong, M.-S., Jang, I., Choi, K.-S., Kim, J.-Y., Lee, H.-J., Kang, M.-S., Jeong, O.-M., Baek, J.-H., Joo, Y.-S., Park, Y.H., Lee, H.-S., 2014. Novel reassortant influenza A(H5N8) viruses, South Korea, 2014. Emerg. Infect. Dis. 20, 1087–1089. https://doi.org/10.3201/eid2006.140233.

Lee, D.-H., Torchetti, M.K., Winker, K., Ip, H.S., Song, C.-S., Swayne, D.E., 2015. Intercontinental spread of Asian-Origin H5N8 to North America through Beringia by migratory birds. J. Virol. 89, 6521–6524. https://doi.org/10.1128/JVI.00728-15.

Li, M., Liu, H., Bi, Y., Sun, J., Wong, G., Liu, D., Li, L., Liu, J., Chen, Q., Wang, H., He, Y., Shi, W., Gao, G.F., Chen, J., 2017. Highly pathogenic avian influenza A(H5N8) virus in wild migratory birds, Qinghai Lake, China. Emerg. Infect. Dis. 23, 637–641. https://doi.org/10.3201/eid2304.161866.

Lipatov, A.S., Evseenko, V.A., Yen, H.-L., Zaykovskaya, A.V., Durimanov, A.G., Zolotykh, S.I., Netesov, S.V., Drozdov, I.G., Onishchenko, G.G., Webster, R.G., Shestopalov, A.M., 2007. Influenza (H5N1) viruses in poultry, Russian Federation, 2005–2006. Emerg. Infect. Dis. 13, 539–546. https://doi.org/10.3201/eid1304.061266.

Lipkind, M., Shihmanter, E., Shoham, D., 1982. Further characterization of H7N7 avian influenza virus isolated from migrating starlings wintering in Israel. Zentralbl. Veterinarmed. B 29, 566–572.

Liu, J., Xiao, H., Lei, F., Zhu, Q., Qin, K., Zhang, X.-W., Zhang, X.-L., Zhao, D., Wang, G., Feng, Y., Ma, J., Liu, W., Wang, J., Gao, G.F., 2005. Highly pathogenic H5N1 influenza virus infection in migratory birds. Science 309, 1206. https://doi.org/10.1126/science.1115273.

Lv, J., Wei, B., Chai, T., Xia, X., Miao, Z., Yao, M., Gao, Y., Huang, R., Yang, H., Roesler, U., 2011. Development of a real-time RT-PCR method for rapid detection of H9 avian influenza virus in the air. Arch. Virol. 156, 1795–1801. https://doi.org/10.1007/s00705-011-1054-4.

Macken, C.A., Webby, R.J., Bruno, W.J., 2006. Genotype turnover by reassortment of replication complex genes from avian influenza A virus. J. Gen. Virol. 87, 2803–2815. https://doi.org/10.1099/vir.0.81454-0.

Mackenzie, J.S., Edwards, E.C., Holmes, R.M., Hinshaw, V.S., 1984. Isolation of ortho- and paramyxoviruses from wild birds in Western Australia, and the characterization of novel influenza A viruses. Aust. J. Exp. Biol. Med. Sci. 62 (Pt. 1), 89–99.

Marchenko, V.Y., Susloparov, I.M., Kolosova, N.P., Goncharova, N.I., Shipovalov, A.V., Durymanov, A.G., Ilyicheva, T.N., Budatsirenova, L.V., Ivanova, V.K., Ignatyev, G.A., Ershova, S.N., Tulyahova, V.S., Mikheev, V.N., Ryzhikov, A.B., 2015. Influenza A(H5N8) virus isolation in Russia, 2014. Arch. Virol. 160, 2857–2860. https://doi.org/10.1007/s00705-015-2570-4.

Marchenko, V.Y., Susloparov, I.M., Komissarov, A.B., Fadeev, A., Goncharova, N.I., Shipovalov, A.V., Svyatchenko, S.V., Durymanov, A.G., Ilyicheva, T.N., Salchak, L.K., Svintitskaya, E.P., Mikheev, V.N., Ryzhikov, A.B., 2017. Reintroduction of highly pathogenic avian influenza A/H5N8 virus of clade 2.3.4.4. in Russia. Arch. Virol. 162, 1381–1385. https://doi.org/10.1007/s00705-017-3246-z.

Marinova-Petkova, A., Georgiev, G., Seiler, P., Darnell, D., Franks, J., Krauss, S., Webby, R.J., Webster, R.G., 2012. Spread of influenza virus A (H5N1) clade 2.3.2.1 to Bulgaria in common buzzards. Emerg. Infect. Dis. 18, 1596–1602. https://doi.org/10.3201/eid1810.120357.

Mase, M., Tsukamoto, K., Imada, T., Imai, K., Tanimura, N., Nakamura, K., Yamamoto, Y., Hitomi, T., Kira, T., Nakai, T., Kiso, M., Horimoto, T., Kawaoka, Y., Yamaguchi, S., 2005. Characterization of H5N1 influenza A viruses isolated during the 2003-2004 influenza outbreaks in Japan. Virology 332, 167–176. https://doi.org/10.1016/j.virol.2004.11.016.

Miller, M., 2006. Spring Migration of Northern Pintails Assessed with Satellite Telemetry. [WWW Document]. URL, www.werc.usgs.gov/OLDsitedata/pubbriefs/millerpbsep2006.html.

More, S., Bicout, D., Bøtner, A., Butterworth, A., Calistri, P., Depner, K., Edwards, S., Garin-Bastuji, B., Good, M., Gortázar Schmidt, C., Michel, V., Miranda, M., Saxmose Nielsen, S., Raj, M., Sihvonen, L., Spoolder, H., Thulke, H., Velarde, A., Willeberg, P., Winckler, C., Adlhoch, C., Baldinelli, F., Breed, A., Brouwer, A., Guillemain, M., Harder, T., Monne, I., Roberts, H., Cortinas Abrahantes, J., Mosbach-Schulz, O., Verdonck, F., Morgado, J., Stegeman, A., 2017. Urgent request on avian influenza. EFSA J. 15. https://doi.org/10.2903/j.efsa.2016.4687.

Morgan, I.R., Kelly, A.P., 1990. Epidemiology of an avian influenza outbreak in Victoria in 1985. Aust. Vet. J. 67, 125–128.

Munster, V.J., Baas, C., Lexmond, P., Waldenström, J., Wallensten, A., Fransson, T., Rimmelzwaan, G.F., Beyer, W.E.P., Schutten, M., Olsen, B., Osterhaus, A.D.M.E., Fouchier, R.A.M., 2007. Spatial, temporal, and species variation in prevalence of Influenza A viruses in wild migratory birds. PLoS Pathog. 3, e61. https://doi.org/10.1371/journal.ppat.0030061.

Nguyen, D.C., Uyeki, T.M., Jadhao, S., Maines, T., Shaw, M., Matsuoka, Y., Smith, C., Rowe, T., Lu, X., Hall, H., Xu, X., Balish, A., Klimov, A., Tumpey, T.M., Swayne, D.E., Huynh, L.P.T., Nghiem, H.K., Nguyen, H.H.T., Hoang, L.T., Cox, N.J., Katz, J.M., 2005. Isolation and characterization of avian influenza viruses, including highly pathogenic H5N1, from poultry in live bird Markets in Hanoi, Vietnam, in 2001. J. Virol. 79, 4201–4212. https://doi.org/10.1128/JVI.79.7.4201-4212.2005.

Nicolai, C.A., Flint, P.L., Wege, M.L., 2005. Annual survival and site fidelity of northern pintails banded on the Yukon-Kuskokwim delta, Alaska. J. Wildl. Manage. 69, 1202–1210. https://doi.org/10.2193/0022-541X(2005)069[1202:ASASFO]2.0. CO;2.

Nishiura, H., Hoye, B., Klaassen, M., Bauer, S., Heesterbeek, H., 2009. How to find natural reservoir hosts from endemic prevalence in a multi-host population: a case study of influenza in waterfowl. Epidemics 1, 118–128. https://doi.org/10.1016/j.epidem.2009. 04.002.

Normile, D., 2006. Avian influenza: wild birds only partly to blame in spreading H5N1. Science 312 (5779), 1451. https://doi.org/10.1126/science.312.5779.1451.

OiE, 2017. Immediate Notification Report. http://www.oie.int/wahis_2/public%5C..%5Ctemp%5Creports/en_imm_0000023927_20170601_141559.pdf. accessed 6.2.17.

Olsen, B., Munster, V.J., Wallensten, A., Waldenström, J., Osterhaus, A.D.M.E., Fouchier, R.A.M., 2006. Global patterns of influenza a virus in wild birds. Science 312, 384–388. https://doi.org/10.1126/science.1122438.

Olsen, B., Lewis, N.S., Stockwell, T.B., Fedorova, N.B., Halpin, R.A., Waldenström, J., Bahl, J., Lexmond, P., Javakhishvili, Z., Smith, G., de Graaf, M., Wentworth, D.E., Verhagen, J.H., Lin, X., Russell, C.A., Bestebroer, T.M., Ransier, A., Fouchier, R.A.M., Westgeest, K.B., Latorre-Margalef, N., 2015. Influenza A virus evolution and spatio-temporal dynamics in Eurasian wild birds: a phylogenetic and phylogeographical study of whole-genome sequence data. J. Gen. Virol. 96, 2050–2060. https://doi.org/10.1099/vir.0.000155.

Pasick, J., Berhane, Y., Joseph, T., Bowes, V., Hisanaga, T., Handel, K., Alexandersen, S., 2015. Reassortant highly pathogenic influenza A H5N2 virus containing gene segments related to Eurasian H5N8 in British Columbia, Canada, 2014. Sci. Rep. 5, 9484. https://doi.org/10.1038/srep09484.

Pearce, J.M., Ramey, A.M., Flint, P.L., Koehler, A.V., Fleskes, J.P., Franson, J.C., Hall, J.S., Derksen, D.V., Ip, H.S., 2009. Avian influenza at both ends of a migratory flyway: characterizing viral genomic diversity to optimize surveillance plans for North America. Evol. Appl. 2, 457–468. https://doi.org/10.1111/j.1752-4571.2009.00071.x.

Pereda, A.J., Uhart, M., Perez, A.A., Zaccagnini, M.E., La Sala, L., Decarre, J., Goijman, A., Solari, L., Suarez, R., Craig, M.I., Vagnozzi, A., Rimondi, A., König, G., Terrera, M.V., Kaloghlian, A., Song, H., Sorrell, E.M., Perez, D.R., 2008. Avian influenza virus isolated in wild waterfowl in Argentina: evidence of a potentially unique phylogenetic lineage in South America. Virology 378, 363–370. https://doi.org/10.1016/j. virol.2008.06.010.

Perez, D.R., Sjaak de Wit, J.J., 2016. Low-pathogenicity avian influenza. In: Swayne, D.E. (Ed.), Animal Influenza John Wiley & Sons, Inc., Hoboken, NJ, pp. 271–301. https://doi.org/10.1002/9781118924341.ch11

Peterson, A.T., Bush, S.E., Spackman, E., Swayne, D.E., Ip, H.S., 2008. Influenza a virus infections in land birds, People's republic of China. Emerg. Infect. Dis. 14, 1644–1646. https://doi.org/10.3201/eid1410.080169.

Philippa, J., Munster, V., Bolhuis, H., Bestebroer, T., Schaftenaar, W., Beyer, W., Fouchier, R., Kuiken, T., Osterhaus, A., 2005. Highly pathogenic avian influenza (H7N7): vaccination of zoo birds and transmission to non-poultry species. Vaccine 23, 5743–5750. https://doi.org/10.1016/j.vaccine.2005.09.013.

Poen, M.J., Verhagen, J.H., Manvell, R.J., Brown, I., Bestebroer, T.M., van der Vliet, S., Vuong, O., Scheuer, R.D., van der Jeugd, H.P., Nolet, B.A., Kleyheeg, E., Müskens, G.J.D.M., Majoor, F.A., Grund, C., Fouchier, R.A.M., 2016. Lack of virological and serological evidence for continued circulation of highly pathogenic avian influenza H5N8 virus in wild birds in the Netherlands, 14 November 2014 to 31 January 2016. Euro Surveill. 21, 30349. https://doi.org/10.2807/1560-7917.ES.2016.21. 38.30349.

Pohlmann, A., Starick, E., Harder, T., Grund, C., Höper, D., Globig, A., Staubach, C., Dietze, K., Strebelow, G., Ulrich, R.G., Schinköthe, J., Teifke, J.P., Conraths, F.J., Mettenleiter, T.C., Beer, M., 2017. Outbreaks among wild birds and domestic poultry caused by reassorted influenza A(H5N8) clade 2.3.4.4 viruses, Germany, 2016. Emerg. Infect. Dis. 23, 633–636. https://doi.org/10.3201/eid2304. 161949.

Prosser, D.J., Cui, P., Takekawa, J.Y., Tang, M., Hou, Y., Collins, B.M., Yan, B., Hill, N.J., Li, T., Li, Y., Lei, F., Guo, S., Xing, Z., He, Y., Zhou, Y., Douglas, D.C., Perry, W.M., Newman, S.H., 2011. Wild bird migration across the Qinghai-Tibetan plateau: a transmission route for highly pathogenic H5N1. PLoS One 6, e17622. https://doi.org/10.1371/journal.pone.0017622.

Ramey, A.M., Poulson, R.L., González-Reiche, A.S., Perez, D.R., Stallknecht, D.E., Brown, J.D., 2014. Genomic characterization of H14 subtype influenza a viruses in new world waterfowl and experimental infectivity in mallards (Anas platyrhynchos). PLoS One 9, e95620. https://doi.org/10.1371/journal.pone.0095620.

Ramey, A.M., Spackman, E., Kim-Torchetti, M., DeLiberto, T.J., 2016. Weak support for disappearance and restricted emergence/persistence of highly pathogenic influenza A in North American waterfowl. Proc. Natl. Acad. Sci. U.S.A. 113, E6551–E6552. https://doi.org/10.1073/pnas.1614530113.

Reid, S.M., Shell, W.M., Barboi, G., Onita, I., Turcitu, M., Cioranu, R., Marinova-Petkova, A., Goujgoulova, G., Webby, R.J., Webster, R.G., Russell, C., Slomka, M.J., Hanna, A., Banks, J., Alton, B., Barrass, L., Irvine, R.M., Brown, I.H., 2011. First reported incursion of highly pathogenic notifiable avian influenza A H5N1 viruses from clade 2.3.2 into European poultry. Transbound. Emerg. Dis. 58, 76–78. https://doi.org/10.1111/j.1865-1682.2010.01175.x.

Reperant, L.A., Fučkar, N.S., Osterhaus, A.D.M.E., Dobson, A.P., Kuiken, T., 2010. Spatial and temporal association of outbreaks of H5N1 influenza virus infection in wild birds with the 0°C isotherm. PLoS Pathog. 6, e1000854. https://doi.org/10.1371/journal. ppat.1000854.

Rohani, P., Breban, R., Stallknecht, D.E., Drake, J.M., 2009. Environmental transmission of low pathogenicity avian influenza viruses and its implications for pathogen invasion. Proc. Natl. Acad. Sci. U.S.A. 106, 10365–10369. https://doi.org/10.1073/pnas. 0809026106.

Sakoda, Y., Sugar, S., Batchluun, D., Erdene-Ochir, T.-O., Okamatsu, M., Isoda, N., Soda, K., Takakuwa, H., Tsuda, Y., Yamamoto, N., Kishida, N., Matsuno, K., Nakayama, E., Kajihara, M., Yokoyama, A., Takada, A., Sodnomdarjaa, R., Kida, H., 2010. Characterization of H5N1 highly pathogenic avian influenza virus strains isolated from migratory waterfowl in Mongolia on the way back from the southern Asia to their northern territory. Virology 406, 88–94. https://doi.org/10.1016/j.virol.2010. 07.007.

Sakoda, Y., Soda, K., Saito, T., Yamamoto, N., Nomura, N., Takada, A., Umemura, T., Usui, T., Kuribayashi, S., Shichinohe, S., Ito, H., Ozaki, H., Murase, T., Uchida, Y., Yamaguchi, T., Kida, H., Sunden, Y., Ito, T., Okamatsu, M., 2012. Reintroduction of H5N1 highly pathogenic avian influenza virus by migratory water birds, causing poultry outbreaks in the 2010–2011 winter season in Japan. J. Gen. Virol. 93, 541–550. https://doi.org/10.1099/vir.0.037572-0.

Senne, D.A., Panigrahy, B., Kawaoka, Y., Pearson, J.E., Süss, J., Lipkind, M., Kida, H., Webster, R.G., 1996. Survey of the hemagglutinin (HA) cleavage site sequence of H5 and H7 avian influenza viruses: amino acid sequence at the HA cleavage site as a marker of pathogenicity potential. Avian Dis. 40, 425–437.

Sharp, G.B., Kawaoka, Y., Wright, S.M., Turner, B., Hinshaw, V., Webster, R.G., 1993. Wild ducks are the reservoir for only a limited number of influenza A subtypes. Epidemiol. Infect. 110, 161–176.

Sharshov, K., Silko, N., Sousloparov, I., Zaykovskaya, A., Shestopalov, A., Drozdov, I., 2010. Avian influenza (H5N1) outbreak among wild birds, Russia, 2009. Emerg. Infect. Dis. 16, 349–351. https://doi.org/10.3201/eid1602.090974.

Shen, H., Wu, B., Chen, Y., Bi, Y., Xie, Q., 2015. Influenza A(H5N6) virus reassortant, Southern China, 2014. Emerg. Infect. Dis. 21, 1261–1262. https://doi.org/10.3201/eid2107.140838.

Shen, Y.-Y., Ke, C.-W., Li, Q., Yuan, R.-Y., Xiang, D., Jia, W.-X., Yu, Y.-D., Liu, L., Huang, C., Qi, W.-B., Sikkema, R., Wu, J., Koopmans, M., Liao, M., 2016. Novel reassortant avian influenza A(H5N6) viruses in humans, Guangdong, China, 2015. Emerg. Infect. Dis. 22, 1507–1509. https://doi.org/10.3201/eid2208.160146.

Shestopalov, A.M., Durimanov, A.G., Evseenko, V.A., Ternovoi, V.A., Rassadkin, Y.N., Razumova, Y.V., Zaykovskaya, A.V., Zolotykh, S.I., Netesov, S.V., 2006. H5N1 influenza virus, domestic birds, Western Siberia, Russia. Emerg. Infect. Dis. 12, 1167–1169. https://doi.org/10.3201/eid1207.051338.

Short, K.R., Richard, M., Verhagen, J.H., van Riel, D., Schrauwen, E.J.A., van den Brand, J.M.A., Mänz, B., Bodewes, R., Herfst, S., 2015. One health, multiple challenges: the inter-species transmission of influenza A virus. One Health 1, 1–13. https://doi.org/10.1016/j.onehlt.2015.03.001.

Smith, G.J.D., Fan, X.H., Wang, J., Li, K.S., Qin, K., Zhang, J.X., Vijaykrishna, D., Cheung, C.L., Huang, K., Rayner, J.M., Peiris, J.S.M., Chen, H., Webster, R.G., Guan, Y., 2006. Emergence and predominance of an H5N1 influenza variant in China. Proc. Natl. Acad. Sci. U.S.A. 103, 16936–16941. https://doi.org/10.1073/pnas.0608157103.

Smith, G.J.D., Vijaykrishna, D., Ellis, T.M., Dyrting, K.C., Leung, Y.H.C., Bahl, J., Wong, C.W., Kai, H., Chow, M.K.W., Duan, L., Chan, A.S.L., Zhang, L.J., Chen, H., Luk, G.S.M., Peiris, J.S.M., Guan, Y., 2009. Characterization of avian influenza viruses a (H5N1) from wild birds, Hong Kong, 2004–2008. Emerg. Infect. Dis. 15, 402–407. https://doi.org/10.3201/eid1503.081190.

Sonnberg, S., Webby, R.J., Webster, R.G., 2013. Natural history of highly pathogenic avian influenza H5N1. Virus Res. 178, 63–77. https://doi.org/10.1016/j.virusres.2013.05.009.

Stallknecht, D.E., Brown, J.D., 2017. Wild bird infections and the ecology of avian influenza viruses. In: Swayne, D.E. (Ed.), Animal Influenza John Wiley & Sons, Inc., Hoboken, NJ, pp. 153–175.

Stallknecht, D.E., Shane, S.M., 1988. Host range of avian influenza virus in free-living birds. Vet. Res. Commun. 12, 125–141.

Swayne, D.E., Pantin-Jackwood, M., 2006. Pathogenicity of avian influenza viruses in poultry. Dev. Biol. (Basel) 124, 61–67.

Tolf, C., Latorre-Margalef, N., Wille, M., Bengtsson, D., Gunnarsson, G., Grosbois, V., Hasselquist, D., Olsen, B., Elmberg, J., Waldenström, J., 2013. Individual variation in influenza A virus infection histories and long-term immune responses in mallards. PLoS One 8, e61201. https://doi.org/10.1371/journal.pone.0061201.

Tong, S., Li, Y., Rivailler, P., Conrardy, C., Castillo, D.A.A., Chen, L.-M., Recuenco, S., Ellison, J.A., Davis, C.T., York, I.A., Turmelle, A.S., Moran, D., Rogers, S., Shi, M., Tao, Y., Weil, M.R., Tang, K., Rowe, L.A., Sammons, S., Xu, X., Frace, M., Lindblade, K.A., Cox, N.J., Anderson, L.J., Rupprecht, C.E., Donis, R.O., 2012. A distinct lineage of influenza A virus from bats. Proc. Natl. Acad. Sci. U.S.A. 109, 4269–4274. https://doi.org/10.1073/pnas.1116200109.

Tong, S., Zhu, X., Li, Y., Shi, M., Zhang, J., Bourgeois, M., Yang, H., Chen, X., Recuenco, S., Gomez, J., Chen, L.-M., Johnson, A., Tao, Y., Dreyfus, C., Yu, W., McBride, R., Carney, P.J., Gilbert, A.T., Chang, J., Guo, Z., Davis, C.T., Paulson, J.C., Stevens, J., Rupprecht, C.E., Holmes, E.C., Wilson, I.A., Donis, R.O., 2013. New world bats harbor diverse influenza A viruses. PLoS Pathog. 9, e1003657. https://doi.org/10.1371/journal.ppat.1003657.

Torchetti, M.K., Killian, M.L., Dusek, R.J., Pedersen, J.C., Hines, N., Bodenstein, B., White, C.L., Ip, H.S., 2015. Novel H5 clade 2.3.4.4 reassortant (H5N1) virus from a green-winged teal in Washington, USA. Genome Announc. 3, e00195-15. https://doi.org/10.1128/genomeA.00195-15.

U.S. Geological Survey (USGS), 2009. USGS Western Ecological Research Center. [WWW Document]. URL, https://www.werc.usgs.gov/ResearchTopicPage.aspx?id=17. accessed 6.1.17.

Uchida, Y., Mase, M., Yoneda, K., Kimura, A., Obara, T., Kumagai, S., Saito, T., Yamamoto, Y., Nakamura, K., Tsukamoto, K., Yamaguchi, S., 2008. Highly pathogenic avian influenza virus (H5N1) isolated from whooper swans, Japan. Emerg. Infect. Dis. 14, 1427–1429. https://doi.org/10.3201/eid1409.080655.

Usui, T., Yamaguchi, T., Ito, H., Ozaki, H., Murase, T., Ito, T., 2009. Evolutionary genetics of highly pathogenic H5N1 avian influenza viruses isolated from whooper swans in northern Japan in 2008. Virus Genes 39, 319–323. https://doi.org/10.1007/s11262-009-0403-9.

Velkers, F.C., Blokhuis, S.J., Veldhuis Kroeze, E.J.B., Burt, S.A., 2017. The role of rodents in avian influenza outbreaks in poultry farms: a review. Vet. Q. 37, 182–194. https://doi.org/10.1080/01652176.2017.1325537.

Verhagen, J.H., Majoor, F., Lexmond, P., Vuong, O., Kasemir, G., Lutterop, D., Osterhaus, A.D.M.E., Fouchier, R.A.M., Kuiken, T., 2014a. Epidemiology of Influenza A virus among black-headed gulls, the Netherlands, 2006–2010. Emerg. Infect. Dis. 20, 138–141. https://doi.org/10.3201/eid2001.130984.

Verhagen, J.H., van Dijk, J.G.B., Vuong, O., Bestebroer, T., Lexmond, P., Klaassen, M., Fouchier, R.A.M., 2014b. Migratory birds reinforce local circulation of avian influenza viruses. PLoS One 9, e112366. https://doi.org/10.1371/journal.pone.0112366.

Verhagen, J.H., Herfst, S., Fouchier, R.A.M., 2015a. Infectious disease. How a virus travels the world. Science 347, 616–617. https://doi.org/10.1126/science.aaa6724.

Verhagen, J.H., Höfle, U., van Amerongen, G., van de Bildt, M., Majoor, F., Fouchier, R.A.M., Kuiken, T., 2015b. Long-term effect of serial infections with H13 and H16 low-pathogenic avian influenza viruses in black-headed gulls. J. Virol. 89, 11507–11522. https://doi.org/10.1128/JVI.01765-15.

Verhagen, J.H., Lexmond, P., Vuong, O., Schutten, M., Guldemeester, J., Osterhaus, A.D.M.E., Elbers, A.R.W., Slaterus, R., Hornman, M., Koch, G., Fouchier, R.A.M., 2017. Discordant detection of avian influenza virus subtypes in time and space between poultry and wild birds; towards improvement of surveillance programs. PLoS One 12, e0173470. https://doi.org/10.1371/journal.pone.0173470.

Vijaykrishna, D., Bahl, J., Riley, S., Duan, L., Zhang, J.X., Chen, H., Peiris, J.S.M., Smith, G.J.D., Guan, Y., 2008. Evolutionary dynamics and emergence of Panzootic H5N1 influenza viruses. PLoS Pathog. 4, e1000161. https://doi.org/10.1371/journal.ppat.1000161.

Wallensten, A., Munster, V.J., Karlsson, M., Lundkvist, A., Brytting, M., Stervander, M., Osterhaus, A.D.M.E., Fouchier, R.A.M., Olsen, B., 2006. High prevalence of influenza A virus in ducks caught during spring migration through Sweden. Vaccine 24, 6734–6735. https://doi.org/10.1016/j.vaccine.2006.05.057.

Wallensten, A., Munster, V.J., Latorre-Margalef, N., Brytting, M., Elmberg, J., Fouchier, R.A.M., Fransson, T., Haemig, P.D., Karlsson, M., Lundkvist, A., Osterhaus, A.D.M.E., Stervander, M., Waldenström, J., Björn, O., 2007. Surveillance of influenza A virus in migratory waterfowl in northern Europe. Emerg. Infect. Dis. 13, 404–411. https://doi.org/10.3201/eid1303.061130.

Wang, J., Vijaykrishna, D., Duan, L., Bahl, J., Zhang, J.X., Webster, R.G., Peiris, J.S.M., Chen, H., Smith, G.J.D., Guan, Y., 2008. Identification of the progenitors of Indonesian and Vietnamese avian influenza A (H5N1) viruses from southern China. J. Virol. 82, 3405–3414. https://doi.org/10.1128/JVI.02468-07.

Webster, R.G., Rott, R., 1987. Influenza virus A pathogenicity: the pivotal role of hemagglutinin. Cell 50, 665–666.

Webster, R.G., Bean, W.J., Gorman, O.T., Chambers, T.M., Kawaoka, Y., 1992. Evolution and ecology of influenza A viruses. Microbiol. Rev. 56, 152–179. https://doi.org/10.1111/j.1541-0420.2008.01180.x.

Wilcox, B.R., Knutsen, G.A., Berdeen, J., Goekjian, V., Poulson, R., Goyal, S., Sreevatsan, S., Cardona, C., Berghaus, R.D., Swayne, D.E., Yabsley, M.J., Stallknecht, D.E., 2011. Influenza-A viruses in ducks in Northwestern Minnesota: fine scale spatial and temporal variation in prevalence and subtype diversity. PLoS One 6, e24010. https://doi.org/10.1371/journal.pone.0024010.

Wu, H., Peng, X., Xu, L., Jin, C., Cheng, L., Lu, X., Xie, T., Yao, H., Wu, N., 2014. Novel reassortant influenza A(H5N8) viruses in domestic ducks, Eastern China. Emerg. Infect. Dis. 20, 1315–1318. https://doi.org/10.3201/eid2008.140339.

Xu, X., Subbarao, Cox, N.J., Guo, Y., 1999. Genetic characterization of the pathogenic influenza A/Goose/Guangdong/1/96 (H5N1) virus: similarity of its hemagglutinin gene to those of H5N1 viruses from the 1997 outbreaks in Hong Kong. Virology 261, 15–19.

Yamane, I., 2006. Epidemics of emerging animal diseases and food-borne infection problems over the last 5 years in Japan. Ann. N. Y. Acad. Sci. 1081, 30–38. https://doi.org/10.1196/annals.1373.003.

Yoon, S.-W., Webby, R.J., Webster, R.G., 2014. Evolution and ecology of influenza A viruses. Curr. Top. Microbiol. Immunol. 385, 359–375. https://doi.org/10.1007/82_2014_396.

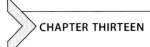

CHAPTER THIRTEEN

Intracellular Antiviral Immunity

Maria Bottermann, Leo C. James[1]

MRC Laboratory of Molecular Biology, Cambridge, United Kingdom
[1]Corresponding author: e-mail address: lcj@mrc-lmb.cam.ac.uk

Contents

Abstract

Innate immunity is traditionally thought of as the first line of defense against pathogens that enter the body. It is typically characterized as a rather weak defense mechanism, designed to restrict pathogen replication until the adaptive immune response generates a tailored response and eliminates the infectious agent. However, intensive research in recent years has resulted in better understanding of innate immunity as well as the discovery of many effector proteins, revealing its numerous powerful mechanisms to defend the host. Furthermore, this research has demonstrated that it is simplistic to strictly separate adaptive and innate immune functions since these two systems often work synergistically rather than sequentially.

Here, we provide a broad overview of innate pattern recognition receptors in antiviral defense, with a focus on the TRIM family, and discuss their signaling pathways and mechanisms of action with special emphasis on the intracellular antibody receptor TRIM21.

Advances in Virus Research, Volume 100
ISSN 0065-3527
https://doi.org/10.1016/bs.aivir.2018.01.002

ABBREVIATIONS

AIM2	absent in melanoma 2
ALR	AIM-like receptor
AP-1	activator protein 1
ARF	ADP-ribosylation like
ASC	apoptosis-associated speck-like protein
BIR	baculoviral inhibitory repeat-like domain
BVDV	bovine viral diarrhea virus
CARD	caspase activation and recruitment domain
CDR	complementarity-determining region
cGAMP	cyclic guanosine monophosphate–adenosine monophosphate
cGAS	cyclic GMP–AMP synthase
CIITA	class II major histocompatibility complex transactivator
CLR	C-type lectin receptors
CpG	deoxycytidylate-phosphate-deoxyguanylate
CypA	cyclophilin A
DAI	DNA-dependent activator of IFN-regulatory factors
DAMP	damage-associated molecular patterns
DAXX	death domain-associated protein
DC	dendritic cell
DC-SIGN	DC-Specific Intercellular adhesion molecule-3-Grabbing Nonintegrin
DDX	DEAD box helicase
DENV	Dengue virus
DExD/H-box	DEAD/DEAH box helicases
DHX	DEAH box helicase
DRP1	dynamin-related protein 1
DUB	deubiquitinase
EBV	Epstein–Barr virus
EIAV	equine infectious anemia virus
EMCV	encephalomyocarditis virus
Fc	fragment crystallizable
FcR	Fc receptor
FcRn	neonatal Fc receptor
FCV	feline calicivirus
FMDV	foot-and-mouth disease virus
FMF	familial Mediterranean fever
FN3	fibronectin type 3
GSK3	glycogen synthase kinase 3
hAdV	human adenovirus
HCMV	human cytomegalovirus
hCoV	human coronavirus
HCV	hepatitis C virus
HIV	human immunodeficiency virus
HRV	human rhinovirus
HSV	herpes simplex virus
HTLV	human T-lymphotropic virus
IAV	influenza A virus

IBV	influenza B virus
IFI16	interferon-γ-inducible protein 16
IFN	interferon
IRF	interferon regulatory factor
ISG	interferon-stimulated gene
IκB	inhibitor of kappa B
JEV	Japanese encephalitis virus
JNK	c-Jun N-terminal kinases
LGP2	laboratory of genetics and physiology 2
LPS	lipopolysaccharide
LRR	leucine-rich repeat
LRRFIP1	leucine-rich repeat flightless-interacting protein 1
MATH	meprin and TRAF homology
MAV-1	mouse adenovirus 1
MAVS	mitochondrial antiviral signaling
MCMV	mouse cytomegalovirus
MDA5	melanoma differentiation-associated gene 5
MEF	mouse embryonic fibroblast
MLV	murine leukemia virus
MMTV	mouse mammary tumor virus
MNDA	myeloid cell nuclear differentiation antigen
MV	measles virus
Myd88	myeloid differentiation primary response gene 88
NAP-1	NF-κB-activating kinase-associated protein
NDV	Newcastle disease virus
NF-κB	nuclear factor κB
NLR	NOD-like receptor
N-MLV	N-tropic murine leukemia virus
NOD	nucleotide-binding and oligomerization domain
OAS	iligoadenylate synthetase
OLR	OAS-like receptor
PAMP	pathogen-associated molecular pattern
PHD	plant homeodomains
PML	promyelocytic leukemia protein
PRR	pattern recognition receptor
PYD	pyrin domain
PYHIN1	pyrin and HIN domain-containing protein 1
RGNNV	red-spotted grouper nervous necrosis virus
RIG-I	retinoic acid-inducible gene I
RING	really interesting new gene
RIP	receptor-interacting serine/threonine protein
RIPK	RIP kinase
RLR	RIG-I-like receptor
ROS	reactive oxygen species
RT	reverse transcription
SeV	Sendai virus
SGIV	Singapore grouper iridovirus

SinV	Sindbis virus
SLE	systemic lupus erythematosus
STAT	signal transducers and activators of transcription
STING	stimulator of IFN genes
SUMO	small ubiquitin-like modifier
TAB	TGF-beta-activated kinase
TANK	TRAF family member-associated NF-κB activator
TBEV	Tick-borne encephalitis virus
TBK1	TANK-binding kinase 1
TGF	transforming growth factor
TIR domain	Toll/interleukin-1 receptor domain
TLR	Toll-like receptor
TNF	tumor necrosis factor
TRAF	TNF receptor-associated factor
TRIF	TIR-domain-containing adapter-inducing interferon-β
TRIM	tripartite motif-containing protein
VSV	vesicular stomatitis virus
VV	vaccinia virus
WNV	West Nile virus
YFV	yellow fever virus
ZAP	zinc finger antiviral protein

1. PATTERN RECOGNITION RECEPTORS IN ANTIVIRAL DEFENSE

Pattern recognition receptors (PRRs) are upstream factors that initiate innate immune signaling in response to viral infection and induce an antiviral state. Rather than recognizing residue-specific epitopes of pathogens, as demonstrated by the adaptive immune response, PRRs bind to conserved patterns uniquely associated with pathogens, termed pathogen–associated molecular patterns (PAMPs) (Odendall and Kagan, 2017). PRRs are currently classified into six families according to structural and domain features: Toll-like receptors (TLRs), NOD-like receptors (NLRs), C-type lectin receptors (CLRs), RIG-I-like receptors (RLRs), OAS-like receptors (OLRs), and AIM-like receptors (ALRs) (Kagan and Barton, 2016). PRRs provide comprehensive immune surveillance as they not only recognize a large number of varied PAMPs but are also widely expressed and localize to the diverse cellular spaces that come into contact with viruses during infection. TLRs can recognize viral envelope constituents at the cell surface and viral genomes in endolysosomes, whereas in the cytosol, the viral genome is detected by NLRs, RLRs, ALRs, and OLRs.

1.1 Toll-Like Receptors

Toll-like receptors were the first PRRs discovered and are thus well studied. We will only give a brief overview as they have been extensively reviewed before (Akira and Takeda, 2004; Kawai and Akira, 2010; Kawasaki and Kawai, 2014; Lester and Li, 2014; Odendall and Kagan, 2017; Takeda and Akira, 2005; Thompson et al., 2011). The TLR family has 10 members in humans, TLR1–10, of which TLR1, TLR2, TLR4, TLR5, and TLR6 are expressed at the plasma membrane, while TLR3, TLR7, TLR8, and TLR9 are located in endosomes (Thompson et al., 2011). Although they can be found in diverse tissues (for instance, in intestinal epithelium) and a variety of immune cells, TLRs are mainly expressed in professional antigen-presenting cells (B cells, DCs, and macrophages). Why they display restricted tissue expression is unclear but may reflect that their role is in immune surveillance rather than the detection of infection per se. As professional cell sensors they are well placed to both activate the innate cellular response and promote adaptive immunity. Many TLRs were first discovered as receptors for bacterial PAMPs. For instance, TLR4 is the primary receptor for bacterial lipopolysaccharide (LPS) (Lu et al., 2008), while TLR2 is activated by bacterial lipoproteins such as lipoteichoic acid (Hashimoto et al., 2006; Oliveira-Nascimento et al., 2012). Signal transduction through TLR2 also requires heterodimerization with either TLR1 or TLR6 and helps broaden ligand specificity (Farhat et al., 2007; Kang et al., 2009; Schenk et al., 2009). TLR5 is largely responsible for the innate immune response to flagellin (Hayashi et al., 2001). This pattern suggests that plasma membrane-associated TLRs are mainly responsible for the detection of invading bacteria. However, more recently, it has been shown that TLR4 and TLR2 can produce a signaling response upon infection with RSV (Murawski et al., 2009; Rallabhandi et al., 2012), and TLR2 with mouse mammary tumor virus (MMTV) and murine leukemia virus (MLV) (Villano et al., 2014), measles virus (MV) (Bieback et al., 2002), and human cytomegalovirus (HCMV) (Compton et al., 2003). These studies demonstrate that plasma membrane-bound TLRs can also sense cell-bound viruses. However, although direct binding is suggested, it is unclear how such diverse ligands are detected and what the mechanism of activation is. Of the endosomal TLRs, TLR3 has been shown to recognize dsRNA and mediate a protective response against poliovirus, coxsackievirus, and herpes simplex virus 1 (HSV1), all of which use dsRNA intermediates in their life cycle (Tatematsu et al., 2014). Additionally, TLR3 is capable of recognizing stem loop structures in ssRNA (Tatematsu et al., 2013).

TLR7 and TLR8 can both sense long ssRNA, with TLR7 also capable of recognizing specific motifs in short dsRNA (Thompson et al., 2011). They have been implicated in the response to RNA viruses such as influenza (Diebold, 2004; Lund et al., 2004), coxsackie B virus (Triantafilou et al., 2005), vesicular stomatitis virus (VSV) (Lund et al., 2004), and hepatitis C virus (HCV) (Lee et al., 2015; Wang et al., 2011a). Finally, TLR9 is capable of recognizing unmethylated deoxycytidylate-phosphate-deoxyguanylate (CpG) motifs, which are common in viral and bacterial DNA, but do not occur in mammalian DNA (Hemmi et al., 2000). TLR9 is important in the defense against DNA viruses such as human adenovirus (hAdV) (Zhu et al., 2007), mouse cytomegalovirus (MCMV) (Krug et al., 2004), and Epstein–Barr virus (EBV) (Fiola et al., 2010). The role of TLR10 has not been elucidated yet; however, there is evidence that it functions as a negative regulator of TLR signaling and thus is an inhibitory TLR (Jiang et al., 2016; Oosting et al., 2014), while one study reported that it is involved in the immune response against influenza virus (Lee et al., 2014).

All activating TLRs, apart from TLR3, signal through the adapter molecule myeloid differentiation primary response gene 88 (MyD88), which results in the activation of NF-κB and AP-1 signaling pathways. Mice deficient in MyD88 primarily succumb to bacterial rather than viral infection, in common with other immunodeficiencies such as agammaglobulinemia (Villano et al., 2014). TLR3 and TLR4 have been shown to signal through a TIR-domain-containing adapter-inducing interferon-β (TRIF)-dependent pathway, which also results in the activation of IRF, NF-κB, and AP-1 signaling pathways (Kawasaki and Kawai, 2014).

1.2 C-Type Lectin Receptors

CLRs are mainly expressed on dendritic cells but also on other myeloid cells. They are characterized by a carbohydrate recognition domain which allows them to bind pathogen-associated carbohydrate motifs (Geijtenbeek and Gringhuis, 2009). This makes them especially important in the defense against bacteria and fungi (Drummond and Brown, 2013). A well-known CLR is DC-Specific Intercellular adhesion molecule-3-Grabbing Nonintegrin (DC-SIGN), which interacts with mannose and fucose residues on pathogen surfaces. It has since been shown that DC-SIGN can act as a receptor for numerous enveloped viruses including HIV (Geijtenbeek et al., 2000), dengue virus (DENV) (Tassaneetrithep et al., 2003), and MV (de Witte et al., 2006), through interactions with their envelope glycoproteins, exemplifying how viruses can directly exploit the host's defense mechanisms. Since CLRs are exclusively expressed on the cell surface, they will not be discussed further here but have been excellently reviewed (Dambuza and Brown, 2015; Drummond and Brown, 2013; Geijtenbeek and Gringhuis, 2009; Hoving et al., 2014; Osorio and Reis e Sousa, 2011; Sancho and Reis e Sousa, 2012).

1.3 NOD-Like Receptors

Nucleotide-binding and oligomerization domain (NOD)-like receptors (NLRs) are cytosolic PPRs that mediate responses to a diverse range of PAMPs such as LPS (Kayagaki et al., 2013), flagellin (Kayagaki et al., 2013), and viral RNA (Allen et al., 2009; Li et al., 2015), but also host cell and environmental factors such as cholesterol crystals (Duewell et al., 2010) and reactive oxygen species (ROS) (Kanneganti, 2010). They are characterized by a central NACHT domain as well as a C-terminal leucine-rich repeat (LRR) and can be divided into five groups based on their N-terminal domain: NLRA (acidic activation domain), NLRB (baculoviral inhibitory repeat-like domain (BIR)), NLRC (caspase activation and recruitment domain (CARD)), NLRP (pyrin domain (PYD)), and NLRX. Activation of NLRs can result in four different effector functions: inflammasome activation, activation of innate immunity signaling pathways, transcriptional regulation, and autophagy. Inflammasome formation is mediated through members of NLRP and NLRC and results in recruitment of Caspase-1 and the release of the inflammatory cytokines IL-1β and IL-18, as well as pyroptosis. Members of NLRP lack a CARD domain; they depend on the adaptor molecule apoptosis-associated speck-like protein (ASC), which contains a C-terminal CARD domain, for recruitment of Caspase-1. While members of the NLRC family, such as NLRC4, have a CARD domain and thus do not require ASC for direct interaction with Caspase-1, ASC is required for full activation and robust IL-1β release (Broz et al., 2010; Lamkanfi and Dixit, 2014). Inflammasomes, especially NLRP3 inflammasomes, play an important role in the immune response to many viruses, including influenza A virus (IAV) (Ichinohe et al., 2009, 2010), hAdV (Barlan et al., 2011), encephalomyocarditis virus (EMCV), VSV (Rajan et al., 2011), and rabies virus (Lawrence et al., 2013). Inflammasome activation by hAdV can be caused by plasma membrane and endosomal damage (Barlan et al., 2011), both of which occur during adenoviral infection (Luisoni et al., 2015), and are known triggers for the NLRP3 inflammasome (Hornung and Latz, 2010; Muñoz-Planillo et al., 2013). Viral RNA (Allen et al., 2009) as well as RNA analogues such as polyI:C (Rajan et al., 2010) can also activate the NLRP3 inflammasome; however, the mechanism is not yet fully elucidated. It has been suggested that recognition of viral RNA results in the activation of the RIPK1–RIPK3 complex which stimulates the mitochondria-associated GTPase DRP1, thus promoting mitochondrial damage and the production of ROS (Wang et al., 2014), another known trigger of the NLRP3 inflammasome (Abais et al., 2015; Heid et al., 2013). Other studies have identified DDX19A (Li et al., 2015) and DHX33 (Mitoma et al., 2013) as cytosolic RNA sensors that can interact with NLRP3, thus bridging viral RNA and the NLRP3 inflammasome. For a comprehensive overview of the role of inflammasomes in viral infection, see the following reviews: Franchi et al. (2008), Guo et al. (2015), Kanneganti (2010), Kim et al. (2016), Lamkanfi and Dixit (2014), and Thompson et al. (2011).

Members of NLRC are capable of activating immune signaling pathways in response to PAMP recognition. The most well known are NOD1 and NOD2 (NLRCs), which recognize bacterial peptidoglycans and activate both NF-κB and AP-1 signaling pathways (Franchi et al., 2009). NOD2 can also recognize viral ssRNA and mediate the production of IFNβ through MAVS (mitochondrial antiviral signaling)–dependent IRF3 activation (Sabbah et al., 2009). NLRC4 is predominately a potent inflammasome activator in response to bacterial ligands. Here, neural apoptosis inhibitory proteins (NAIPs, members of the NLRB family) act as receptors for bacterial PAMPs such as flagellin (NAIP5) or the type three secretion system (NAIP2), with NLRC4 being the adapter recruiting Caspase-1 to the NLRC4 inflammasome (Zhao and Shao, 2015; Zhao et al., 2011).

NLRA has only one member, CIITA, which is unique in that it can act as a transcription factor in the activation of MHC class II genes (Kim et al., 2016).

Finally, NLRX has also only one member, NLRX1, whose N-terminal domain does not fall within the four existing groups but instead carries a mitochondrial targeting sequence (Moore et al., 2008). While its role has not been fully elucidated yet, there is evidence that it is involved in negatively regulating innate immune signaling pathways (Allen et al., 2011; Moore et al., 2008; Parvatiyar and Cheng, 2011; Xia et al., 2011); however, there are also data, implicating that NLRX-1 increases ROS and thus increases NF-κB- and JNK-dependent signaling.

1.4 RIG-I-Like Receptors

Retinoic acid-inducible gene I (RIG-I)-like receptors (RLRs) are PRRs present in all nucleated cells, where they are poised to detect cytosolic viral

RNAs (Ireton and Gale, 2011). This expression pattern is in clear contrast to TLRs, CLRs, and NLRs and may reflect that RLRs are true sensors of infection rather than part of immune sampling and surveillance. This can also be discerned from the species of viral ligand that they detect. It has been clearly shown for influenza that it is progeny rather than incoming genomes that are detected by the RLR RIG-I (Rehwinkel et al., 2010). Thus, it is replicating virus and not merely inert particles that are being sensed. The RLR family has two other known members: melanoma differentiation-associated gene 5 (MDA5), and laboratory of genetics and physiology 2 (LGP2), which, like RIG-I, possess a central ATPase-containing DExD/H-box helicase domain (Dixit and Kagan, 2013). However, only RIG-I and MDA5 have N-terminal CARDs which are essential for initiation of signal transduction. LGP2 is thus thought to modulate RIG-I and MDA5 signaling instead of initiating signaling itself (Thompson et al., 2011). RIG-I and MDA5 both recognize viral RNA; however, while RIG-I senses small dsRNA that is characterized by a 5′-triphosphate group and a 3′-polyuridine-rich region, MDA5 binds long ssRNA and oligomerizes along its length (Kagan and Barton, 2014; Wu et al., 2013a). Binding of RNA to MDA5 or RIG-I leads to interaction of the N-terminal CARD with the CARD of MAVS, which is mainly located in the outer mitochondrial membrane. Upon activation, MAVS multimerizes, forming the "MAVS signalosome" and initiating downstream activation of NF-κB and IRF3 (Koshiba, 2013). Both MDA5 and RIG-I are tightly regulated through constitutive phosphorylation of their CARDs, which prevents interaction with MAVS. Upon viral infection, both sensors are rapidly dephosphorylated which results in downstream immune signaling (Gack, 2014; Maharaj et al., 2012; Sun et al., 2011; Wies et al., 2013). Ligand-free RIG-I adopts an autorepressed conformation in which the CARDs are sequestered. Binding of RNA results in a conformational change that liberates the CARDs (Kowalinski et al., 2011; Liu et al., 2017a); however, this liberation is not thought to be sufficient for RIG-I activation and thus additional activation mechanisms exist. These include ubiquitin conjugation by the E3-ligase TRIM25 to the CARDs (Gack et al., 2007), binding of unanchored K63-linked ubiquitin chains to the CARDs (Jiang et al., 2012; Zeng et al., 2010) and ATP-dependent filamentous oligomerization of RIG-I along the dsRNA (Peisley et al., 2013). All of these mechanism allow for subsequent MAVS aggregation and it has been suggested that ubiquitin promotes the formation of a RIG-I tetramer that acts as a primer for MAVS oligomerization (Peisley et al., 2014).

RLRs have been implicated in the sensing of multiple RNA viruses, with RIG-I sensing viruses such as influenza (Loo et al., 2008; Mäkelä et al., 2015), rhabdoviruses (Furr et al., 2010), HCV (Saito et al., 2008), and other flaviviruses (Chang et al., 2006), and MDA5 recognizing mainly picornaviruses (Chang et al., 2006; Gitlin et al., 2006) and caliciviruses (McCartney et al., 2008). RIG-I is also capable of detecting picornavirus infection but is antagonized by the viral 3C protease (Barral et al., 2009; Papon et al., 2009). Enveloped viruses such as West Nile virus (WNV), MV, and Sendai virus (SeV) can be sensed by both MDA5 and RIG-I (Schlee, 2013). These sensing events are not necessarily redundant as it has been shown that during WNV infection MDA5 and RIG-I cooperate in sensing RNA of the replicating virus, likely by operating at different times during the viral life cycle (Errett et al., 2013). Interestingly, RIG-I can also be activated by dsDNA viruses such as HSV-1 (Rasmussen et al., 2009) or hAdV (Minamitani et al., 2011). Here, it relies on the RNA polymerase III-dependent transcription of AT-rich regions of the viral genome into dsRNA that contain a $5'$-triphosphate (Ablasser et al., 2009; Chiu et al., 2009). As further evidence that RLRs detect replicating pathogens, many viruses have evolved to antagonize RIG-I-dependent immune activation, as reviewed in Kell and Gale (2015).

1.5 AIM-Like Receptors

Absent in melanoma (AIM)-like receptors are a relatively recently discovered family of cytosolic and nuclear DNA sensors. In humans, it consists of four members: AIM-2, interferon-γ-inducible protein 16 (IFI16), myeloid cell nuclear differentiation antigen (MNDA), and pyrin and HIN domain–containing protein 1 (PYHIN1) (Gray et al., 2016). Like NLRPs, they have an N-terminal pyrin domain, but their C-terminal nucleotide-binding site is an HIN domain rather than an NACHT domain (Ratsimandresy et al., 2013). AIM2 and IFI16 are thus far the best-characterized family members. AIM2 is a potent inflammasome activator in response to cytosolic DNA. It binds DNA with its HIN domain and ASC with its pyrin domain, which results in recruitment of Caspase-1. This leads to release of IL-1β and IL-18 as well as cell death by pyroptosis (Fernandes-Alnemri et al., 2009; Hornung et al., 2009). It has been shown to promote host defense against DNA viruses such as MCMV, vaccinia virus (VV) (Rathinam et al., 2010), and hAdV (Eichholz et al., 2016; Stein and Falck-Pedersen, 2012). IFI16 activates an alternative immune response via the ER-associated stimulator of IFN genes (STING) upon binding of dsDNA. Activation of STING promotes TBK1 activity, resulting in the induction of type I interferon (Unterholzner et al., 2010). A recent study by Gray et al. using ALR knockout mice has demonstrated that ALRs are dispensable for the IFN response to synthetic DNA as well as infection with DNA viruses and further do not contribute to the autoimmune phenotype found in Trex-1 knockout mouse models of Aicardi–Goutières syndrome (Gray et al., 2016). However, the mouse and human ALR families are significantly divergent, with 13 members in mice and only 4 known in humans (Brunette et al., 2012; Cridland et al., 2012). Furthermore, AIM2 is the only member of the family showing true orthology between mice and humans, while IFI204, initially considered to be the murine equivalent of IFI16, is not now thought to be a true orthologue of IFI16 (Brunette et al., 2012), as two independent studies have shown that IFI16 is required for efficient DNA sensing in both human macrophages (Jønsson et al., 2017) and human keratinocytes (Almine et al., 2017) and that it cooperates with cGAS to achieve full activation of the type I IFN response.

1.6 OAS-Like Receptors

The oligoadenylate synthetase (OAS)-like receptors (OLRs) are a family of viral dsRNA and dsDNA sensors, which generate immune second messengers. They are characterized by a core nucleotidyl transferase domain, but have divergent C-terminal domains that explain their different ligand specificity (Kranzusch et al., 2013). OAS 1, OAS 2, and OAS 3 are the founding members of the family. Upon recognition of viral dsRNA, they produce the secondary messenger $2'-5'$-linked oligoadenylate, which results in dimerization and thus activation of the endoribonuclease RNaseL. RNaseL then recognizes viral (and cellular) dsRNA and degrades it (Hornung et al., 2014). This directly interferes with the viral life cycle and the generated RNA cleavage products can be recognized by RLRs, which initiates the induction of type I IFN (Malathi et al., 2007). OAS proteins have been shown to be protective against a number of RNA viruses, such as flaviviruses like HCV (Kwon et al., 2013), DENV, and WNV (Ferguson et al., 2008; Lin et al., 2009). The function of OAS-like proteins is not well elucidated as they lack an active nucleotidyl transferase domain. They have been implicated to compete with OAS proteins and thus negatively regulate the RNaseL pathway (Choi et al., 2015; Rogozin et al., 2003), although one study has shown that they positively regulate the RIG-I pathway (Choi et al., 2015; Zhu et al., 2014, 2015).

Although only discovered in 2013 (Sun et al., 2013), cyclic GMP–AMP synthase (cGAS) is now considered the pivotal dsDNA sensor in the cytosol, since it has been shown to be absolutely required for IFN signaling in response to dsDNA. Binding of cGAS to dsDNA results in the production of cyclic guanosine monophosphate–adenosine monophosphate (cGAMP), which binds STING (Wu et al., 2013b). STING then dimerizes and interacts with TBK1, which phosphorylates IRF3 and thus leads to the induction of IFNβ. TBK1 also activates the IKK complex, resulting in the transcription of NF-κB target genes (Burdette and Vance, 2013; Sun et al., 2013). To date, cGAS has been implicated in the host's immune defense against multiple viruses, including DNA viruses such as HSV-1 (Reinert et al., 2016), hAdV (Lam et al., 2014), and HCMV (Paijo et al., 2016), and retroviruses such as HIV (Gao et al., 2014), and surprisingly the RNA virus WNV as cGAS KO mice were more susceptible to it (Cai et al., 2014; Schoggins et al., 2014). Basal ISG (interferon-stimulated gene) expression is altered upon cGAS knockout, so this apparent ability to sense an RNA virus is almost certainly an indirect effect due to the reduction in expression levels of other sensors such as RIG-I. Constitutive cGAS activity may occur through stimulation by DNA from damaged mitochondria, sequences generated from viral RNA by cellular reverse transcriptases (Lazear and Diamond, 2016; Shimizu et al., 2014), or microbial infection (Cai et al., 2014; Gough et al., 2012). It has also been shown that cGAMP can be incorporated into nascent viral particles and thus be transferred between cells, leading to a rapid type I IFN response in newly infected cells (Bridgeman et al., 2015). Presumably this occurs in parallel with the paracrine interferon response itself. Aside from cGAS, there are several other cytosolic DNA sensors that have been identified, which do not belong to the OLR family. These include DDX41, DHDX36, DHX9, DAI, and LRRFIP1; however, there is increasing evidence that many of them are dispensable for the IFN induction in response to dsDNA (Burdette and Vance, 2013; Vance, 2016).

2. TRIM PROTEINS IN INNATE IMMUNITY

Tripartite motif-containing proteins (TRIMs) are a family which consists of up to 100 members in humans. They are ancient proteins, with orthologues of TRIM37 being found in species such as *Dictyostelium discoideum* and *Trichomonas vaginalis* (Marín, 2012); however, the family has greatly expanded in mammals to become the largest group of E3 ubiquitin ligases. In recent years, it has become clear that many TRIMs have a function in innate immunity. Unusually for PRRs, they have been shown to function as both viral restriction factors and modulators of innate immune signaling.

2.1 Structure of TRIM Proteins

Almost all TRIMs are characterized by the presence of an RBCC motif, which consists of a RING domain, a B-box domain, and a coiled-coil domain. While some proteins might lack one of the domains, the spacing and order in which the domains occur is highly conserved (Ozato et al., 2008).

The N-terminal RING (Really Interesting New Gene) domain is a zinc-binding motif that is associated with E3-ligase activity (Metzger et al., 2012). In TRIMs, it can not only mediate ubiquitination with various linkage types but also transfer the small ubiquitin-like modifier (SUMO) and the ubiquitin like molecule ISG15 (Ozato et al., 2008).

C-terminally of the RING domain, TRIM proteins carry one or two B-box domains. B-box domains are also zinc finger domains. While all TRIM proteins have one B-box domain (B-box 2), some carry a second B-box (B-box 1) (Ozato et al., 2008). The function of the B-box in TRIM proteins is poorly understood; however, it is required for higher order assembly of some family members (Wagner et al., 2016) and is crucial for function (Koliopoulos et al., 2016).

The last constituent of the tripartite motif is the coiled-coil domain, which is also involved in maintaining quaternary structure where it mediates homodimerization and possibly tetramerization of TRIM proteins (Ozato et al., 2008).

While the N-terminal RBCC motif is conserved among all TRIM proteins, the C-terminal domains differ depending on the downstream effector functions of the TRIM protein. The most common C-terminal domain is the PRYSPRY domain, which is found in 39 human TRIM proteins and consists of an ancient PRY element and a juxtaposed SPRY element. The PRYSPRY domain mediates interactions with various ligands, such as antibody in the case of TRIM21 and retroviruses in the case of TRIM5α. Structural studies on the TRIM21 PRYSPRY domain have shown that ligand interactions occur through a canonical binding site, which consists of six variable loops, similar to antibody CDRs, whose rapid diversification may have driven the evolution of PRYSPRY domains (James et al., 2007). Other

C-terminal domains include the COS-box, which has been shown to mediate interaction with microtubules; FN3 domains, which contain a DNA-binding site; PHDs, which are usually associated with chromatin-mediated transcriptional regulation; and ARF domains, which partake in intracellular trafficking; and finally MATH domains, which have been shown to be involved in receptor binding and oligomerization (Ozato et al., 2012).

2.2 Functions of TRIM Proteins in Viral Restriction

The most widely studied antiviral TRIM is TRIM5α, which restricts HIV-1 in old world monkeys such as rhesus macaque (Stremlau et al., 2004). TRIM5α binds to the HIV-1 capsid via its PRYSPRY domain and is thought to form a hexagonal lattice around the virus (Ganser-Pornillos et al., 2011; Li et al., 2016) via B-box oligomerization (Wagner et al., 2016). TRIM5α restriction involves stepwise autoubiquitination (Fletcher et al., 2015) and subsequent proteasomal degradation of the viral capsid (Lukic et al., 2011; Rold and Aiken, 2008; Stremlau et al., 2006), a block to infection which occurs prior to reverse transcription. If the proteasome is inhibited or TRIM5α's RING domain, which mediates E3-ligase activity, is deleted, RT is restored; however, HIV-1 infection is still efficiently prevented (Anderson et al., 2006; Kutluay et al., 2013; Roa et al., 2012; Wu et al., 2006). Why the two separate blocks to viral infection exist is not understood. Simultaneous with restriction of HIV-1, TRIM5α also elicits potent immune signaling via AP-1 and NF-κB, which is also dependent on its E3-ligase activity (Pertel et al., 2011). Crucially, human TRIM5α cannot restrict HIV-1, which may help to explain why the virus is so pathogenic in man. Human TRIM5α is capable of restricting N-tropic MLV (N-MLV) and equine infectious anemia virus (EIAV) (Nisole et al., 2005; Yap et al., 2004), suggesting that it is nevertheless an active antiviral. Interestingly, in new world owl monkeys, whose TRIM5α is also unable to restrict HIV, a retrotransposition of cyclophilin A (CypA), which binds the HIV-1 capsid, into the TRIM5 loci has generated the fusion protein TRIM-Cyp that renders owl monkeys resistant to HIV-1 infection (Sayah et al., 2004). TRIM-Cyp has also independently evolved in old world monkeys, in the macaque lineage via an exon-skipping mutation (Wilson et al., 2008). This highlights the intensive selective pressure that retroviral infection has on primate species and the selective advantage a functional TRIM protein can provide. Indeed, TRIM5α is thought to be the fastest evolving primate gene.

Another TRIM that has been implicated in the restriction of HIV-1 is TRIM19 (Turelli et al., 2001). While the mechanism has not been elucidated, it has been suggested that it interferes with viral replication (Turelli et al., 2001), silences gene expression (Lusic et al., 2013; Masroori et al., 2016), or indirectly interferes with reverse transcription (Dutrieux et al., 2015). Indeed, TRIM19 has been implicated in the restriction of multiple viruses, including human HCMV, VSV, and IAV (Nisole et al., 2005). The importance of TRIM19 in viral restriction is highlighted by the fact that HSV encodes a specific antagonist in the form of ICP0, which causes the degradation of TRIM19 (PML) bodies (Boutell et al., 2003). For VSV, it has been shown that TRIM19 is able to directly restrict virus by blocking viral protein expression, while HCMV and IAV are only restricted through TRIM19's effect on type I IFN signaling. This highlights another similarity between TRIM5α and TRIM19, namely that they are able to both restrict viral infection directly and initiate innate immune signaling. However, while the signaling activity of TRIM5α is directly coupled to its mechanism of viral restriction, since both require K63-linked ubiquitination upon capsid recognition (Pertel et al., 2011), TRIM19 potentiates signaling indirectly, for instance, by recruiting Pin1 into nuclear bodies and interfering with Pin1-mediated degradation of IRF3 to positively regulate type I IFN signaling (El Asmi et al., 2014).

Several TRIM proteins have been shown to be involved in the restriction of nonretroviruses, such as flaviviruses and orthomyxoviruses. TRIM22 has been shown to restrict IAV, by mediating proteasomal degradation of the viral nucleoprotein (Di Pietro et al., 2013), HBV, and HCV (Yang et al., 2016). Another TRIM which is capable of restricting flaviviruses is TRIM79α, with one study demonstrating its importance in restricting tick-borne encephalitis virus by degrading the viral RNA polymerase (Taylor et al., 2012).

2.3 Functions of TRIM Proteins in Innate Immune Regulation

In addition to directly inhibiting viral replication, TRIMs have also been shown to alter viral infectivity through modulation of innate immune signaling pathways, via their E3-ligase activity. One example of this is the potentiation of RIG-I signaling through N-terminal CARD ubiquitination by TRIM25 (Gack et al., 2007; Zeng et al., 2010). RIG-I undergoes a conformational change in response to ligand binding and dephosphorylation (see Section 1.4), which enables TRIM25 binding. It is thought that

TRIM25-mediated ubiquitination of the CARDs facilitates the interaction of RIG-I and MAVS and thus modulates downstream IFNβ induction (Gack, 2014; Gack et al., 2007; Sanchez et al., 2016; Zeng et al., 2010). In this context, two studies have also found a role of TRIM4 in the ubiquitination of RIG-I in cooperation with TRIM25 (Sun et al., 2016; Yan et al., 2014).

TRIM6 has been shown to interact with IKKε via its PRYSPRY, mediate its K48-linked ubiquitination, and thus activate IKKε for STAT-1 phosphorylation (Rajsbaum et al., 2014), which is thought to be important in the IRF3 signaling pathway (Fitzgerald et al., 2003; Perwitasari et al., 2011). This pathway can be antagonized by Nipah virus through TRIM6 degradation by its matrix structural protein (Bharaj et al., 2016).

Similarly, TRIM14 has been implicated in the regulation of both RIG-I and cGAS signaling pathways. TRIM14 has been reported to interact with cGAS via its PRYSPRY domain and upon DNA virus infection recruit the proteasome-associated deubiquitinase (DUB) USP14 to deubiquitinate cGAS, preventing recruitment of p62 and autophagy-dependent degradation of cGAS (Jia et al., 2017). TRIM14 has also been shown to interact with MAVS and upon viral infection undergo K63-linked ubiquitination, thereby recruiting NEMO to the MAVS signalosome and activating IRF3 and NF-κB signaling pathways (Zhou et al., 2014).

TRIM proteins have also been implicated in immune cell signaling pathways. For instance, TRIM20, also referred to as Pyrin, is a key player in inflammasome activation. Interestingly, TRIM20 does not have a RING domain but instead has an N-terminal Pyrin domain and thus acts as an inflammasome activator through recruitment of ASC and subsequent activation of Caspase-1, analogous to NLRP3 and AIM2 (Latz et al., 2013; Richards et al., 2001; Yu et al., 2006). Mutations in *MEFV*, the gene encoding TRIM20, are associated with the autoinflammatory disease familial Mediterranean fever (FMF) (Latsoudis et al., 2017; Manukyan and Aminov, 2016; Masters et al., 2016; Park et al., 2016). The pyrin inflammasome can be activated by Rho GTPases that have been modified and inactivated by bacterial toxins (Xu et al., 2014). It is thought that Rho GTPases constitutively activate pyrin phosphorylation, which leads to the binding of inhibitory 14-3-3 proteins (Park et al., 2016). When Rho GTPases are inhibited, TRIM20 is no longer phosphorylated and becomes active. Notably, one mutation associated with FMF is S242R, which results in a loss of inhibitory 14-3-3 binding at phosphorylated S242 and might thus result in constitutive TRIM20 activation (Masters et al., 2016).

The above examples illustrate that TRIM proteins are often found synergizing with and potentiating the activity of well-established immune pathways. This highlights the notion that it is important to consider immune responses in their totality rather than focusing on the contribution of any one pathway or component. In addition to the detailed cases earlier, further examples include TRIM30α, which has been shown to negatively regulate TLR-mediated TRAF6-induced NF-κB activation by degrading TAB2 and TAB3 (Shi et al., 2008). A study by Hu et al. has also shown that TRIM30 negatively regulates the NLRP3 inflammasome. Knockdown of TRIM30 resulted in higher levels of IL-1β secretion in J774 cells as well as BMDMs in response to several NLRP3 agonists. Since there is no direct interaction of TRIM30 with members of the NLRP3 inflammasome, the authors suggest that TRIM30 attenuates the production of ROS and thus NLRP3 inflammasome activation.

TRIM23 has been implicated in the activation of NF-κB signaling in response to viral infection through polyubiquitination of NEMO (Arimoto et al., 2010). Likewise, TRIM56 has been shown to play a role in dsDNA-mediated type I IFN induction through K63 ubiquitination of STING, which promotes STING dimerization and the recruitment of TBK1 (Tsuchida et al., 2010). TRIM27 has also been suggested to regulate NF-κB signaling, via the K48-linked ubiquitination and subsequent proteasomal degradation of NOD2, thereby acting as a negative regulator of NOD2-induced NF-κB signaling (Zurek et al., 2012). TRIM38 is another TRIM that has been proposed as a negative regulation of innate immune pathways through its E3-ligase activity. Several studies have shown that TRIM38 attenuates TLR signaling pathways through K48-linked ubiquitination and degradation of TRIF (Hu et al., 2015; Xue et al., 2012), TRAF6 (Zhao et al., 2012a), and NAP1 (Zhao et al., 2012b). For a detailed review of the role of TRIM38 in innate immunity, see Hu and Shu (2017).

Consistent with a broad role of TRIM proteins in innate immune regulation, one study by Uchil et al. demonstrated that numerous TRIMs are capable of activating the innate immune signaling pathways NF-κB and AP-1 upon overexpression. The same study implicated TRIM62 as part of the TLR4 signaling pathway and TRIM15 in regulating the RIG-I signaling pathway, upstream or at the level of MAVS (Uchil et al., 2013). However, as TRIM proteins are E3 ligases that efficiently catalyze the synthesis of ubiquitin chains, this study could also be interpreted as a warning that overexpression of these enzymes may result in gain-of-function phenotypes.

These are only some examples of the diverse functions TRIM proteins, which are currently understood to have in the innate immune response. Table 1 provides a comprehensive overview of studies so far analyzing the role of individual TRIM proteins in innate immunity. Research into the antiviral roles of TRIM proteins is still in its infancy and this list is likely to grow substantially in the coming years. In many cases, current data establish a phenotype but not a molecular mechanism. An understanding of how less-studied TRIMs exert their function may be gained by considering the activity of specific TRIMs for which there are molecular, cellular, and organismal data available. The cytosolic antibody receptor TRIM21 provides an excellent such exemplar for both signaling and effector TRIM function as it simultaneously restricts antibody-coated viruses and elicits potent innate immune signaling (Mallery et al., 2010; McEwan et al., 2013); hence, its mechanism will be discussed in depth in the following sections.

2.4 The Role of TRIM21 in Innate Immunity

Human TRIM21 is a 52-kDa cytosolic protein that consists of the classical N-terminal RBCC motif and a C-terminal PRYSPRY domain. It is located on chromosome 11 in a cluster of nine TRIM proteins, all of which contain PRYSPRY regions, indicating the important role of chromosomal duplications in expanding the TRIM family (Han et al., 2011). The TRIM21 gene consists of seven exons, with exons 2–5 encoding the RBCC motif and exon 7 giving rise to the PRYSPRY domain.

TRIM21 is the only known cytosolic IgG receptor in mammals. All other known IgG receptors capture IgG via their Fc at the plasma membrane (FcγRs) or within an endosome (FcRn). TRIM21 is structurally unrelated to FcγRs and engages a different region of IgG Fc. The PRY element of TRIM21 forms a binding pocket for the C_{H2} domain of the Fc region, while the SPRY domain forms a pocket for the C_{H3} region. Binding of the antibody molecule occurs within the canonical PRYSPRY-binding site defined by its six variable loops (see Section 2.1). There are four hot spot residues in TRIM21 that are crucial for antibody interaction and their mutation abrogates all binding: D355 proximal to VL2, W381 and W383 in VL4, and F450 in VL6. They contact three hot spot residues in the IgG-Fc, located near the C-terminus of C_{H3}: H433, N434, and H435. The PRYSPRY residues in VL4 and VL6 form a hydrophobic ring around a bifurcated hydrogen bond that D355 forms with H433 and N434, shielding it from solvent (James et al., 2007; Keeble et al., 2008). Interestingly, while this binding site

Table 1 The Role of TRIM Proteins in Innate Immunity

TRIM Protein	Function in Innate Immunity	Viruses Affected	Mechanism	References
TRIM1	Restriction of retroviruses through initiation of innate immune signaling	N-MLV		Yap et al. (2004)
TRIM4	Ubiquitination of RIG-I in cooperation with TRIM25	SeV, VSV		Yan et al. (2014); Sun et al. (2016)
TRIM5	Restriction of retroviruses and innate immune signaling upon capsid recognition	HIV-1, N-MLV, EIAV	Capsid binding via the PRYSPRY domain, autoubiquitination and proteasomal recruitment, stimulation of signaling pathways through unanchored K63 ubiquitin chains	Lukic et al. (2011); Pertel et al. (2011); Stremlau et al. (2004); Grütter and Luban (2012)
TRIM6	Regulation of the IRF3 signaling pathway	SeV, IAV, ECMV	Generation of unanchored K48-linked ubiquitin chains that activate IKKε for STAT1 phosphorylation	Rajsbaum et al. (2014); Bharaj et al. (2016)
TRIM8	Positive regulation of NF-κB target genes IL-1β and TNFα		K63-linked ubiquitination and subsequent activation of TAK-1	Okumura et al. (2010)
	Epinephelus coioides TRIM8 restricts Singapore grouper iridovirus (SGIV)	SGIV		Huang et al. (2016a)
TRIM9 short isoform	Positive regulation of IRF3 signaling pathway	VSV, HSV-1	Autoubiquitination of TRIM9 facilitates GSK3β-mediated activation of TBK1	Qin et al. (2016)
TRIM11	Restriction of retroviruses	HIV-1	Acceleration of HIV-1 uncoating which results in reduced reverse transcription	Yuan et al. (2014); Yuan et al. (2016)
	Negative regulation of IFNβ production	HSV-1, VSV	Interaction with TBK1	Lee et al. (2013)
	Negative regulation of the AIM2 inflammasome	HSV-1, MCMV	Interaction with AIM2 via the PRYSPRY domain, autoubiquitination and recruitment of p62 which results in AIM2 degradation by autophagy	Liu et al. (2016a)

Continued

Table 1 The Role of TRIM Proteins in Innate Immunity—cont'd

TRIM Protein	Function in Innate Immunity	Viruses Affected	Mechanism	References
TRIM13	Negative regulation of MDA5 signaling pathway, positive regulation of RIG-I pathway	ECMV, SeV		Narayan et al. (2014)
	Positive regulation of the TLR2-stimulated NF-κB signaling pathway		K29-linked polyubiquitination of TRAF6	Huang and Baek (2017)
	Negative regulation of NF-κB activation		Regulation of NEMO ubiquitination	Tomar and Singh (2014)
	Epinephelus coioides TRIM13 negatively regulates IRF3 and MDA5 signaling pathways	RGNNV		Huang et al. (2016b)
TRIM14	Positive regulation of the RLR signaling pathway	SeV	K63-linked polyubiquitination of TRIM14 after viral infection likely through interaction with MAVS results in recruitment of NEMO to the MAVS signalosome	Zhou et al. (2014)
	Positive regulation of cGAS-dependent type I IFN response	HSV-1, VSV	Recruitment of USP14 which deubiquitinates cGAS, thus preventing its p62-dependent autophagic degradation	Chen et al. (2016)
	Restriction of flaviviruses	HCV	Degradation of viral NS5A protein	Wang et al. (2016); Nenasheva et al. (2015)
TRIM15	Regulation of the RIG-I signaling pathway	VSV		Uchil et al. (2013)
	Restriction of retroviruses	HIV-1, N-MLV	Inhibition of viral release through interaction of the B-box with the Gag precursor protein	Uchil et al. (2008)

	Function	Virus/target	Description	Reference
TRIM19 (PML)	Restriction of retroviruses	HIV-1	Interference with early steps of replication	Turelli et al. (2001)
			Cell type-specific restriction early in the viral life cycle	Kahle et al. (2016)
			Repression of viral transcription	Lusic et al. (2013); Masroori et al. (2016)
			Stabilization of Daxx which then inhibits reverse transcription	Dutrieux et al. (2015)
	Restriction of parvoviruses	AAV		Mitchell et al. (2014)
	Restriction of herpesviruses	HCMV		Schilling et al. (2017); Wagenknecht et al. (2015)
	Restriction of rhabdoviruses	VSV	Inhibition of viral protein synthesis	Chelbi-Alix et al. (1998)
	Positive regulation of IFNβ	VSV, SeV, ECMV, HTLV-1, IAV, VV	Recruitment of Pin1 into nuclear bodies which prevents degradation of IRF3 (Saitoh et al., 2006)	El Asmi et al. (2014)
TRIM20 (pyrin)	Inflammasome activation		Inactivation of Rho GTPases results in loss of downstream pyrin phosphorylation. Phosphorylated pyrin is usually bound by inhibitory 14-3-3 proteins, and thus a loss of phosphorylation might result in activation	Richards et al. (2001); Yu et al. (2006); Masters et al. (2016); Manukyan and Aminov (2016); Park et al. (2016); Latsoudis et al. (2017); Xu et al. (2014); Vajjhala et al. (2014)
	Regulation of NF-κB signaling		Caspase-1 cleaves an N-terminal fragment of TRIM20 that results in ASC-dependent NF-κB activation	Chae et al. (2008)

Continued

Table 1 The Role of TRIM Proteins in Innate Immunity—cont'd

TRIM Protein	Function in Innate Immunity	Viruses Affected	Mechanism	References
TRIM21	Restriction of adenoviruses	hAdV5, MAV-1	Binding of the PRYSPRY domain to antibody-coated virus results in autoubiquitination and recruitment of the proteasome	Mallery et al. (2010); Vaysburd et al. (2013); Watkinson et al. (2013); Fletcher and James (2016)
	Restriction of picornaviruses	FMDV		Fan et al. (2016a)
	Innate immune sensing of viruses	hAdV5, HRV14, FCV	Release of K63-linked ubiquitin chains by proteasome-associated DUB Poh-1	McEwan et al. (2013); Watkinson et al. (2015); Watkinson et al. (2013); Fletcher et al. (2014)
	Negative regulation of dsDNA cellular response	HSV-1	K48-linked polyubiquitination and degradation of DDX41	Zhang et al. (2012a)
	Negative regulation of IRF signaling pathways	SeV	Polyubiquitination and degradation of IRF3, IRF5, and IRF7	Higgs et al. (2008); Lazzari et al. (2014); Higgs et al. (2010)
	Positive regulation of IRF signaling pathways		Preventing interaction between Pin1 and IRF3, thus preventing Pin1-dependent IRF3 degradation	Kong et al. (2007)
			Ubiquitination of IRF8 results in increased ability to stimulate IL-12p40 expression	Kong et al. (2007)

TRIM22	Restriction of retroviruses	HIV-1		Singh et al. (2011); Barr et al. (2008)
			Transcriptional silencing	Turrini et al. (2015); Kajaste-Rudnitski et al. (2011)
	Restriction of flaviviruses	HCV	Ubiquitination of NS5A	Yang et al. (2016)
		HBV	Transcriptional repression mediated by the RING and PRYSPRY domains	Yang et al. (2016)
	Restriction of orthomyxoviruses	IAV	Degradation of the viral nucleoprotein	Di Pietro et al. (2013)
TRIM23	Regulation of NF-κB signaling	SeV	K27-linked polyubiquitination of NEMO	Arimoto et al. (2010)
	Positive regulation of viral infectivity	YFV	Polyubiquitination of YFV NS5 promotes binding to STAT2 and suppresses type I IFN signaling	Laurent-Rolle et al. (2014)
		HCMV	Interaction with HCMV UL144 facilitates association with TRAF6, which activates NF-κB signaling	Poole et al. (2009)
TRIM25	Positive regulation of the RIG-I pathway	NDV, VSV, SeV	Ubiquitination of the RIG-I CARDs, which facilitates the interaction with MAVS	Gack et al. (2007); Zeng et al. (2010); Sanchez et al. (2016)
	Modulation of antiviral activity of zinc finger antiviral protein (ZAP)	SinV		Zheng et al. (2017); Li et al. (2017)

Continued

Table 1 The Role of TRIM Proteins in Innate Immunity—cont'd

TRIM Protein	Function in Innate Immunity	Viruses Affected	Mechanism	References
TRIM26	Positive regulation of the RLR signaling pathway	NDV, VSV	Direct interaction with TBK and likely recruitment of NEMO through autoubiquitination bridges NEMO and TBK1 and positively regulates IFNβ	Ran et al. (2016)
	Negative regulation of type I IFN signaling pathway	VSV	Polyubiquitination and degradation of IRF3 resulting in diminished IFNβ response	Wang et al. (2015a)
TRIM27	Negative regulation of NOD2-mediated NF-κB signaling		K48-linked ubiquitination and subsequent proteasomal degradation of NOD2	Zurek et al. (2012)
TRIM28	Restriction of retroviruses	M-MLV	Transcriptional repression	Wolf and Goff (2007); Wolf and Goff (2007)
		HIV-1	Inhibition of HIV-1 integration	Allouch et al. (2011); Figueiredo and Hope (2011)
	Negative regulation of the IRF7 signaling pathway	VSV	SUMOylation of IRF7	Liang et al. (2011)
TRIM29	Negative regulation of NF-κB and type I IFN signaling pathways	IAV	Ubiquitination and subsequent degradation of NEMO in alveolar macrophages	Xing et al. (2016)
TRIM30	Negative regulation of NF-κB signaling		TRIM30α facilitates degradation of TAB2 and TAB3	Shi et al. (2008)
	Negative regulation of NLRP3 inflammasome activation		Attenuation of ROS production	Hu et al. (2010)
TRIM31	Negative regulation of NLRP3 inflammasome activation		K48-linked ubiquitination and proteasomal degradation of NLRP3	Song et al. (2016)
	Positive regulation of the RLR signaling pathway	SeV	K63-linked polyubiquitination of MAVS which promotes MAVS aggregation	Liu et al. (2017b)

TRIM32	Restriction of orthomyxoviruses	IAV	Ubiquitination and degradation of IAV PB1 polymerase	Fu et al. (2015)
	Positive regulation of type I IFN signaling	VSV, NDV	K63-linked ubiquitination of STING which promotes interaction with TBK1	Zhang et al. (2012b)
TRIM33	Activation of NLRP3 inflammasome in response to dsRNA		K63-linked ubiquitination of dsRNA sensor DHX33 (Gallouet et al., 2017) which results in DHX33–NLRP3 complex formation	Weng et al. (2014)
	Regulation of *Ifnb1* expression in macrophages		Regulatory element at the *Ifnb1* enhancer	Ferri et al. (2015)
TRIM35	Negative regulation of type I IFN signaling in response to TLR9 and TLR7 activation	VSV, HSV-1	K48-linked ubiquitination of IRF7 which results in proteasomal degradation	Wang et al. (2015b)
TRIM37	Restriction of retroviruses	HIV-1		Tabah et al. (2014)
TRIM38	Negative regulation of TLR3/4 signaling pathways		K48-linked polyubiquitination and subsequent proteasomal degradation of TRIF	Hu et al. (2015); Xue et al. (2012)
			K48-linked polyubiquitination and subsequent proteasomal degradation of TRAF6	Zhao et al. (2012a)
		VSV	K48-linked polyubiquitination and subsequent proteasomal degradation of NAP1	Zhao et al. (2012b)
	Negative regulation of IL-1β and TNFα induction		Proteasomal degradation of TAB2/3	Hu et al. (2014)
	Regulation of the cGAS signaling pathway		SUMOylation of cGAS and STING which results in increased stability	Hu et al. (2016)

Continued

Table 1 The Role of TRIM Proteins in Innate Immunity—cont'd

TRIM Protein	Function in Innate Immunity	Viruses Affected	Mechanism	References
TRIM40	Negative regulation of NF-κB signaling		Inhibition of NEMO through its neddylation in the gastrointestinal tract	Noguchi et al. (2011)
TRIM41	Inhibition of flaviviruses	HBV	Inhibition of HBV transcription	Zhang et al. (2013)
TRIM44	Positive regulation of RLR signaling pathway	SeV	Stabilization of MAVS	Yang et al. (2013)
TRIM45	Negative regulation of NF-κB signaling			Shibata et al. (2012)
TRIM52	Positive regulation of NF-κB signaling			Fan et al. (2017)
	Restriction of flaviviruses	JEV	Ubiquitination and subsequent degradation of viral NS2A protein	Fan et al. (2016b)
TRIM56	Positive regulation of the STING signaling pathway		K63-linked ubiquitination of STING which facilitates dimerization and TBK1 recruitment	Tsuchida et al. (2010)
	Restriction of flaviviruses and coronaviruses	BVDV, YFV, DENV2, hCoV-OC43		Wang et al. (2011b); Liu et al. (2014)
	Positive regulation of TLR3 signaling pathway	HCV		Shen et al. (2012)
	Restriction of orthomyxoviruses	IAV, IBV	Inhibition of viral RNA synthesis	Liu et al. (2016b)
	Restriction of retroviruses	HIV-1		Kane et al. (2016)

TRIM	Function	Virus	Reference
TRIM59	Negative regulation of NF-κB and IRF3/7 signaling pathways		Kondo et al. (2012)
TRIM62	Restriction of retroviruses and involvement in the TLR4 signaling pathway	N-MLV	Uchil et al. (2013)
TRIM65	Positive regulator of the MDA5 signaling pathway	ECMV	Lang et al. (2016)
TRIM68	K63-linked ubiquitination of MDA5, thus promoting MDA5 oligomerization and activation		
TRIM68	Polyubiquitination and degradation of TGF which interacts with NEMO		Wynne et al. (2014)
TRIM79α	Negative regulation of type I IFN signaling		
TRIM79α	Degradation of the viral RNA polymerase	TBEV	Taylor et al. (2012)

is distant from the binding site of classic FcγRs, it overlaps with the FcRn-binding site. FcRn is important for prolonging the half-life of IgG molecules through recycling of internalized antibodies as well as transfer of IgG from mother to fetus across the placenta. The binding of FcRn to IgG can only occur at the endosomal pH of 6.5 and is markedly reduced at pH 7.4 since FcRn binding relies on the protonation of H433 and H435, which only occurs at acidic pH (Roopenian and Akilesh, 2007; Stapleton et al., 2011). In contrast, the binding of TRIM21 is pH independent and does not require protonation. TRIM21 is capable of binding all IgG subclasses with nM affinity (Keeble et al., 2008) and has also been shown to bind IgM (Mallery et al., 2010) and IgA (Bidgood et al., 2014), however with lower affinities of 17 and 50 μM, respectively.

2.5 TRIM21 Effector Mechanism

TRIM21 is an IFN-inducible, cytosolic high-affinity IgG receptor that detects antibody-coated viruses or bacteria that have entered the cytosol. In response, it mediates dual effector and sensor functions by facilitating simultaneous proteasomal degradation of virions and innate immune signaling (Fig. 1). The two critical prerequisites for this mechanism are virus penetration of the cytosol and exposure of antibody molecules to the cytosol. This means that not all virus/antibody combinations will be able to stimulate TRIM21; the antibody cannot block viral entry into the cells, e.g., through binding viral epitopes crucial for receptor engagement and the virus cannot gain access to the cytosol through a fusion mechanism that will result in shedding of the antibody. Therefore, most experiments elucidating viral neutralization and innate immune signaling mediated by TRIM21 have used either hAdV or mouse adenovirus 1 (MAV-1) as well as human rhinovirus 14 (HRV14), as they are nonenveloped viruses that penetrate the endosome during entry, carrying bound antibodies with them. In this review the term neutralization is used as defined by P.J. Klasse: "Neutralization [....] is defined as the reduction in viral infectivity by the binding of antibodies to the surface of viral particles (virions), thereby blocking a step in the viral replication cycle that precedes virally encoded transcription or synthesis" (Klasse, 2014).

Once the virus has accessed the cytosol, TRIM21 binds the Fc region of an antibody with a 1:1 stoichiometry (one TRIM21 dimer to one heterodimeric IgG), with the coiled-coil domain mediating TRIM21 dimerization. Binding of the antibody activates the E3-ligase activity of

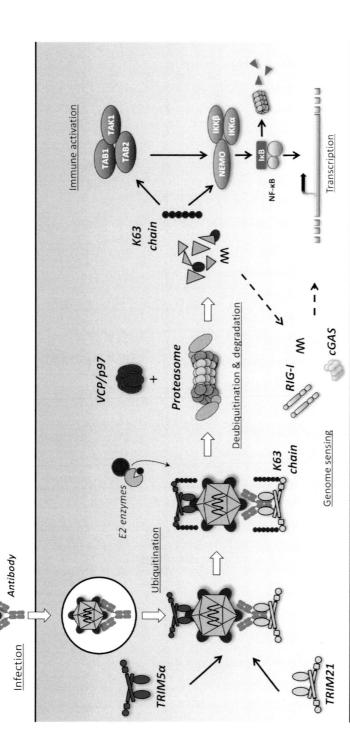

Fig. 1 The antibody-coated virus enters the cell and accesses the cytosol, where TRIM21 can bind the Fc region of the antibody; in case of a retrovirus, TRIM5α is able to bind to the viral capsid. Both TRIM21 and TRIM5α will recruit Ube2W resulting in N-terminal monoubiquitination. The E2 enzyme complex Ube2N/Ube2V2 then extends the N-terminal ubiquitin through K63-linked chains. Ubiquitination results in recruitment of the proteasome, the virus, or virus/antibody complex become degraded, while the proteasome-associated DUB Poh1 simultaneously releases the K63-linked ubiquitin chains, which can stimulate innate immune pathways downstream. TRIM21 has been shown to stimulate NF-κB, AP-1, as well as IRF3, IRF5, and IRF7 pathways, while TRIM5α only stimulates NF-κB and AP-1 signaling pathways. In the case of TRIM21 it has been shown that viral degradation of hAdV and HRV results in exposure of the viral DNA or RNA genome which can be sensed further downstream by cGAS or RIG-I, respectively, initiating a second wave of innate immune signaling.

TRIM21 through a still unknown mechanism. It is thought that TRIM21 first recruits the E2 enzyme Ube2W, which monoubiquitinates the N-terminus of TRIM21. Subsequently, the E2 enzyme complex Ube2N/Ube2V2 polyubiquitinates TRIM21 through K63 chain extension of the N-terminal ubiquitin. This mechanism of autoubiquitination is analogous to the mechanism the TRIM5α uses (Fletcher et al., 2015). Cellular depletion of Ube2N also results in loss of TRIM21 K48 ubiquitination, suggesting that there may be additional E2 enzymes recruited to TRIM21 resulting in mixed or branched chains. It is not known whether the antibody or the virus also becomes ubiquitinated. Following ubiquitination, it has been shown that PohI, a proteasome-associated DUB, is required for the removal of K63-linked ubiquitin chains, which is pivotal for both TRIM21-mediated neutralization and signaling. The virus:antibody:TRIM21 complex is then degraded by the proteasome in cooperation with the AAA ATPase p97/VCP (Hauler et al., 2012), while the liberated K63 chains activate innate immune signaling through NF-κB, AP-1 as well as IRF3, IRF5, and IRF7 signaling pathways (McEwan et al., 2013). This results in the induction of proinflammatory cytokines such as IL-6, CCL4, and TNFα as well as IFNβ. Interestingly, while TRIM21-dependent neutralization has only been demonstrated for hAdV (and recently for foot-and-mouth disease virus (FMDV) in swines (Fan et al., 2016a)), TRIM21-dependent signaling could be demonstrated for hAdV, HRV14, feline calicivirus (FCV), as well as *Salmonella enterica*. Furthermore, TRIM21 is important in exposing the respective dsDNA and ssRNA genomes of hAdV and HRV, through degradation of the viral capsid, thus making them accessible to sensing by cGAS and RIG-I, and driving a second wave of signal induction after the first wave initiated by TRIM21 (Watkinson et al., 2015).

While the neutralization and signaling activities of TRIM21 are coupled, they have different response thresholds. Neutralization of hAdV could be observed with as little as 1.6 antibodies per virus in IFNα-treated MEF cells (McEwan et al., 2012). Similarly, TRIM21's neutralization activity is tolerant to mutations in the Fc region that decrease the antibody's affinity for TRIM21 to the point that it is even capable of neutralizing virus with an H433K mutant, which displays a 100-fold decrease in affinity for TRIM21. Conversely, signaling is highly sensitive to changes in affinity. In cells where Fc mutant I253A (which has approximately a twofold lower affinity for TRIM21 than the wild-type (WT) antibody) does not impact neutralization, signaling is almost completely lost. This phenotype can be partially rescued by increasing antibody concentration, but this mutant's signaling activity is always significantly lower than WT (McEwan et al., 2012). In line with this observation, it has been shown that TRIM21 effector functions strongly correlate with antibody off-rate, more so than simply affinity for the antigen, a trend that is again more pronounced for TRIM21's signaling output than its neutralization function (Bottermann et al., 2016). It is intuitive that signaling would be regulated more strictly and have thresholds, since TRIM21's neutralization activity cannot be harmful for the host, while the initiation of potent immune signaling can have potentially severe consequences. During an immune response, this may ensure that TRIM21 signaling only activates immune transcription in the presence of high-affinity IgG or significant viral challenge. However, this separate threshold allows for neutralization function during the early stages of an immune response where viremia is lower and where antibodies are derived from the natural or low-affinity IgM repertoire. This is supported by the fact that in vivo, TRIM21 can protect naïve mice from fatal MAV-1 infection, where the protective antibody effect can only result from natural or low-affinity IgM that is produced prior to affinity maturation. Moreover, immune signaling in naïve mice after challenge with MAV-1 shows no TRIM21 dependence (Vaysburd et al., 2013). Conversely, mice that received MAV-1 immune sera prior to challenge with MAV-1 were not only better protected from fatal infection in a TRIM21-dependent manner (Vaysburd et al., 2013), but they also showed strong TRIM21-dependent upregulation of proinflammatory cytokines (Watkinson et al., 2013).

Recently, it has been shown that TRIM21 can also inhibit tau seeds, which is the source of pathological tau that exhibits prion-like properties (Iqbal et al., 2015), in a manner similar to neutralizing antibody-bound viruses (McEwan et al., 2017). This suggests that the protection mediated by TRIM21 extends to nonclassical pathogens, such as proteopathic agents. This also highlights that TRIM21 is agnostic to the nature of the infectious agent. TRIM21 is essentially a DAMP sensor for antibodies that mislocalize to the cytosol—something that should only happen if normal cellular compartmentalization has been compromised.

2.6 The Role of TRIM21 in Innate Immune Regulation and Autoimmunity

Systemic lupus erythematosus (SLE) is an autoimmune disorder that is characterized by erythematosus, fatigue as well as joint pain and swelling. While its cause and origin are still unknown, it is often associated with autoantibodies against TRIM21. The same is true for the autoimmune disorder

Sjögren's syndrome, where the presence of TRIM21 autoantibodies has served as a diagnostic tool for decades (Fujimoto et al., 1997). One hypothesis of how TRIM21 may contribute to these autoimmune disorders is that autoantibodies against it might undergo bipolar bridging, involving simultaneous engagement of their Fc and Fab regions. This could result in the formation of large aggregated immune complexes that cannot be cleared by Fcγ-mediated phagocytosis, thereby contributing to pathogenesis (James et al., 2007). Another study has shown that macrophages from SLE-prone mice do not fully mature their lysosomes, which has been suggested to result in a defect in clearance of apoptotic cells, an accumulation of nuclear antigens and leakage of DNA and IgG into the cytosol, which then activates AIM2 and TRIM21 (Monteith et al., 2016). Furthermore, there has been evidence that TRIM21 is involved in not only the initiation of immune signaling but also its regulation. TRIM21 has been implicated in the polyubiquitination and subsequent degradation of IRF transcription factors IRF3, IRF5, and IRF7 and thus in the negative regulation of IFNβ signaling (Higgs et al., 2008, 2010; Lazzari et al., 2014; Oke and Wahren-Herlenius, 2012). However, other studies contradict a negative regulatory role and have shown that TRIM21 positively upregulates type I IFN signaling through interference with the Pin1–IRF3 interaction (Yang et al., 2009), which usually results in IRF3 degradation (Saitoh et al., 2006), or through ubiquitination and thus stabilization of IRF8 (Kong et al., 2007). One study using TRIM21 KO mice has suggested that while mice are phenotypically normal when left unmanipulated, they develop symptoms consistent with autoimmune disorders upon metal eartagging. In mice that spontaneously become autoimmune, proinflammatory cytokines such as IL-6 and IL-17 (Espinosa et al., 2009) are upregulated. However, one drawback of this study was that the TRIM21 KO generated in these mice was not complete, but through homologous recombination targeted to exon 5. This means that the RING, B-box, and coiled-coil domains of TRIM21 are still intact and in frame with the native promoter, while the PRYSPRY domain has been knocked out, meaning that the catalytic part of TRIM21 is still present. On the other hand, Yoshimi et al. generated TRIM21 KO mice where the entire sequence encoding the TRIM21 mRNA was replaced by eGFP. In this study, it was shown that TRIM21 expression is prevalent in many tissues, while particularly high expression levels are observed in immune cells. Interestingly, these mice did not display any autoimmune phenotypes upon eartagging (Yoshimi et al., 2010). However, MEF cells from these TRIM21 KO mice displayed higher levels of proinflammatory cytokines after TNFα stimulation than MEFs from WT animals as well as enhanced NF-κB promoter activity. The ubiquitination of IRF3 and IRF8 was reduced in the TRIM21 KO MEFs, but ISG expression in BMDMs was not affected. This suggests that knockout of TRIM21 can impact the regulation of proinflammatory cytokines; however, it is not clear whether this plays a role in autoimmune disease.

In summary, TRIM21 is a unique innate immune sensor in that it is a cytosolic IgG receptor that is capable of both neutralization and initiation of innate immune signaling. Unlike other innate immune sensors, which often recognize PAMPs associated with the pathogen itself, TRIM21 is not specific to a particular pathogen or antigen as its activation depends on the presence of antigen-bound antibody rather than the antigen itself. Future work will seek to further elucidate the activation and regulatory mechanisms of TRIM21, which will hopefully also give further insights into its role in autoimmune disease.

ACKNOWLEDGMENTS

M.B. and L.C.J. received funding from the Medical Research Council (UK; U105181010) and through a Wellcome Trust Investigator Award.

REFERENCES

Abais, J.M., Xia, M., Zhang, Y., Boini, K.M., Li, P.-L., 2015. Redox regulation of NLRP3 inflammasomes: ROS as trigger or effector? Antioxid. Redox Signal. 22, 1111–1129.

Ablasser, A., et al., 2009. RIG-I-dependent sensing of poly(dA:dT) through the induction of an RNA polymerase III-transcribed RNA intermediate. Nat. Immunol. 10, 1065–1072.

Akira, S., Takeda, K., 2004. Toll-like receptor signalling. Nat. Rev. Immunol. 4, 499–511.

Allen, I.C., et al., 2009. The NLRP3 inflammasome mediates in vivo innate immunity to influenza A virus through recognition of viral RNA. Immunity 30, 556–565.

Allen, I.C., et al., 2011. NLRX1 protein attenuates inflammatory responses to infection by interfering with the RIG-I-MAVS and TRAF6-NF-κB signaling pathways. Immunity 34, 854–865.

Allouch, A., et al., 2011. The TRIM family protein KAP1 inhibits HIV-1 integration. Cell Host Microbe 9, 484–495.

Almine, J.F., et al., 2017. IFI16 and cGAS cooperate in the activation of STING during DNA sensing in human keratinocytes. Nat. Commun. 8, 14392.

Anderson, J.L., et al., 2006. Proteasome inhibition reveals that a functional preintegration complex intermediate can be generated during restriction by diverse TRIM5 proteins. J. Virol. 80, 9754–9760.

Arimoto, K., et al., 2010. Polyubiquitin conjugation to NEMO by triparite motif protein 23 (TRIM23) is critical in antiviral defense. Proc. Natl. Acad. Sci. U.S.A. 107, 15856–15861.

Barlan, A.U., Griffin, T.M., McGuire, K.A., Wiethoff, C.M., 2011. Adenovirus membrane penetration activates the NLRP3 inflammasome. J. Virol. 85, 146–155.

Barr, S.D., Smiley, J.R., Bushman, F.D., 2008. The interferon response inhibits HIV particle production by induction of TRIM22. PLoS Pathog. 4, 1–11.

Barral, P.M., Sarkar, D., Fisher, P.B., Racaniello, V.R., 2009. RIG-I is cleaved during picornavirus infection. Virology 39, 171–176.

Bharaj, P., et al., 2016. The matrix protein of nipah virus targets the E3–ubiquitin ligase TRIM6 to inhibit the IKKε kinase-mediated type-I IFN antiviral response. PLoS Pathog. 12, 1–27.

Bidgood, S.R., Tam, J.C.H., McEwan, W.A., Mallery, D.L., James, L.C., 2014. Translocalized IgA mediates neutralization and stimulates innate immunity inside infected cells. Proc. Natl. Acad. Sci. U.S.A. 111, 13463–13468.

Bieback, K., et al., 2002. Hemagglutinin protein of wild-type measles virus activates toll-like receptor hemagglutinin protein of wild-type measles virus activates toll-like receptor 2 signaling. J. Virol. 76, 8729–8736.

Bottermann, M., et al., 2016. Antibody-antigen kinetics constrain intracellular humoral immunity. Sci. Rep. 6, 37457.

Boutell, C., Orr, A., Everett, R.D., 2003. PML residue lysine 160 is required for the degradation of PML induced by herpes simplex virus type 1 regulatory protein ICP0 PML residue lysine 160 is required for the degradation of PML induced by herpes simplex virus type 1 regulatory protein ICP0. Society 77, 8686–8694.

Bridgeman, A., et al., 2015. Viruses transfer the antiviral second messenger cGAMP between cells. Science 349, 1228–1232.

Broz, P., Von Moltke, J., Jones, J.W., Vance, R.E., Monack, D.M., 2010. Differential requirement for caspase-1 autoproteolysis in pathogen-induced cell death and cytokine processing. Cell Host Microbe 8, 471–483.

Brunette, R.L., et al., 2012. Extensive evolutionary and functional diversity among mammalian AIM2-like receptors. J. Exp. Med. 209, 1969–1983.

Burdette, D.L., Vance, R.E., 2013. STING and the innate immune response to nucleic acids in the cytosol. Nat. Immunol. 14, 19–26.

Cai, X., Chiu, Y.H., Chen, Z.J., 2014. The cGAS-cGAMP-STING pathway of cytosolic DNA sensing and signaling. Mol. Cell 54, 289–296.

Chae, J.J., Wood, G., Richard, K., Jaffe, H., Colburn, N.T., Masters, S.L., Gumucio, D.L., Shoham, N.G., Kastner, D.L., 2008. The familial Mediterranean fever protein, pyrin, is cleaved by caspase-1 and activates NF-kB through its N-terminal fragment. Blood 12, 6–7.

Chang, T.H., Liao, C.L., Lin, Y.L., 2006. Flavivirus induces interferon-beta gene expression through a pathway involving RIG-I-dependent IRF-3 and PI3K-dependent NF-κB activation. Microbes Infect. 8, 157–171.

Chelbi-Alix, M.K., Quignon, F., Pelicano, L., Koken, M.H., de Thé, H., 1998. Resistance to virus infection conferred by the interferon-induced promyelocytic leukemia protein. J. Virol. 72, 1043–1051.

Chen, M., et al., 2016. TRIM14 inhibits cGAS degradation mediated by selective autophagy receptor p62 to promote innate immune responses. Mol. Cell 64, 105–119.

Chiu, Y.-H., MacMillan, J.B., Chen, Z.J., 2009. RNA polymerase III detects cytosolic DNA and induces type-I interferons through the RIG-I pathway. Cell 138, 576–591.

Choi, U.Y., Kang, J.S., Hwang, Y.S., Kim, Y.J., 2015. Oligoadenylate synthase-like (OASL) proteins: dual functions and associations with diseases. Exp. Mol. Med. 47, e144.

Compton, T., et al., 2003. Human cytomegalovirus activates inflammatory cytokine responses via CD14 and toll-like receptor 2. J. Virol. 77, 4588–4596.

Cridland, J.A., et al., 2012. The mammalian PYHIN gene family: phylogeny, evolution and expression. BMC Evol. Biol. 12, 140.

Dambuza, I.M., Brown, G.D., 2015. C-type lectins in immunity: recent developments. Curr. Opin. Immunol. 32, 21–27.

de Witte, L., Abt, M., Schneider-Schaulies, S., van Kooyk, Y., Geijtenbeek, T.B.H., 2006. Measles virus targets DC-SIGN to enhance dendritic cell infection. J. Virol. 80, 3477–3486.

Diebold, S.S., 2004. Innate antiviral responses by means of TLR7-mediated recognition of single-stranded RNA. Science 303, 1529–1531.

Di Pietro, A., et al., 2013. TRIM22 inhibits influenza A virus infection by targeting the viral nucleoprotein for degradation. J. Virol. 87, 4523–4533.

Dixit, E., Kagan, J.C., 2013. Intracellular pathogen detection by RIG-I-like receptors. Adv. Immunol. 117, 99–125.

Drummond, R.A., Brown, G.D., 2013. Signalling C-type lectins in antimicrobial immunity. PLoS Pathog. 9, 9–11.

Duewell, P., et al., 2010. NLRP3 inflammasomes are required for atherogenesis and activated by cholesterol crystals. Nature 464, 1357–1361.

Dutrieux, J., et al., 2015. PML/TRIM19-dependent inhibition of retroviral reverse-transcription by Daxx. PLoS Pathog. 11, 1–22.

Eichholz, K., et al., 2016. Immune-complexed adenovirus induce AIM2-mediated pyroptosis in human dendritic cells. PLoS Pathog. 12, e1005871.

El Asmi, F., et al., 2014. Implication of PMLIV in both intrinsic and innate immunity. PLoS Pathog. 10 (2), e1003975. https://doi.org/10.1371/journal.ppat.1003975.

Errett, J.S., Suthar, M.S., McMillan, A., Diamond, M.S., Gale, M., 2013. The essential, non-redundant roles of RIG-I and MDA5 in detecting and controlling west nile virus infection. J. Virol. 87, 11416–11425.

Espinosa, A., et al., 2009. Loss of the lupus autoantigen Ro52/Trim21 induces tissue inflammation and systemic autoimmunity by disregulating the IL-23-Th17 pathway. J. Exp. Med. 206, 1661–1671.

Fan, W., et al., 2016a. Swine TRIM21 restricts FMDV infection via an intracellular neutralization mechanism. Antiviral Res. 127, 32–40.

Fan, W., et al., 2016b. TRIM52 inhibits Japanese encephalitis virus replication by degrading the viral NS2A. Sci. Rep. 6, 33698.

Fan, W., et al., 2017. TRIM52: a nuclear TRIM protein that positively regulates the nuclear factor-kappa B signaling pathway. Mol. Immunol. 82, 114–122.

Farhat, K., et al., 2007. Heterodimerization of TLR2 with TLR1 or TLR6 expands the ligand spectrum but does not lead to differential signaling. J. Leukoc. Biol. 83, 692–701.

Ferguson, W., Dvora, S., Gallo, J., Orth, A., Boissinot, S., 2008. Long-term balancing selection at the West Nile virus resistance gene, Oas1b, maintains transspecific polymorphisms in the house mouse. Mol. Biol. Evol. 25, 1609–1618.

Fernandes-Alnemri, T., et al., 2009. AIM2 activates the inflammasome and cell death in response to cytoplasmic DNA. Nature 458, 509–513.

Ferri, F., et al., 2015. TRIM33 switches off Ifnb1 gene transcription during the late phase of macrophage activation. Nat. Commun. 6, 8900.

Figueiredo, A., Hope, T.J., 2011. KAPs off for HIV-1 integration. Cell Host Microbe 9, 447–448.

Fiola, S., Gosselin, D., Takada, K., Gosselin, J., 2010. TLR9 contributes to the recognition of EBV by primary monocytes and plasmacytoid dendritic cells. J. Immunol. 185, 3620–3631.

Fitzgerald, K.A., et al., 2003. IKKε and TBK1 are essential components of the IRF3 signaling pathway. Nat. Immunol. 4, 491–496.

Fletcher, A.J., James, L.C., 2016. Coordinated neutralization and immune activation by the cytosolic antibody receptor TRIM21. J. Virol. 90, 4856–4859.

Fletcher, A.J., Mallery, D.L., Watkinson, R.E., Dickson, C.F., James, L.C., 2014. Sequential ubiquitination and deubiquitination enzymes synchronise the dual sensor and effector functions of TRIM21. Proc. Natl. Acad. Sci. U.S.A. 112, 10014–10019.

Fletcher, A.J., et al., 2015. TRIM5α requires Ube2W to anchor Lys63-linked ubiquitin chains and restrict reverse transcription. EMBO J. 34, 1–18.

Franchi, L., et al., 2008. Intracellular NOD-like receptors in innate immunity, infection and disease. Cell. Microbiol. 10, 1–8.

Franchi, L., Warner, N., Viani, K., Nuñez, G., 2009. Function of Nod-like receptors in microbial recognition and host defense. Immunol. Rev. 227, 106–128.

Fu, B., et al., 2015. TRIM32 senses and restricts influenza A virus by ubiquitination of PB1 polymerase. PLoS Pathog. 11, 1–23.

Fujimoto, M., et al., 1997. Prevalence and clinical relevance of 52-kDa and 60-kDa Ro/ SS-A autoantibodies in Japanese patients with systemic sclerosis. Ann. Rheum. Dis. 56, 667–670.

Furr, S.R., Moerdyk-Schauwecker, M., Grdzelishvili, V.Z., Marriott, I., 2010. RIG-I mediates nonsegmented negative-sense RNA virus-induced inflammatory immune responses of primary human astrocytes. Glia 58, 1620–1629.

Gack, M.U., 2014. Mechanisms of RIG-I-like receptor activation and manipulation by viral pathogens. J. Virol. 88, 5213–5216.

Gack, M.U., et al., 2007. TRIM25 RING-finger E3 ubiquitin ligase is essential for RIG-I-mediated antiviral activity. Nature 446, 916–920.

Gallouet, A.-S., et al., 2017. Macrophage production and activation are dependent on TRIM33. Oncotarget 8, 5111–5122.

Ganser-Pornillos, B.K., et al., 2011. Hexagonal assembly of a restricting TRIM5 protein. Proc. Natl. Acad. Sci. U.S.A. 108, 534–539.

Gao, D., et al., 2014. Cyclic GMP-AMP synthase is an innate immune sensor of HIV and other retroviruses. Science 341, 903–906.

Geijtenbeek, T.B.H., Gringhuis, S.I., 2009. Signalling through C-type lectin receptors: shaping immune responses. Nat. Rev. Immunol. 9, 465–479.

Geijtenbeek, T.B., et al., 2000. DC-SIGN, a dendritic cell-specific HIV-1-binding protein that enhances trans-infection of T cells. Cell 100, 587–597.

Gitlin, L., et al., 2006. Essential role of mda-5 in type I IFN responses to polyriboinosinic: polyribocytidylic acid and encephalomyocarditis picornavirus. Proc. Natl. Acad. Sci. U.S.A. 103, 8459–8464.

Gough, D.J., Messina, N.L., Clarke, C.J.P., Johnstone, R.W., Levy, D.E., 2012. Constitutive type I interferon modulates homeostatic balance through tonic signaling. Immunity 36, 759–785.

Gray, E.E., et al., 2016. The AIM2-like receptors are dispensable for the interferon response to intracellular DNA. Immunity 45, 255–266.

Grütter, M.G., Luban, J., 2012. TRIM5 structure, HIV-1 capsid recognition, and innate immune signaling. Curr. Opin. Virol. 2, 142–150.

Guo, H., Callaway, J.B., Ting, J.P.-Y., 2015. Inflammasomes: mechanism of action, role in disease and therapeutics. Nat. Med. 21, 677–687.

Han, K., Lou, D.I., Sawyer, S.L., 2011. Identification of a genomic reservoir for new trim genes in primate genomes. PLoS Genet. 7 (12), e1002388.

Hashimoto, M., et al., 2006. Lipoprotein is a predominant toll-like receptor 2 ligand in staphylococcus aureus cell wall components. Int. Immunol. 18, 355–362.

Hauler, F., Mallery, D.L., McEwan, W.A., Bidgood, S.R., James, L.C., 2012. AAA ATPase p97/VCP is essential for TRIM21-mediated virus neutralization. Proc. Natl. Acad. Sci. U.S.A. 109, 19733–19738.

Hayashi, F., et al., 2001. The innate immune response to bacterial flagellin is mediated by Toll-like receptor 5. Nature 410, 1099–1103.

Heid, M.E., et al., 2013. Mitochondrial reactive oxygen species induces NLRP3-dependent lysosomal damage and inflammasome activation. J. Immunol. 191, 5230–5238.

Hemmi, H., et al., 2000. A toll-like receptor recognizes bacterial DNA. Nature 408, 740–745.

Higgs, R., Gabhann, J.N., Larbi, N.B., Breen, E.P., Fitzgerald, K.A., Jefferies, C.A., 2008. The E3 ubiquitin ligase Ro52 negatively regulates IFN-β production post-pathogen recognition by polyubiquitin-mediated degradation of IRF3. J. Immunol. 181, 1780–1786.

Higgs, R., et al., 2010. Self protection from anti-viral responses—Ro52 promotes degradation of the transcription factor IRF7 downstream of the viral toll-like receptors. PLoS One 5, 1–7.

Hornung, V., Latz, E., 2010. Critical functions of priming and lysosomal damage for NLRP3 activation. Eur. J. Immunol. 6, 620–623.

Hornung, V., et al., 2009. AIM2 recognizes cytosolic dsDNA and forms a caspase-1 activating inflammasome with ASC. Nature 458, 514–518.

Hornung, V., Hartmann, R., Ablasser, A., Hopfner, K.-P., 2014. OAS proteins and cGAS: unifying concepts in sensing and responding to cytosolic nucleic acids. Nat. Rev. Immunol. 14 (8), 521.

Hoving, J.C., Wilson, G.J., Brown, G.D., 2014. Signalling C-type lectin receptors, microbial recognition and immunity. Cell. Microbiol. 16, 185–194.

Hu, M.-M., Shu, H.-B., 2017. Multifaceted roles of TRIM38 in innate immune and inflammatory responses. Cell. Mol. Immunol. 14, 331–338.

Hu, Y., et al., 2010. Tripartite-motif protein 30 negatively regulates NLRP3 inflammasome activation by modulating reactive oxygen species production. J. Immunol. 185, 7699–7705.

Hu, M.-M., et al., 2014. TRIM38 inhibits TNFα- and IL-1β-triggered NF-κB activation by mediating lysosome-dependent degradation of TAB2/3. Proc. Natl. Acad. Sci. U.S.A. 111, 1509–1514.

Hu, M.-M., et al., 2015. TRIM38 negatively regulates TLR3/4-mediated innate immune and inflammatory responses by two sequential and distinct mechanisms. J. Immunol. 195, 4415–4425.

Hu, M.M., et al., 2016. Sumoylation promotes the stability of the DNA sensor cGAS and the adaptor STING to regulate the kinetics of response to DNA virus. Immunity 45, 555–569.

Huang, B., Baek, S., 2017. Trim13 potentiates toll-like receptor 2-mediated nuclear factor κB activation via K29-linked polyubiquitination of tumor necrosis factor receptor-associated factor 6. Mol. Pharmacol. 91, 307–316.

Huang, Y., et al., 2016a. Fish TRIM8 exerts antiviral roles through regulation of the proinflammatory factors and interferon signaling. Fish Shellfish Immunol. 54, 435–444.

Huang, Y., et al., 2016b. Grouper TRIM13 exerts negative regulation of antiviral immune response against nodavirus. Fish Shellfish Immunol. 55, 106–115.

Ichinohe, T., Lee, H.K., Ogura, Y., Flavell, R., Iwasaki, A., 2009. Inflammasome recognition of influenza virus is essential for adaptive immune responses. J. Exp. Med. 206, 79–87.

Ichinohe, T., Pang, I.K., Iwasaki, A., 2010. Influenza virus activates inflammasomes via its intracellular M2 ion channel. Nat. Immunol. 11, 404–410.

Iqbal, K., Liu, F., Gong, C.-X., 2015. Tau and neurodegenerative disease: the story so far. Nat. Rev. Neurol. 12, 15–27.

Ireton, R.C., Gale, M., 2011. RIG-I like receptors in antiviral immunity and therapeutic applications. Virus 3, 906–919.

James, L.C., Keeble, A.H., Khan, Z., Rhodes, D.a., Trowsdale, J., 2007. Structural basis for PRYSPRY-mediated tripartite motif (TRIM) protein function. Proc. Natl. Acad. Sci. U.S.A. 104, 6200–6205.

Jia, X., et al., 2017. The ubiquitin ligase RNF125 targets innate immune adaptor protein TRIM14 for ubiquitination and degradation. J. Immunol. 198, 1601322. https://doi.org/10.4049/jimmunol.1601322.

Jiang, X., et al., 2012. Ubiquitin-induced oligomerization of the RNA sensors RIG-I and MDA5 activates antiviral innate immune response. Immunity 36, 959–973.

Jiang, S., Li, X., Hess, N.J., Guan, Y., Tapping, R.I., 2016. TLR 10 is a negative regulator of both MyD88-dependent and -independent TLR signaling. J. Immunol. 196, 3834–3841.

Jønsson, K.L., et al., 2017. IFI16 is required for DNA sensing in human macrophages by promoting production and function of cGAMP. Nat. Commun. 8, 14391.

Kagan, J.C., Barton, G.M., 2014. Transduction by pattern-recognition receptors, Cold Spring Harb. Perspect. Biol. 1–16.

Kagan, J.C., Barton, G.M., 2016. Emerging principles governing signal transduction by pattern-recognition receptors. Cold Spring Harb. Perspect. Biol. 33, 395–401.

Kahle, T., et al., 2016. TRIM19/PML restricts HIV infection in a cell type-dependent manner. Virus 8, 1–18.

Kajaste-Rudnitski, A., et al., 2011. TRIM22 inhibits HIV-1 transcription independently of its E3 ubiquitin ligase activity, tat, and NF-κB-responsive long terminal repeat elements. J. Virol. 85, 5183–5196.

Kane, M., et al., 2016. Identification of interferon-stimulated genes with antiretroviral activity. Cell Host Microbe 20, 392–405.

Kang, J.Y., et al., 2009. Recognition of lipopeptide patterns by toll-like receptor 2-toll-like receptor 6 heterodimer. Immunity 31, 873–884.

Kanneganti, T.-D., 2010. Central roles of NLRs and inflammasomes in viral infection. Nat. Rev. Immunol. 10, 688–698.

Kawai, T., Akira, S., 2010. The role of pattern-recognition receptors in innate immunity: update on Toll-like receptors. Nat. Immunol. 11, 373–384.

Kawasaki, T., Kawai, T., 2014. Toll-like receptor signaling pathways. Front. Immunol. 5, 1–8.

Kayagaki, N., et al., 2013. Noncanonical inflammasome activation by intracellular lps independent of tlr4. Science 130, 1246–1249.

Keeble, A.H., Khan, Z., Forster, A., James, L.C., 2008. TRIM21 is an IgG receptor that is structurally, thermodynamically, and kinetically conserved. Proc. Natl. Acad. Sci. U.S.A. 105, 6045–6050.

Kell, A.M., Gale Jr., M., 2015. RIG-I in RNA virus recognition. Virology 479–480, 110–121. https://doi.org/10.1016/j.virol.2015.02.017.RIG-I.

Kim, Y.K., Shin, J.S., Nahm, M.H., 2016. NOD-like receptors in infection, immunity, and diseases. Yonsei Med. J. 57, 5–14.

Klasse, P.J., 2014. Review article neutralization of virus infectivity by antibodies: old problems in new perspectives. Adv. Biol. 2014. pii: 157895.

Koliopoulos, M.G., Esposito, D., Christodoulou, E., Taylor, I.A., Rittinger, K., 2016. Functional role of TRIM E 3 ligase oligomerization and regulation of catalytic activity. EMBO J. 35, 1–15.

Kondo, T., Watanabe, M., Hatakeyama, S., 2012. TRIM59 interacts with ECSIT and negatively regulates NF-κB and IRF-3/7-mediated signal pathways. Biochem. Biophys. Res. Commun. 422, 501–507.

Kong, H.J., et al., 2007. Cutting edge: autoantigen Ro52 is an interferon inducible E3 ligase that ubiquitinates IRF-8 and enhances cytokine expression in macrophages. J. Immunol. 179, 26–30.

Koshiba, T., 2013. Mitochondrial-mediated antiviral immunity. Biochim. Biophys. Acta 1833, 225–232.

Kowalinski, E., et al., 2011. Structural basis for the activation of innate immune pattern-recognition receptor RIG-I by viral RNA. Cell 147, 423–435.

Kranzusch, P.J., Lee, A.S., Berger, J.M., Jennifer, A., 2013. Structure of human cGAS reveals a conserved family of second-messenger enzymes in innate immunity. Cell Rep. 3, 1362–1368.

Krug, A., et al., 2004. TLR9-dependent recognition of MCMV by IPC and DC generates coordinated cytokine responses that activate antiviral NK cell function. Immunity 21, 107–119.

Kutluay, S.B., Perez-Caballero, D., Bieniasz, P.D., 2013. Fates of retroviral core components during unrestricted and TRIM5-restricted infection. PLoS Pathog. 9 (3), e1003214. https://doi.org/10.1371/journal.ppat.1003214.

Kwon, Y.-C., Kang, J.-I., Hwang, S.B., Ahn, B.-Y., 2013. The ribonuclease L-dependent antiviral roles of human 2',5'-oligoadenylate synthetase family members against hepatitis C virus. FEBS Lett. 587, 156–164.

Lam, E., Stein, S., Falck-Pedersen, E., 2014. Adenovirus detection by the cGAS/STING/TBK1 DNA sensing cascade. J. Virol. 88, 974–981.

Lamkanfi, M., Dixit, V.M., 2014. Review mechanisms and functions of inflammasomes. Cell 157, 1013–1022.

Lang, X., et al., 2016. TRIM65-catalized ubiquitination is essential for MDA5-mediated antiviral innate immunity. J. Exp. Med. 214, 459–473. https://doi.org/10.1084/jem.20160592.

Latsoudis, H., et al., 2017. Differential expression of miR-4520a associated with pyrin mutations in familial mediterranean fever (FMF). J. Cell. Physiol. 232, 1326–1336.

Latz, E., Xiao, T.S., Stutz, A., 2013. Activation and regulation of the inflammasomes. Nat. Rev. Immunol. 13, 397–411.

Laurent-Rolle, M., et al., 2014. The interferon signaling antagonist function of yellow fever virus NS5 protein is activated by type I interferon. Cell Host Microbe 16, 314–327.

Lawrence, T.M., Hudacek, A.W., de Zoete, M.R., Flavell, R.A., Schnell, M.J., 2013. Rabies virus is recognized by the NLRP3 inflammasome and activates interleukin-1 release in murine dendritic cells. J. Virol. 87, 5848–5857.

Lazear, H.M., Diamond, M.S., 2016. New insights into innate immune restriction of west nile virus infection. Curr. Opin. Virol. 1848, 3047–3054.

Lazzari, E., et al., 2014. TRIpartite motif 21 (TRIM21) differentially regulates the stability of interferon regulatory factor 5 (IRF5) isoforms. PLoS One 9, 1–10.

Lee, Y., Song, B., Park, C., Kwon, K.S., 2013. TRIM11 negatively regulates IFNβ production and antiviral activity by targeting TBK1. PLoS One 8, 1–12.

Lee, S.M.Y., et al., 2014. Toll-like receptor 10 is involved in induction of innate immune responses to influenza virus infection. Proc. Natl. Acad. Sci. U.S.A. 111, 3793–3798.

Lee, J., et al., 2015. TNF-α induced by hepatitis C virus via TLR7 and TLR8 in hepatocytes supports interferon signaling via an autocrine mechanism. PLoS Pathog. 11, 1–19.

Lester, S.N., Li, K., 2014. Toll-like receptors in antiviral innate immunity. J. Mol. Biol. 426, 1246–1264.

Li, J., et al., 2015. DDX19A senses viral RNA and mediates NLRP3-dependent inflammasome activation. J. Immunol. 195, 5732–5749.

Li, Y.L., et al., 2016. Primate TRIM5 proteins form hexagonal nets on HIV-1 capsids. eLife 5, 1–33.

Li, M.M.H., et al., 2017. TRIM25 enhances the antiviral action of zinc-finger antiviral protein (ZAP). PLoS Pathog. 13, 1–25.

Liang, Q., et al., 2011. Tripartite motif-containing protein 28 is a small ubiquitin-related modifier E3 ligase and negative regulator of IFN regulatory factor 7. J. Immunol. 187, 4754–4763.

Lin, R.J., et al., 2009. Distinct antiviral roles for human 2',5'-oligoadenylate synthetase family members against dengue virus infection. J. Immunol. 183, 8035–8043.

Liu, B., et al., 2014. Overlapping and distinct molecular determinants dictating the antiviral activities of TRIM56 against flaviviruses and coronavirus. J. Virol. 88, 13821–13835.

Liu, T., et al., 2016a. TRIM11 suppresses AIM2 inflammasome by degrading AIM2 via p62-dependent selective autophagy. Cell Rep. 16, 1988–2002.

Liu, B., et al., 2016b. The C-terminal tail of TRIM56 dictates antiviral restriction of influenza A and B viruses by impeding viral RNA synthesis. J. Virol. 90, 4369–4382.

Liu, Y., Olagnier, D., Lin, R., 2017a. Host and viral modulation of RIG-I-mediated antiviral immunity. Front. Immunol. 7, 1–12.

Liu, B., et al., 2017b. The ubiquitin E3 ligase TRIM31 promotes aggregation and activation of the signaling adaptor MAVS through Lys63-linked polyubiquitination. Nat. Immunol. 18, 214–224.

Loo, Y.-M., et al., 2008. Distinct RIG-I and MDA5 signaling by RNA viruses in innate immunity. J. Virol. 82, 335–345.

Lu, Y.C., Yeh, W.C., Ohashi, P.S., 2008. LPS/TLR4 signal transduction pathway. Cytokine 42, 145–151.

Luisoni, S., et al., 2015. Co-option of membrane wounding enables virus penetration into cells. Cell Host Microbe 18, 75–85.

Lukic, Z., et al., 2011. TRIM5α associates with proteasomal subunits in cells while in complex with HIV-1 virions. Retrovirology 8, 93.

Lund, J.M., et al., 2004. Recognition of single-stranded RNA viruses by Toll-like receptor 7. Proc. Natl. Acad. Sci. U.S.A. 101, 5598–5603.

Lusic, M., et al., 2013. Proximity to PML nuclear bodies regulates HIV-1 latency in CD4 + T cells. Cell Host Microbe 13, 665–677.

Maharaj, N.P., Wies, E., Stoll, A., Gack, M.U., 2012. Conventional protein kinase C-α (PKC-α) and PKC-β negatively regulate RIG-I antiviral signal transduction. J. Virol. 86, 1358–1371.

Mäkelä, S.M., et al., 2015. RIG-I signaling is essential for influenza B virus-induced rapid interferon gene expression. J. Virol. 89, 12014–12025.

Malathi, K., Dong, B., Gale, M.J., Silverman, R.H., 2007. Small self-RNA generated by RNase L amplifies antiviral innate immunity. Nature 448, 816–819.

Mallery, D.L., et al., 2010. Antibodies mediate intracellular immunity through tripartite motif-containing 21 (TRIM21). Proc. Natl. Acad. Sci. U.S.A. 107, 19985–19990.

Manukyan, G., Aminov, R., 2016. Update on pyrin functions and mechanisms of familial mediterranean fever. Front. Microbiol. 7, 1–8.

Marín, I., 2012. Origin and diversification of TRIM ubiquitin ligases. PLoS One 7 (11), e50030. https://doi.org/10.1371/journal.pone.0050030.

Masroori, N., Merindol, N., Berthoux, L., 2016. The interferon-induced antiviral protein PML (TRIM19) promotes the restriction and transcriptional silencing of lentiviruses in a context-specific, isoform-specific fashion. Retrovirology 13, 19.

Masters, S.L., et al., 2016. Familial autoinflammation with neutrophilic dermatosis reveals a regulatory mechanism of pyrin activation. Sci. Transl. Med. 8, 332ra45.

McCartney, S.A., et al., 2008. MDA-5 recognition of a murine norovirus. PLoS Pathog. 4, 1–7.

McEwan, W.A., et al., 2012. Regulation of virus neutralization and the persistent fraction by TRIM21. J. Virol. 86, 8482–8491.

McEwan, W.A., et al., 2013. Intracellular antibody-bound pathogens stimulate immune signaling via the Fc receptor TRIM21. Nat. Immunol. 14, 327–336.

McEwan, W.A., et al., 2017. Cytosolic Fc receptor TRIM21 inhibits seeded tau aggregation. Proc. Natl. Acad. Sci. U.S.A. 114, 201607215.

Metzger, M.B., Hristova, V.A., Weissman, A.M., 2012. HECT and RING finger families of E3 ubiquitin ligases at a glance. J. Cell Sci. 125, 531–537.

Minamitani, T., Iwakiri, D., Takada, K., 2011. Adenovirus virus-associated RNAs induce type I interferon expression through a RIG-I-mediated pathway. J. Virol. 85, 4035–4040.

Mitchell, A.M., Hirsch, M.L., Li, C., Samulski, R.J., 2014. Promyelocytic leukemia protein is a cell-intrinsic factor inhibiting parvovirus DNA replication. J. Virol. 88, 925–936.

Mitoma, H., et al., 2013. The DHX33 RNA helicase senses cytosolic RNA and activates the NLRP3 inflammasome. Immunity 39, 123–135.

Monteith, A.J., et al., 2016. Defects in lysosomal maturation facilitate the activation of innate sensors in systemic lupus erythematosus. Proc. Natl. Acad. Sci. U.S.A. 113, E2142–E2151.

Moore, C.B., et al., 2008. NLRX1 is a regulator of mitochondrial antiviral immunity. Nature 451, 573–577.

Muñoz-Planillo, R., Kuffa, P., Giovanny Martínez-Colón, B.L.S., Rajendiran, T.M., Núñez, G., 2013. K + efflux is the common trigger of NLRP3 inflammasome activation by bacterial toxins and particulate matter. Immunity 38, 1142–1153.

Murawski, M.R., et al., 2009. Respiratory syncytial virus activates innate immunity through Toll-like receptor 2. J. Virol. 83, 1492–1500.

Narayan, K., et al., 2014. TRIM13 is a negative regulator of MDA5-mediated type I interferon production. J. Virol. 88, 10748–10757.

Nenasheva, V.V., et al., 2015. Enhanced expression of trim14 gene suppressed Sindbis virus reproduction and modulated the transcription of a large number of genes of innate immunity. Immunol. Res. 62, 255–262.

Nisole, S., Stoye, J.P., Saïb, A., 2005. TRIM family proteins: retroviral restriction and antiviral defence. Nat. Rev. Microbiol. 3, 799–808.

Noguchi, K., et al., 2011. Trim40 promotes neddylation of IKKγ and is downregulated in gastrointestinal cancers. Carcinogenesis 32, 995–1004.

Odendall, C., Kagan, J.C., 2017. Activation and pathogenic manipulation of the sensors of the innate immune system. Microbes Infect. 19, 229–237. https://doi.org/10.1016/j.micinf.2017.01.003.

Oke, V., Wahren-Herlenius, M., 2012. The immunobiology of Ro52 (TRIM21) in autoimmunity: a critical review. J. Autoimmun. 39, 77–82.

Okumura, F., Matsunaga, Y., Katayama, Y., Nakayama, K.I., Hatakeyama, S., 2010. TRIM8 modulates STAT3 activity through negative regulation of PIAS3. J. Cell Sci. 123, 2238–2245.

Oliveira-Nascimento, L., Massari, P., Wetzler, L.M., 2012. The role of TLR2 in infection and immunity. Front. Immunol. 3, 1–17.

Oosting, M., et al., 2014. Human TLR10 is an anti-inflammatory pattern-recognition receptor. Proc. Natl. Acad. Sci. U.S.A. 111, E4478–E4484.

Osorio, F., Reis e Sousa, C., 2011. Myeloid C-type lectin receptors in pathogen recognition and host defense. Immunity 34, 651–664.

Ozato, K., Shin, D.-M., Chang, T.-H., Morse, H.C., 2008. TRIM family proteins and their emerging roles in innate immunity. Nat. Rev. Immunol. 8, 849–860.

Ozato, K., Shin, D., Chang, T., Morse, H., 2012. TRIM family proteins and their emerging roles in innate immunity. Nat. Rev. Immunol. 8, 849–860.

Paijo, J., et al., 2016. cGAS senses human cytomegalovirus and induces type I interferon responses in human monocyte-derived cells. PLoS Pathog. 12, 1–24.

Papon, L., et al., 2009. The viral RNA recognition sensor RIG-I is degraded during encephalomyocarditis virus (EMCV) infection. Virology 393, 311–318.

Park, Y.H., Wood, G., Kastner, D.L., Chae, J.J., 2016. Pyrin inflammasome activation and RhoA signaling in the autoinflammatory diseases FMF and HIDS. Nat. Immunol. 17, 914–921.

Parvatiyar, K., Cheng, G., 2011. NOD so fast: NLRX1 puts the brake on inflammation. Immunity 34, 821–822.

Peisley, A., Wu, B., Yao, H., Walz, T., Hur, S., 2013. RIG-I forms signaling-competent filaments in an ATP-dependent, ubiquitin-independent manner. Mol. Cell 51, 573–583.

Peisley, A., Wu, B., Xu, H., Chen, Z.J., Hur, S., 2014. Structural basis for ubiquitin-mediated antiviral signal activation by RIG-I. Nature 509, 110–114.

Pertel, T., et al., 2011. TRIM5 is an innate immune sensor for the retrovirus capsid lattice. Nature 472, 361–365.

Perwitasari, O., Cho, H., Diamond, M.S., Gale, M., 2011. Inhibitor of kB kinase ε (IKKε), STAT1, and IFIT2 proteins define novel innate immune effector pathway against West Nile virus infection. J. Biol. Chem. 286, 44412–44423.

Poole, E., et al., 2009. Identification of TRIM23 as a cofactor involved in the regulation of NF-kB by human cytomegalovirus. J. Virol. 83, 3581–3590.

Qin, Y., et al., 2016. TRIM9 short isoform preferentially promotes DNA and RNA virus-induced production of type I interferon by recruiting GSK3β to TBK1. Cell Res. 26, 613–628.

Rajan, J.V., Warren, S.E., Miao1, E.A., Aderem, A., 2010. Activation of the NLRP3 inflammasome by intracellular poly I:C. FEBS Lett. 584, 4627–4632.

Rajan, J.V., Rodriguez, D., Miao, E.A., Aderem, A., 2011. The NLRP3 inflammasome detects encephalomyocarditis virus and vesicular stomatitis virus infection. J. Virol. 85, 4167–4172.

Rajsbaum, R., Versteeg, G.A., Schmid, S., Maestre, A.M., Belicha-Villanueva, A., Martínez-Romero, C., Patel, J.R., Morrison, J., Pisanelli, G., Miorin, L., Laurent-Rolle, M., Moulton, H.M., Stein, D.A., Fernandez-Ses, A., Sastre, A.G., 2014. Unanchored K48-linked poly-ubiquitin synthesized by the E3-ubiquitin ligase TRIM6 stimulates the interferon-IKKε kinase mediated antiviral response. Immunity 40, 880–895.

Rallabhandi, P., et al., 2012. Respiratory syncytial virus fusion protein-induced toll-like receptor 4 (TLR4) signaling is inhibited by the TLR4 antagonists Rhodobacter sphaeroides lipopolysaccharide and eritoran (E5564) and requires direct interaction with MD-2. mBio 3 (4), e00218-12. https://doi.org/10.1128/mBio.00218-127.

Ran, Y., et al., 2016. Autoubiquitination of TRIM 26 links TBK 1 to NEMO in RLR-mediated innate antiviral immune response. J. Mol. Cell Biol. 8, 31–43.

Rasmussen, S.B., et al., 2009. Herpes simplex virus infection is sensed by both toll-like receptors and RIG-like receptors, which synergize to induce type I interferon production. J. Gen. Virol. 90, 74–78.

Rathinam, V.A.K., et al., 2010. The AIM2 inflammasome is essential for host defense against cytosolic bacteria and DNA viruses. Nat. Immunol. 11, 395–402.

Ratsimandresy, R.A., Dorfleutner, A., Stehlik, C., 2013. An update on PYRIN domain-containing pattern recognition receptors: from immunity to pathology. Front. Immunol. 4, 1–20.

Rehwinkel, J., et al., 2010. RIG-I detects viral genomic RNA during negative-strand RNA virus infection. Cell 140, 397–408.

Reinert, L.S., et al., 2016. Sensing of HSV-1 by the cGAS-STING pathway in microglia orchestrates antiviral defence in the CNS. Nat. Commun. 7, 13348.

Richards, N., et al., 2001. Interaction between pyrin and the apoptotic speck protein (ASC) modulates ASC-induced apoptosis. J. Biol. Chem. 276, 39320–39329.

Roa, A., et al., 2012. RING domain mutations uncouple TRIM5 restriction of HIV-1 from inhibition of reverse transcription and acceleration of uncoating. J. Virol. 86, 1717–1727.

Rogozin, I.B., Aravind, L., Koonin, E.V., 2003. Differential action of natural selection on the N and C-terminal domains of 2'-5' oligoadenylate synthetases and the potential nuclease function of the C-terminal domain. J. Mol. Biol. 326, 1449–1461.

Rold, C.J., Aiken, C., 2008. Proteasomal degradation of TRIM5α during retrovirus restriction. PLoS Pathog. 4 (5), e1000074. https://doi.org/10.1371/journal.ppat.1000074.

Roopenian, D.C., Akilesh, S., 2007. FcRn: the neonatal Fc receptor comes of age. Nat. Rev. Immunol. 7, 715–725.

Sabbah, A., et al., 2009. Activation of innate immune antiviral responses by Nod2. Nat. Immunol. 10, 1073–1080.

Saito, T., Owen, D.M., Jiang, F., Marcotrigiano, J., Gale Jr., M., 2008. Innate immunity induced by composition-dependent RIG-I recognition of hepatitis C virus RNA. Nature 454, 523–527.

Saitoh, T., et al., 2006. Negative regulation of interferon-regulatory factor 3-dependent innate antiviral response by the prolyl isomerase Pin1. Nat. Immunol. 7, 598–605.

Sanchez, J.G., et al., 2016. Mechanism of TRIM25 catalytic activation in the antiviral RIG-I pathway. Cell Rep. 16, 1315–1325.

Sancho, D., Reis e Sousa, C., 2012. Signaling by myeloid C-type lectin receptors in immunity and homeostasis. Annu. Rev. Immunol. 30, 491–529.

Sayah, D.M., Sokolskaja, E., Berthoux, L., Luban, J., 2004. Cyclophilin A retrotransposition into TRIM5 explains owl monkey resistance to HIV-1. Nature 430, 569–573.

Schenk, M., Belisle, J.T., Modlin, R.L., 2009. TLR2 looks at lipoproteins. Immunity 31, 847–849.

Schilling, E.-M., Scherer, M., Reuter, N., Schweininger, J., Muller, Y.A., Stamminger, T., 2017. The human cytomegalovirus IE1 protein antagonizes PML nuclear body-mediated intrinsic immunity via the inhibition of PML de novo SUMOylation. J. Virol. 91, 1–17.

Schlee, M., 2013. Master sensors of pathogenic RNA-RIG-I like receptors. Immunobiology 218, 1322–1335.

Schoggins, J.W., et al., 2014. Pan-viral specificity of IFN-induced genes reveals new roles for cGAS in innate immunity. Nature 505, 691–695.

Shen, Y., et al., 2012. TRIM56 is an essential component of the TLR3 antiviral signaling pathway. J. Biol. Chem. 287, 36404–36413.

Shi, M., et al., 2008. TRIM30α negatively regulates TLR-mediated NF-κB activation by targeting TAB2 and TAB3 for degradation. Nat. Immunol. 9, 369–377.

Shibata, M., Sato, T., Nukiwa, R., Ariga, T., Hatakeyama, S., 2012. TRIM45 negatively regulates NF-kB-mediated transcription and suppresses cell proliferation. Biochem. Biophys. Res. Commun. 423, 104–109.

Shimizu, A., et al., 2014. Characterisation of cytoplasmic DNA complementary to non-retroviral RNA viruses in human cells. Sci. Rep. 4, 1–9.

Singh, R., et al., 2011. Association of TRIM22 with the type 1 interferon response and viral control during primary HIV-1 infection. J. Virol. 85, 208–216.

Song, H., et al., 2016. The E3 ubiquitin ligase TRIM31 attenuates NLRP3 inflammasome activation by promoting proteasomal degradation of NLRP3. Nat. Commun. 7, 13727.

Stapleton, N.M., et al., 2011. Competition for FcRn-mediated transport gives rise to short half-life of human IgG3 and offers therapeutic potential. Nat. Commun. 2, 599.

Stein, S.C., Falck-Pedersen, E., 2012. Sensing adenovirus infection: activation of interferon regulatory factor 3 in RAW 264.7 cells. J. Virol. 86, 4527–4537.

Stremlau, M., et al., 2004. The cytoplasmic body component TRIM5alpha restricts HIV-1 infection in Old World monkeys. Nature 427, 848–853.

Stremlau, M., et al., 2006. Specific recognition and accelerated uncoating of retroviral capsids by the TRIM5 restriction factor. Proc. Natl. Acad. Sci. U.S.A. 103, 5514–5519.

Sun, Z., Ren, H., Liu, Y., Teeling, J.L., Gu, J., 2011. Phosphorylation of RIG-I by casein kinase II inhibits its antiviral response. J. Virol. 85, 1036–1047.

Sun, L., Wu, J., Du, F., Chen, X., Chen, Z.J., 2013. Cyclic GMP-AMP synthase is a cytosolic DNA sensor that activates the type-I interferon pathway. Science 257, 2432–2437.

Sun, X., et al., 2016. A hierarchical mechanism of RIG-I ubiquitination provides sensitivity, robustness and synergy in antiviral immune responses. Sci. Rep. 6, 29263.

Tabah, A.A., Tardif, K., Mansky, L.M., 2014. Anti-HIV-1 activity of trim 37. J. Gen. Virol. 95, 960–967.

Takeda, K., Akira, S., 2005. Toll-like receptors in innate immunity. Int. Immunol. 17, 1–14.

Tassaneetrithep, B., et al., 2003. DC-SIGN (CD209) mediates dengue virus infection of human dendritic cells. J. Exp. Med. 197, 823–829.

Tatematsu, M., Nishikawa, F., Seya, T., Matsumoto, M., 2013. Toll-like receptor 3 recognizes incomplete stem structures in single-stranded viral RNA. Nat. Commun. 4, 1833.

Tatematsu, M., Seya, T., Matsumoto, M., 2014. Beyond dsRNA: toll-like receptor 3 signalling in RNA-induced immune responses. Biochem. J. 458, 195–201.

Taylor, R.T., et al., 2012. TRIM79α, an interferon-stimulated gene product, restricts tickborne encephalitis virus replication by degrading the viral RNA polymerase. Cell Host Microbe 10, 185–196.

Thompson, M.R., Kaminski, J.J., Kurt-Jones, E.A., Fitzgerald, K.A., 2011. Pattern recognition receptors and the innate immune response to viral infection. Virus 3, 920–940.

Tomar, D., Singh, R., 2014. TRIM13 regulates ubiquitination and turnover of NEMO to suppress TNF induced NF-κB activation. Cell. Signal. 26, 2606–2613.

Triantafilou, K., et al., 2005. Human cardiac inflammatory responses triggered by coxsackie B viruses are mainly toll-like receptor (TLR) 8-dependent. Cell. Microbiol. 7, 1117–1126.

Tsuchida, T., et al., 2010. The ubiquitin ligase TRIM56 regulates innate immune responses to intracellular double-stranded DNA. Immunity 33, 765–776.

Turelli, P., et al., 2001. Cytoplasmic recruitment of INI1 and PML on incoming HIV preintegration complexes: interference with early steps of viral replication. Mol. Cell 7, 1245–1254.

Turrini, F., et al., 2015. HIV-1 transcriptional silencing caused by TRIM22 inhibition of Sp1 binding to the viral promoter. Retrovirology 12, 104.

Uchil, P.D., Quinlan, B.D., Chan, W.T., Luna, J.M., Mothes, W., 2008. TRIM E3 ligases interfere with early and late stages of the retroviral life cycle. PLoS Pathog. 4 (2), e16. https://doi.org/10.1371/journal.ppat.0040016.

Uchil, P.D., et al., 2013. TRIM protein-mediated regulation of inflammatory and innate immune signaling and its association with antiretroviral activity. J. Virol. 87, 257–272.

Unterholzner, L., et al., 2010. IFI16 is an innate immune sensor for intracellular DNA. Nat. Immunol. 11, 997–1004.

Vajjhala, P.R., et al., 2014. Identification of multifaceted binding modes for pyrin and ASC pyrin domains gives insights into pyrin inflammasome assembly. J. Biol. Chem. 289, 23504–23519.

Vance, R.E., 2016. Cytosolic DNA sensing: the field narrows. Immunity 45, 227–228.

Vaysburd, M., et al., 2013. Intracellular antibody receptor TRIM21 prevents fatal viral infection. Proc. Natl. Acad. Sci. U.S.A. 110, 12397–12401.

Villano, J.S., Rong, F., Cooper, T.K., 2014. Bacterial infections in Myd88-deficient mice. Comp. Med. 64, 110–114.

Wagenknecht, N., et al., 2015. Contribution of the major ND10 proteins PML, hDaxx and sp100 to the regulation of human cytomegalovirus latency and lytic replication in the monocytic cell line THP-1. Virus 7, 2884–2907.

Wagner, J.M., et al., 2016. Mechanism of B-box 2 domain-mediated higher-order assembly of the retroviral restriction factor TRIM5α. eLife 5, 1–26.

Wang, C.H., et al., 2011a. TLR7 and TLR8 gene variations and susceptibility to hepatitis C virus infection. PLoS One 6, 6–13.

Wang, J., et al., 2011b. TRIM56 is a virus- and interferon-inducible E3 ubiquitin ligase that restricts pestivirus infection. J. Virol. 85, 3733–3745.

Wang, X., et al., 2014. RNA viruses promote activation of the NLRP3 inflammasome through a RIP1-RIP3-DRP1 signaling pathway. Nat. Immunol. 15, 1126–1133.

Wang, P., Zhao, W., Zhao, K., Zhang, L., Gao, C., 2015a. TRIM26 negatively regulates interferon beta production and antiviral response through polyubiquitination and degradation of nuclear IRF3. PLoS Pathog. 11, e1004726.

Wang, Y., et al., 2015b. TRIM35 negatively regulates TLR7- and TLR9-mediated type I interferon production by targeting IRF7. FEBS Lett. 589, 1322–1330.

Wang, S., et al., 2016. TRIM14 inhibits hepatitis C virus infection by SPRY domain-dependent targeted degradation of the viral NS5A protein. Sci. Rep. 6, 32336.

Watkinson, R.E., Tam, J.C., Vaysburd, M.J., James, L.C., 2013. Simultaneous neutralization and innate immune detection of a replicating virus by TRIM21. J. Virol. 87, 7309–7313.

Watkinson, R.E., McEwan, W.A., Tam, J.C.H., Vaysburd, M., James, L.C., 2015. TRIM21 promotes cGAS and RIG-I sensing of viral genomes during infection by antibody-opsonized virus. PLoS Pathog. 11 (10), e1005253. https://doi.org/10.1371/journal.ppat.1005253.

Weng, L., et al., 2014. The E3 ubiquitin ligase tripartite motif 33 is essential for cytosolic RNA-induced NLRP3 inflammasome activation. J. Immunol. 193, 3676–3682.

Wies, E., Wang, M.K., Maharaj, N.P., Chen, K., Shenghua Zhou, R., Finberg, W., Gack, M.U., 2013. Dephosphorylation of the RNA sensors RIG-I and MDA5 by the phosphatase PP1 is essential for innate immune signaling. Immunity 38, 437–449.

Wilson, S.J., et al., 2008. Independent evolution of an antiviral TRIMCyp in rhesus macaques. Proc. Natl. Acad. Sci. U.S.A. 105, 3557–3562.

Wolf, D., Goff, S.P., 2007. TRIM28 mediates primer binding site-targeted silencing of murine leukemia virus in embryonic cells. Cell 131, 46–57.

Wu, X., Anderson, J.L., Campbell, E.M., Joseph, A.M., Hope, T.J., 2006. Proteasome inhibitors uncouple rhesus TRIM5alpha restriction of HIV-1 reverse transcription and infection. Proc. Natl. Acad. Sci. U.S.A. 103, 7465–7470.

Wu, B., et al., 2013a. Structural basis for dsRNA recognition, filament formation, and antiviral signal activation by MDA5. Cell 152, 276–289.

Wu, J., Sun, L., Chen, X., Du, F., Shi, H., Chen, C., Chen, Z.J., 2013b. Cyclic-GMP-AMP is an endogenous second messenger in innate immune signaling by cytosolic DNA. Science 339, 826–830.

Wynne, C., et al., 2014. TRIM68 negatively regulates IFN beta production by degrading TRK fused gene, a novel driver of IFN beta downstream of anti-viral detection systems. PLoS One 9 (7), e101503.

Xia, X., Cui, J., Wang, H.Y., Liang, Z., Matsueda, S., Wang, Q., Yang, X., Hong, J., Songyang, Z., Chen, Z.J., Wang, R.-F., 2011. NLRX1 negatively regulates TLR-induced NF-κB signaling by targeting. Immunity 34, 843–853.

Xing, J., et al., 2016. Identification of a role for TRIM29 in the control of innate immunity in the respiratory tract. Nat. Immunol. 17, 1373–1380.

Xu, H., et al., 2014. Innate immune sensing of bacterial modifications of Rho GTPases by the Pyrin inflammasome. Nature 513, 237–241.

Xue, Q., et al., 2012. TRIM38 negatively regulates TLR3-mediated IFN-β signaling by targeting TRIF for degradation. PLoS One 7 (10), e46825.

Yan, J., Li, Q., Mao, A., Hu, M., Shu, H., 2014. TRIM 4 modulates type I interferon induction and cellular antiviral response by targeting RIG-I for K 63-linked ubiquitination. J. Mol. Cell Biol. 6, 154–163.

Yang, K., et al., 2009. TRIM21 is essential to sustain IFN regulatory factor 3 activation during antiviral response. J. Immunol. 182, 3782–3792.

Yang, B., et al., 2013. Novel function of Trim44 promotes an antiviral response by stabilizing VISA. J. Immunol. 190, 3613–3619.

Yang, C., et al., 2016. Interferon alpha (IFNα)-induced TRIM22 interrupts HCV replication by ubiquitinating NS5A. Cell. Mol. Immunol. 13, 94–102.

Yap, M.W., Nisole, S., Lynch, C., Stoye, J.P., 2004. Trim5alpha protein restricts both HIV-1 and murine leukemia virus. Proc. Natl. Acad. Sci. U.S.A. 101, 10786–10791.

Yoshimi, R., et al., 2010. Gene disruption study reveals a non-redundant role for TRIM21/Ro52 in NF-κB-dependent cytokine expression in fibroblasts. J. Immunol. 182, 7527–7538.

Yu, J.-W., et al., 2006. Cryopyrin and pyrin activate caspase-1, but not NF-κB, via ASC oligomerization. Cell Death Differ. 13, 236–249.

Yuan, T., Yao, W., Huang, F., Sun, B., Yang, R., 2014. The human antiviral factor TRIM11 is under the regulation of HIV-1 Vpr. PLoS One 9 (8), e104269. https://doi.org/10.1371/journal.pone.0104269.

Yuan, T., Yao, W., Tokunaga, K., Yang, R., Sun, B., 2016. An HIV-1 capsid binding protein TRIM11 accelerates viral uncoating. Retrovirology 13, 72.

Zeng, W., et al., 2010. Reconstitution of the RIG-I pathway reveals a signaling role of unanchored polyubiquitin chains in innate immunity. Cell 141, 315–330.

Zhang, Z., et al., 2012a. The E3 ubiquitin ligase TRIM21 negatively regulates the innate immune response to intracellular double-stranded DNA. Nat. Immunol. 14, 172–178.

Zhang, J., Hu, M.M., Wang, Y.Y., Shu, H.B., 2012b. TRIM32 protein modulates type I interferon induction and cellular antiviral response by targeting MITA/STING protein for K63-linked ubiquitination. J. Biol. Chem. 287, 28646–28655.

Zhang, S., Guo, J.T., Wu, J.Z., Yang, G., 2013. Identification and characterization of multiple TRIM proteins that inhibit hepatitis B virus transcription. PLoS One 8 (8), e70001. https://doi.org/10.1371/journal.pone.0070001.

Zhao, Y., Shao, F., 2015. The NAIP-NLRC4 inflammasome in innate immune detection of bacterial flagellin and type III secretion apparatus. Immunol. Rev. 265, 85–102.

Zhao, Y., et al., 2011. The NLRC4 inflammasome receptors for bacterial flagellin and type III secretion apparatus. Nature 477, 596–600.

Zhao, W., Wang, L., Zhang, M., Yuan, C., Gao, C., 2012a. E3 ubiquitin ligase tripartite motif 38 negatively regulates TLR-mediated immune responses by proteasomal degradation of TNF receptor-associated factor 6 in macrophages. J. Immunol. 188, 2567–2574.

Zhao, W., et al., 2012b. Tripartite motif-containing protein 38 negatively regulates TLR3/4- and RIG-I-mediated IFN- production and antiviral response by targeting NAP1. J. Immunol. 188, 5311–5318.

Zheng, X., et al., 2017. TRIM25 is required for the antiviral activity of zinc-finger antiviral protein (ZAP). J. Virol. 91, JVI.00088–17.

Zhou, Z., et al., 2014. TRIM14 is a mitochondrial adaptor that facilitates retinoic acid-inducible gene-I-like receptor-mediated innate immune response. Proc. Natl. Acad. Sci. U.S.A. 111, E245–E254.

Zhu, J., Huang, X., Yang, Y., 2007. Innate immune response to adenoviral vectors is mediated by both toll-like receptor-dependent and -independent pathways. J. Virol. 81, 3170–3180.

Zhu, J., Zhang, Y., Ghosh, A., Cuevas, R.A., Forero, A., Dhar, J., Ibsen, M.S., Schmid-Burgk, J.L., Schmidt, T., Ganapathiraju, M.K., Fujita, T., Hartmann, R., Barik, S., Hornung, V., Coyne, C.B., Sarkar, S.N., 2014. Antiviral activity of human oligoadenylate synthetases-like (OASL) is mediated by enhancing retinoic acid-inducible gene I (RIG-I) signaling. Immunity 40, 936–948.

Zhu, J., Ghosh, A., Sarkar, S.N., 2015. OASL—a new player in controlling antiviral innate immunity. Curr. Opin. Virol. 12, 15–19.

Zurek, B., et al., 2012. TRIM27 negatively regulates NOD2 by ubiquitination and proteasomal degradation. PLoS One 7 (7), e41255. https://doi.org/10.1371/journal.pone.0041255.

CHAPTER FOURTEEN

How Does Vaccinia Virus Interfere With Interferon?

Geoffrey L. Smith[1], Callum Talbot-Cooper, Yongxu Lu
University of Cambridge, Cambridge, United Kingdom
[1]Corresponding author: e-mail address: gls37@cam.ac.uk

Contents

Abstract

Interferons (IFNs) are secreted glycoproteins that are produced by cells in response to virus infection and other stimuli and induce an antiviral state in cells bearing IFN receptors. In this way, IFNs restrict virus replication and spread before an adaptive immune response is developed. Viruses are very sensitive to the effects of IFNs and consequently have evolved many strategies to interfere with interferon. This is particularly well illustrated by poxviruses, which have large dsDNA genomes and encode hundreds of proteins. Vaccinia virus is the prototypic poxvirus and expresses many proteins that interfere with IFN and are considered in this review. These proteins act either inside or outside the cell and within the cytoplasm or nucleus. They function by restricting the production of IFN by blocking the signaling pathways leading to transcription of IFN genes, stopping IFNs binding to their receptors, blocking IFN-induced signal transduction leading to expression of interferon-stimulated genes (ISGs), or inhibiting the antiviral activity of ISG products.

Advances in Virus Research, Volume 100
ISSN 0065-3527
https://doi.org/10.1016/bs.aivir.2018.01.003

355

1. INTRODUCTION TO VACCINIA VIRUS

Vaccinia virus (VACV) is the only vaccine to have eradicated a human disease, smallpox, yet its origin and natural host are unknown (Baxby, 1981). VACV is the prototypic member of the *Orthopoxvirus* genus of the *Poxviridae*, a family of large and complex viruses with big double-stranded (ds)DNA genomes that replicate in the cytoplasm of infected cells (Moss, 2007). Cytoplasmic replication is unusual for DNA viruses and poses challenges because the nuclear enzymes required for transcription and replication of DNA are not available and so poxviruses encode their own. Additionally, cytoplasmic replication of DNA creates an easily recognizable pathogen-associated molecular pattern (PAMP) that can be detected by cytosolic pattern-recognition receptors (PRRs), leading to activation of innate immunity. To combat this, poxviruses encode many proteins that suppress activation of innate immune signaling pathways such as those leading to expression of interferon (IFN).

1.1 Origin of Vaccinia Virus

VACV was the vaccine used to eradicate smallpox but is distinct from cowpox virus (CPXV) the vaccine thought to have been used by Jenner in 1796 when he introduced vaccination against smallpox with a virus taken from the hand of a milkmaid. The distinction between CPXV and the 20th century smallpox vaccines was recognized in 1939 (Downie, 1939). Subsequently, it was suggested that the current smallpox vaccines might be derived from an orthopoxvirus that infects horses (horsepox virus, HSPV) (Baxby, 1981), and this is supported by: (i) reports that early vaccinators, including Jenner, obtained smallpox vaccine from horses when cowpox was scare; (ii) sequence comparisons of VACV with a virus isolated from a horse in Mongolia that show a closer relationship than with other orthopoxviruses (Tulman et al., 2006); (iii) the observation that the IFNγ receptor encoded by VACV can bind and inhibit equine IFNγ (Symons et al., 2002); and (iv) the recent finding that a strain of smallpox vaccine from 1902 is most closely related to HSPV (Schrick et al., 2017). VACV, CPXV, and HSPV share considerable immunological cross-reactivity with each other and with other orthopoxviruses including variola virus (VARV), the cause of smallpox; monkeypox virus (MPXV); camelpox virus; and ectromelia virus, the cause of mousepox. This immunological cross-reactivity is the basis for the protection that infection with members of this genus provides against subsequent infection by other members of this genus. Thus both VACV and CPXV were effective at preventing smallpox.

If Jenner used CPXV in 1796 and all the smallpox vaccines in use in 1939 were VACV, then sometime between 1796 and 1939 VACV replaced CPXV as the smallpox vaccine. It is uncertain when this happened, but there are anecdotes suggesting this occurred early in the 19th century. First, Jenner and other early vaccinators were reported to have used virus taken from horses (called the grease) when the supply of CPXV was limiting. Second, the smallpox vaccine taken from England to the United States in the 1850s and which became the New York City Board of Health vaccine is VACV not CPXV. Third, pathologists who examined cells infected by the smallpox vaccine in the late 19th century described the eosinophilic cytoplasmic inclusion bodies made by both VACV and CPXV, but failed to mention the more obvious A-type inclusion bodies that are formed by CPXV but not VACV. Fourth, the genome sequence of a smallpox vaccine from 1902 shows this virus is very similar to the virus isolated from a horse in Mongolia (Schrick et al., 2017). Collectively, these observations are consistent with VACV being the smallpox vaccine by the first half of the 19th century.

1.2 Vaccinia Virus Replication Cycle

VACV has a complex replication cycle and each infected cell produces multiple forms of infectious progeny that differ in their surface proteins, the number of membranes surrounding the core, and their immunological and biological properties (Appleyard et al., 1971). There are two infectious forms of VACV called intracellular mature virus (IMV) and extracellular enveloped virus (EEV) that are surrounded by one or two membranes, respectively (Hollinshead et al., 1999). Entry into a new cell therefore presents these virions with differing challenges (Vanderplasschen et al., 1998). The IMV form with a single envelope can enter the cytosol by fusion of its envelope with either the plasma membrane or the membrane of an intracellular vesicle after the virion is taken up by endocytosis or macropinocytosis (Carter et al., 2005; Mercer and Helenius, 2008; Townsley et al., 2006), and there is evidence that different strains of VACV may use these different pathways preferentially (Bengali et al., 2009). Fusion is driven by a complex of 10 virus proteins on the IMV surface, which are all essential for fusion (Moss, 2016; Senkevich et al., 2005). This is quite different from the fusion machinery of many other enveloped viruses such as influenza virus or human immunodeficiency virus that consists of a single protein that is cleaved into two subunits and is sufficient for fusion. Entry of EEV presents a topological challenge because fusion of the outer membrane of EEV with the plasma membrane or intracellular vesicle would release an IMV surrounded by its single membrane into the cytosol. However, both virus membranes must be shed for replication to commence. To shed the EEV outer membrane VACV has evolved an unusual nonfusogenic mechanism that involves rupture of the outer membrane at the site of contact between the virus and cell, thereby exposing the IMV membrane that can then fuse as described above (Law et al., 2006). The nonfusogenic dissolution requires negatively charged molecules, such as glycosaminoglycans, on the cell surface and the B5 protein on the EEV surface (Roberts et al., 2009).

After entry, the naked virus core is transported on microtubules deeper into the cell (Carter et al., 2003), where it is uncoated and replication starts forming a virus factory. Within this cytoplasmic replication site the three classes of virus genes (early, intermediate, and late) are expressed in a temporal cascade (Broyles, 2003). DNA replication is a trigger for late gene expression and thereafter virus proteins and genomes assemble to form new virions via distinct morphogenic stages (Morgan et al., 1954). IMV represent the majority of infectious progeny. Most IMV remain within the cell until cell lysis and spread slowly from cell to cell. However, some IMV are transported away from factories on microtubules (Sanderson et al., 2000; Ward, 2005) to sites where they are wrapped by a double membrane derived from early endosomes (Tooze et al., 1993) or the trans-Golgi network (Schmelz et al., 1994) to form a triple-enveloped virus called intracellular enveloped virus (IEV), or wrapped virus. This virion is then transported by kinesin-1 on microtubules (Geada et al., 2001; Hollinshead et al., 2001; Rietdorf et al., 2001; Ward and Moss, 2001) to the cell periphery where the outer membrane fuses with the plasma membrane to expose a double-enveloped virus on the cell surface. If the virion remains on the cell surface, it is called cell-associated enveloped virus (CEV), and if it is released, it is called EEV. EEV mediate long-range virus spread, whereas CEV induce the polymerization of actin beneath the plasma membrane where the virion sits (Cudmore et al., 1995), and this growing actin tail propels the virus away to find new cells to infect. Actin tails are also induced upon superinfection of an infected cell by CEV/EEV that bind to the A33/A36 protein complex on the cell surface and repel superinfecting virions to find uninfected cells (Doceul et al., 2010, 2012).

1.3 Vaccinia Virus Genes

VACV strain Copenhagen was the first poxvirus genome sequenced and is 191 kb (Goebel et al., 1990). VACV genes are organized with those essential for virus replication in the central region of the genome and those nonessential and more variable present near each terminus (Gubser et al., 2004; Upton et al., 2003). It is estimated that approximately half the VACV genes are nonessential for virus replication in cell culture. Many of them encode proteins that affect host range, virulence, or immune evasion. The latter group of genes and specifically those that encode proteins that interfere with IFN are the subject of this chapter.

2. INTERFERONS

Interferons (IFNs) are a group of soluble glycoproteins that are produced and released from cells in response to virus infection (and other stimuli). They bind to specific IFN receptors on cells to trigger signaling pathways that result in the expression of IFN-stimulated genes (ISGs). The ISG products render the cell resistant to subsequent virus infection. Isaacs and Lindenmann are often cited as discovering IFN while working with influenza virus (Isaacs and Lindenmann, 1957; Isaacs et al., 1957), but a few years earlier Japanese scientists working with VACV reported that infection of rabbit skin with ultraviolet light-inactivated VACV induced production of a "facteur inhibiteur" (inhibitory factor) that prevented subsequent virus infection (Nagano and Kojima, 1954; Nagano et al., 1954).

IFNs are categorized into three distinct classes known as type I, type II, and type III IFNs (Pestka et al., 1987, 2004; Platanias, 2005). In humans, the type I IFN family consists of IFNα, IFNβ, IFNε, IFNκ, and IFNω, all of which share a high degree of structural similarity (Platanias, 2005). By contrast, IFNγ constitutes the sole member of the type II IFN family, and is structurally distinct from the type I IFNs (Farrar and Schreiber, 1993). The type III IFNs are the most recently discovered class of IFNs and include IFNλ1, IFNλ2, IFNλ3, and IFNλ4 (Kotenko et al., 2003; Prokunina-Olsson et al., 2013; Sheppard et al., 2003). It should be noted the while IFNλ1, IFNλ2, and IFNλ3 are also referred to as IL-29, IL-28A, and IL-28B, respectively, the IFNλ nomenclature was favored and is now accepted (Fox et al., 2009).

2.1 Induction of IFNβ Expression

The expression of type I IFNs (mainly IFNβ) is induced rapidly after the sensing of virus infection by PRRs engaging their cognate PAMPs. This activates the IFN regulatory factor 3 (IRF3) pathway (Fig. 1), leading to transcription from the IFNβ gene. PRRs that can trigger the activation of IRF3 include TLR3, TLR4, RIG-I, MDA5, and multiple DNA sensing proteins. These PRRs activate different signaling pathways that ultimately converge at the TANK binding kinase (TBK1) and IκB kinase-ε (IKKε) (Fitzgerald et al., 2003). These kinases, in association with adapter proteins TANK (Pomerantz and Baltimore, 1999), nuclear factor kappa B (NF-κB)-activating kinase-associated protein 1 (NAP1) (Fujita et al., 2003), similar to

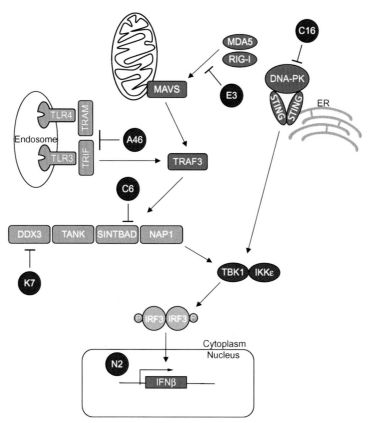

Fig. 1 Diagram showing a simplified version of the pathway leading to activation of the transcription factor IRF3. IRF3 together with the NF-κB and AP-1 forms the enhanceosome that drives transcription of the IFNβ gene. *Red circles* depict individual VACV proteins that inhibit activation of this pathway.

NAP1 TBK1 adaptor SINTBAD (Ryzhakov and Randow, 2007), and DEAD box protein 3 (DDX3) (Soulat et al., 2008), cause phosphorylation of IRF3.

In addition to IRF3 phosphorylation, IRF7 can also be phosphorylated by the same pathway. Unlike IRF3, which is expressed in a ubiquitous manner, expression of IRF7 is relatively low in unstimulated cells, but activation of the pathway leads to an upregulation of IRF7 expression, thereby inducing a positive feedback loop (Honda et al., 2005; Sato et al., 2000). Phosphorylation of IRF3/7 leads to the formation of homo/heterodimers that are translocated into the nucleus.

In addition to the activation of IRF3/7, PRR-induced signaling activates the NF-κB pathway and the mitogen-activated protein kinase (MAPK) pathway, and causes translocation of transcription factors NF-κB and AP-1 into the nucleus. Within the nucleus, these three transcription factors associate to form a complex known as the enhanceosome, driving the transcription of the IFNβ gene (Maniatis et al., 1998; Thanos and Maniatis, 1995).

2.2 IFN-Induced Signaling

After transcription of IFN genes, IFN mRNAs are translated in the cytoplasm and IFNs are secreted from the cell. To exert their effects, IFNs bind to transmembrane, cell surface IFN receptors (IFNRs). The three classes of IFNs bind to distinct IFNRs known as the IFNα/β receptor (IFNAR), the IFNγ receptor (IFNGR), and the IFNλ receptor (IFNLR) (de Weerd and Nguyen, 2012). These receptors can be further divided into two distinct components: IFNAR1 and IFNAR2, IFNGR1 and IFNGR2, and IFNLR1 and IL-10R2 (Fig. 2).

IFNAR and IFNGR are expressed on most cell types, and therefore, both type I and type II IFNs exert their effects in a ubiquitous manner (de Weerd and Nguyen, 2012). In contrast, IFNLR has a far more limited distribution and is expressed predominantly on mucosal epithelial cells (Muir et al., 2010). Type III IFNs therefore promote an increased antiviral state in epithelial tissues vulnerable to frequent and recurrent viral infection, while limiting the risk of systemic inflammation associated with the other IFNs (Wack et al., 2015).

Engagement of IFNs with their cognate receptors induces a signaling cascade known as the Janus-associated kinase (JAK) and signal transducer and activator of transcription (STAT) pathway (Aaronson and Horvath, 2002).

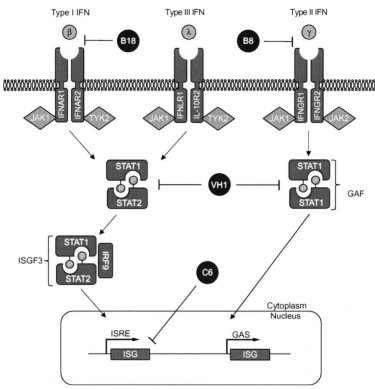

Fig. 2 Diagram showing the JAK–STAT signaling pathways induced by binding of type I, II, or III IFNs to their cognate receptors. These pathways result in assembly of transcription factors in the nucleus that drive transcription from genes bearing the ISRE or GAS promoter elements. *Red circles* depict individual VACV proteins that inhibit activation of this pathway and the positions at which they function.

Although type I and type III IFNs act through distinct receptors, the JAK–STAT pathway is thought to be the same (Crotta et al., 2013; Doyle et al., 2006; Zhou et al., 2007). In contrast, type II IFN activates a subtly different subset of JAKs and STATs (Platanias, 2005).

Upon receptor binding, the IFNR subunits undergo structural rearrangements and dimerize. This brings the receptor-associated JAKs within close proximity, leading to their cross-activation (Leonard, 2001). Each of the subunits from the different IFNRs interacts with a specific member of the JAK family (Fig. 2). The activated JAKs then phosphorylate the cytoplasmic region of the IFNRs, leading to the formation of docking sites to which inactive STAT proteins are recruited (Aaronson and Horvath, 2002; Li, 2008). Once recruited, the JAKs phosphorylate the STAT molecules at specific tyrosine residues near their C terminus, thereby induc-ing the formation of STAT dimers (Aaronson and Horvath, 2002; Li, 2008). In type I and type III IFN signaling, both STAT1 and STAT2 are recruited to form STAT1 and STAT2 heterodimers (Aaronson and Horvath, 2002). In turn, they further associate with IFN regulatory factor 9 (IRF9), to form a trimeric complex known as the IFN-stimulated gene factor 3 (ISGF3) (Aaronson and Horvath, 2002; Schindler et al., 1992). Subsequently, ISGF3 translocates into the nucleus where it associates with the IFN-stimulated responsive element (ISRE) promoter to drive the transcription of ISGs (Aaronson and Horvath, 2002). In type II IFN signaling, only STAT1 is rec-ruited to form STAT1 homodimers (Aaronson and Horvath, 2002; Shuai et al., 1992). These homodimers known as IFNγ-associated factor (GAF) then translocate into the nucleus where they associate with the IFNγ-associated sequence (GAS) promoter, leading to the transcription of ISGs (Aaronson and Horvath, 2002).

2.3 IFN-Stimulated Genes

IFNs induce the transcription of hundreds of ISGs. While some are upregulated by all IFNs, others are upregulated selectively by distinct IFNs. For example, IRF1 is upregulated preferentially in response to IFNγ (Der et al., 1998). This type of specificity in IFN-induced responses is critical for a highly coordinated and fine-tuned innate immune response as well as a heightened antiviral state within cells, thereby halting the spread of infection. Of the many hundreds of ISGs, well-characterized examples include ISG15, protein kinase R (PKR), and 2′-5′-oligoadenylate synthase (OAS).

ISG15 is a 15-kDa protein that has sequence similarity to ubiquitin and is one of the most strongly induced genes upon viral infection (Blomstrom et al., 1986; Haas et al., 1987). ISG15 can become conjugated to both cyto-plasmic and nuclear proteins via an isopeptidase bond in a process known as ISGylation. Conjugation of ISG15 to target proteins such as IRF3, RIG-I, human MxA, and PKR can increase their stability preventing their degradation (Villarroya-Beltri et al., 2017). Additionally, ISGylation through attachment of ISG15 can modulate JAK–STAT signaling (Malakhova et al., 2003).

PKR becomes activated by autophosphorylation upon binding dsRNA, a product often formed during infection by both RNA and DNA viruses. Subsequently, PKR phosphorylates the eukaryotic translational initiation factor 2 alpha (eIF2α) at serine 51, thereby preventing recycling of eIF2α and preventing further protein synthesis (Meurs et al., 1990).

2′-5′-OAS is also activated upon binding to dsRNA. Once activated, 2′-5′-OAS synthesizes 2′-5′-oligoadenylates using ATP as a substrate. In turn, 2′-5′-oligoadenylates activate the ribonuclease RNAaseL, which degrades both viral and cellular mRNAs as well as cellular tRNAs and rRNAs, leading to inhibition of translation (Silverman, 2007).

The importance of the IFN system for protection against viruses has been demonstrated in many ways, not least by the presence of many IFN antagonists in virus genomes. This is illustrated particularly well with VACV that has been known for decades to be relatively resistant to IFN and to confer resistance to IFN to other viruses such as vesicular stomatitis virus (Thacore and Youngner, 1973; Whitaker-Dowling and Youngner, 1983). The observation that large deletions in terminal regions of the VACV genome could arise spontaneously during passage of virus in tissue culture and that this was prevented in the presence of IFN suggested that genes conferring resistance to IFN were present in these terminal regions (Paez and Esteban, 1985). We now know that VACV interferes with the production and action of IFNs in many ways.

3. PREVENTING PRODUCTION OF IFN

3.1 Inhibition of Protein Synthesis in Virus-Infected Cells

IFNs are cellular proteins whose production is blocked by inhibition of host protein synthesis induced by infection with VACV (Moss, 1968). In recent years some of the virus genes involved have been identified. These include the decapping enzymes D9 and D10 that recognize and remove the cap structures from the 5′ end of mRNAs (Parrish and Moss, 2007; Parrish et al., 2007). It might seem counterintuitive for a virus that has capped mRNAs to encode decapping enzymes, but there are advantages to the virus in doing this. First, virus mRNAs may be more abundant than cellular mRNAs and therefore decapping enzymes will cause a preferential inhibition of cellular rather than viral protein synthesis. Second, decapping of virus mRNAs provides a mechanism to achieve an efficient shift from expression of early virus proteins to intermediate and then late proteins by removing the mRNAs of the earlier class. Another VACV protein, called 169, also inhibits protein synthesis, and since this protein is excluded from virus factories, the site of virus protein synthesis, it may target cellular mRNAs preferentially. Loss of protein 169 causes an increased expression of cellular inflammatory proteins during infection in cultured cells and in vivo (Strnadova et al., 2015).

3.2 Limiting the Formation or Availability of Virus Nucleic Acid PAMPs

Viral nucleic acids such as dsRNA, 5′-triphosphate RNA, or cytoplasmic DNA are recognized by specific PRRs, leading to activation of signaling pathways and the production of cytokines, chemokines, and IFNs. A strategy employed by VACV to prevent IFN production is therefore to minimize the production or recognition of these nucleic acid PAMPs by PRRs.

3.2.1 Limiting dsRNA Formation by Gene Arrangement

Production of dsRNAs is minimized early during VACV infection by gene arrangement (Smith et al., 1998). The genes at the left and right end of the genome are, with very few exceptions, transcribed outward from only one DNA strand (Goebel et al., 1990). Therefore, these transcripts lack complementary RNA to form dsRNA. In the central region of the genome, genes are encoded approximately equally on each DNA strand, but here genes are often arranged in blocks with several going left to right followed by an inversion with a block of genes transcribed right to left (Goebel et al., 1990). Furthermore, for pairs of adjacent genes that are transcribed toward each other early during infection, it is notable that the production of overlapping transcripts is minimized by the presence of transcriptional termination sequences (often multiple termination signals) on both DNA strands between these genes (Smith et al., 1998). This arrangement is unlikely to be accidental and may help reduce dsRNA formation and thereby IFN production.

3.2.2 Expression of a dsRNA Binding Protein E3

Late during VACV infection long transcripts are formed that run through several open reading frames due to a failure to terminate at specific sequences. Consequently, much dsRNA is formed late during infection. However, the availability of this PAMP is minimized by the VACV E3 protein that binds dsRNA and so restricts the activation of PRRs by dsRNA (Chang et al., 1992). Notably protein E3 is made early during infection and so is present before most virus dsRNA is formed. A mutant virus lacking the E3 protein is more sensitive to IFN and this sensitivity could be reversed by the expression of other dsRNA binding proteins (Beattie et al., 1995). Viruses lacking E3 are also attenuated in vivo and both the N-terminal domain, which has similarity to Z DNA binding proteins, and the C-terminal domain, which binds dsRNA, are required for virus virulence (Brandt and Jacobs, 2001). The E3 protein also serves to minimize RNA polymerase III-mediated dsDNA sensing and the consequential activation of innate immunity (Marq et al., 2009; Valentine and Smith, 2010).

3.2.3 Targeting DNA-PK by Protein C16

During replication VACV can produce thousands of copies of its ~200-kb dsDNA molecule in the cytoplasm. Given that cytoplasmic DNA is abnormal, DNA sensors such as cGAS (Gao et al., 2013; Li et al., 2013), DNA-PK (Ferguson et al., 2012; Morchikh et al., 2017), and several others (for review, see Paludan, 2015) recognize this and activate an innate response via the STING-TBK1-IRF3 pathway (Fig. 1). To counteract the role of DNA-PK in DNA sensing, VACV encodes a protein called C16 that is made early during infection, contributes to virulence (Fahy et al., 2008), and binds to the Ku proteins that are part of the DNA-PK complex (Peters et al., 2013). By binding to Ku, C16 restricts the binding of DNA by Ku, resulting in reduced recruitment of DNA-PK and reduced activation of IRF3 via the STING-TBK1 pathway. Both in cell culture and in vivo C16 restricts the inflammatory response to transfected DNA or infection by DNA viruses (Fahy et al., 2008; Peters et al., 2013).

3.3 Inhibition of Signaling Pathways Leading to Expression of IFNβ

The IFNβ gene promoter contains binding sites for IRF3, NF-κB, and AP-1 that form the enhanceosome enabling efficient transcription of the IFNβ gene (Maniatis et al., 1998; Thanos and Maniatis, 1995). VACV expresses a remarkable number of proteins that shut down IRF3 or NF-κB activation (Smith et al., 2013) and also expresses proteins that both positively and negatively influence activation of MAP kinases (Torres et al., 2016).

3.3.1 Inhibition of IRF3 Activation

VACV expresses multiple proteins that inhibit IRF3 activation. These proteins and their mechanisms of action (where known) were described in a review of VACV immune evasion (Smith et al., 2013) and so are described only briefly here. They include A46, K7, C6, and N2 that are all known or predicted to be members of the VACV Bcl-2 family. A46 binds to TRIF, TRAM, MAL, and Myd88 and therefore blocks activation of IRF3 early in the pathway downstream of TLRs (Stack et al., 2005) (Fig. 1). K7 binds to the DEAD box helicase DDX3, and this interaction revealed that DDX3 is an adaptor protein for the TBK1/IKKε complex that promotes IRF3 phosphorylation (Schroder et al., 2008). Protein C6 also interferes with the production of IFNβ by binding to other TBK1 adaptor proteins, TANK, SINTBAD, and NAP1 (Unterholzner et al., 2011). Protein N2 acts further downstream in the pathway after IRF3 phosphorylation and translocation into the nucleus, although its precise mechanism remains to be determined (Ferguson et al., 2013). Collectively, these proteins provide a coordinated assault on this pathway and their actions are nonredundant because deletion of any of these proteins causes a reduction in virus virulence in vivo (Benfield et al., 2013; Ferguson et al., 2013; Stack et al., 2005; Unterholzner et al., 2011).

3.3.2 Inhibition of NF-κB Activation

VACV expresses a remarkable number of proteins that target NF-κB activation. Many of these were reviewed previously (Smith et al., 2013), but at least 10 inhibitors have been identified and, as for the IRF3 inhibitors, these proteins are nonredundant because deletion of A46 (Stack et al., 2005), A52 (Harte et al., 2003), N1 (Bartlett et al., 2002), K7 (Benfield et al., 2013), B14 (Chen et al., 2006), C4 (Ember et al., 2012), A49 (Mansur et al., 2013), and E3 (Brandt and Jacobs, 2001) individually each causes an in vivo phenotype despite the presence of the other inhibitors. These proteins act at different stages in the pathway. For instance, A46, K7, and A52 act early by binding to IRAKs and TRAFs (Bowie et al., 2000; Harte et al., 2003; Schroder et al., 2008; Stack et al., 2005), B14 binds to IKKβ part of the IKK complex where the IL-1- and TNF-activated pathways converge (Chen et al., 2008), and A49 binds to the E3 ubiquitin ligase β-TrCP to block p-IκBα ubiquitylation and degradation (Mansur et al., 2013). Binding of A49 to β-TrCP also prevents ubiquitylation and degradation of other β-TrCP substrates such as β-catenin and consequently results in activation of the Wnt signaling pathway (Maluquer de Motes and Smith, 2017). Protein K1 acts further downstream within the nucleus to prevent the acetylation of RelA (Bravo Cruz and Shisler, 2016). Remarkably, a VACV deletion mutant lacking all known NF-κB inhibitors was still able to inhibit NF-κB activation and did so after p65 translocation into the nucleus, indicating the presence of further inhibitors that act within the nucleus (Sumner et al., 2014). Unpublished work from our laboratory has identified several other inhibitors of this pathway.

3.3.3 Modulation of AP-1 Activation

VACV modulates MAPK pathways during infection (Andrade et al., 2004; de Magalhaes et al., 2001; Pereira et al., 2012; Silva et al., 2006). Recently some proteins responsible for this have been identified and these are all Bcl-2 family members. VACV proteins A52, B14, and K7 promote activation of the pathway during infection and when expressed individually ectopically, and of these B14 gave the strongest activation. In contrast, protein A49 was inhibitory (Torres et al., 2016). The biological consequences of these effects remain incompletely understood.

4. BLOCKING BINDING OF IFNs TO IFN RECEPTORS

As illustrated above, VACV has many strategies to reduce the production of IFNs from infected cells, but unless these defenses are deployed immediately after infection the inhibition of IFN production may be incomplete. In addition, these intracellular defenses offer no protection against IFNs produced by activated uninfected cells that are recruited to the site of infection. To combat IFNs outside the cell VACV expresses two proteins called B8 and B18 that are secreted and bind and inhibit IFNs extracellularly (Fig. 2).

Protein B8 was identified by virtue of its similarity to protein M-T7 from the leporipoxvirus myxoma virus that is the cause of myxomatosis in the European rabbit (Upton et al., 1992). M-T7 and VACV B8 share amino acid similarity to the extracellular ligand binding domain of the mouse and human IFNGR but lack the transmembrane anchor of the host protein and the intracellular domain that mediates signal transduction after ligand–receptor interaction (Upton et al., 1992). Direct analysis of the B8 protein confirmed that it is secreted from cells and acts a soluble antagonist of IFNγ (Alcami and Smith, 1995; Mossman et al., 1995). B8 showed an unusually broad specificity for IFNγs from different species, unlike the cellular IFNGRs that are generally species specific. B8 bound human, bovine, rat, and rabbit IFNγ well, but had much lower affinity for mouse IFNγ (Alcami and Smith, 1995; Mossman et al., 1995). Further studies showed that the B8 protein was a homodimer (Alcami and Smith, 2002) and also bound equine IFNγ (consistent with an equine origin of VACV) (Symons et al., 2002). In vivo loss of the B8 protein did not affect VACV virulence in mice, consistent with the low affinity for mouse IFNγ; however, it did affect lesion formation in rabbit skin (Symons et al., 2002).

Protein B18 from VACV strain Western Reserve (WR) functions as a soluble inhibitor of type I IFNs. This protein was identified as a soluble inhibitor of type I IFNs in the culture medium of cells infected with VACV, and subsequently was mapped to the *B18R* gene (Symons et al., 1995). B18 is a member of the immunoglobulin superfamily and has a signal peptide and three Ig domains, but no transmembrane anchor or cytosolic signal transduction domain (Smith and Chan, 1991). The B18 protein functions as a type I IFN inhibitor and prevents type I IFN-induced signaling (Colamonici et al., 1995; Symons et al., 1995). Like B8, B18 showed a broad species specificity and inhibited type I IFNs from human, rabbit, bovine, rat, and mouse and contributed to virulence in mouse models of infection (Symons et al., 1995). B18 has another important property not shared by B8 and can also bind to glycosaminoglycans on the surface of cells (Montanuy et al., 2011) and still bind and inhibit IFNs (Alcami et al., 2000).

Although B18 does not inhibit type III IFNs, a protein encoded by a yatapoxvirus, Yaba-like disease virus (YLDV), called Y136, shares amino acid similarity to B18 (Lee et al., 2001) and is able to bind and inhibit both type I and type III IFNs (Huang et al., 2007).

5. BLOCKING IFN-INDUCED SIGNALING PATHWAYS

Two VACV proteins are known to inhibit IFN signaling. VH1 is a tyrosine phosphatase and is packaged into the virus particle within the lateral bodies of the IMV particle that flank the biconcave virion core. Therefore, VH1 is delivered into cells immediately after infection. VH1 dephosphorylates STAT1 and STAT2 that are phosphorylated upon type I, II, or III IFNs binding to their receptors (Mann et al., 2008; Najarro et al., 2001). Thus VH1 provides a very rapid defense to IFN-induced signaling and can function within the infected cell immediately after the lateral bodies have been disassembled to release the proteins carried therein. Surprisingly, VH1 is essential for virus replication.

C6 also blocks IFN-induced signaling. It was characterized first as an inhibitor of IRF3 signaling (Unterholzner et al., 2011), but further work showed that it also inhibits JAK–STAT signaling in response to type I IFN (Stuart et al., 2016). Mapping its site of action showed that it did not prevent STAT phosphorylation or nuclear translocation, nor binding of the ISGF3 complex to the ISRE promoter, but it prevented transcription from promoters bearing the ISRE. C6 interacts with STAT2 and this interaction requires the last 104 amino acids of STAT2 representing the transactivation domain (Stuart et al., 2016). Whether C6 can inhibit type II IFN signaling is unknown.

6. BLOCKING THE ANTIVIRAL ACTION OF ISGs

VACV encodes several proteins that antagonize the antiviral effects of ISGs. Well-characterized examples are the E3 and K3 proteins. The dsRNA binding protein E3 (Chang et al., 1992) is able to sequester dsRNA produced during infection and thereby prevent activation of ISGs, such as PKR and 2'-5'-OAS. Activation of PKR and 2'-5'-OAS by binding dsRNA leads to an inhibition of protein synthesis (Fig. 3). PKR phosphorylates eIF2α rendering it inactive thus preventing protein biosynthesis. The activation of 2'-5'-OAS leads to the synthesis of oligoadenylates and these activate RNAaseL that then cleaves all forms of RNA and so also results in the inhibition of protein synthesis.

Protein K3 also prevents the inhibition of protein synthesis. This 88-amino acid protein shows sequence similarity to the N-terminal region of eIF2α including serine 51 that is phosphorylated by PKR. Consequently, K3 acts as a mimic and blocks the phosphorylation of eIF2α even if PKR has been activated (Beattie et al., 1991).

VACV proteins K1 and C7 were identified as factors that extended the range of host cells in which VACV could replicate (Perkus et al., 1990) and in their absence virus virulence was reduced (Liu et al., 2013). This host range restriction is related to the stimulation of ISG expression by type I IFN. VACV lacking K1 and C7 could replicate in Huh7 and MCF-7 cells

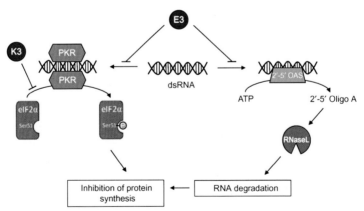

Fig. 3 Diagram showing the activation of ISGs protein kinase R (PKR) and 2'-5'-oligoadenylate synthetase (2'-5'-OAS) by binding dsRNA and how this leads to inhibition of protein synthesis. *Red circles* depict VACV proteins E3 and K3 and the positions at which they inhibit these pathways to ensure that protein synthesis continues.

but not if these cells were pretreated with IFNβ. This blockage was reversed by the reintroduction of K1 or C7 (Meng et al., 2009). Screening of an ISG library identified IRF1 as the ISG targeted by K7- and C1-mediated suppression of antiviral activity (Meng et al., 2012). Proteins K1 and C7 can also prevent the phosphorylation of eIF2α in VACV strain MVA-infected cells (Backes et al., 2010).

7. SUMMARY

VACV has acquired a remarkable arsenal of proteins that inhibit the production of IFNs, the binding of IFNs to their receptors, IFN-induced signaling, and the antiviral activity of ISGs. The existence of these VACV proteins provides not only evidence of the importance of the IFN system for protection against viruses but also illustrates how the IFN system functions. It is likely that additional VACV proteins that target the IFN system remain to be discovered and, equally, it is possible that VACV proteins that target the IFN system will lead to the discovery of additional cellular proteins that function in the IFN system. Viruses are wonderful tools for learning about innate immunity and cell biology and so, although VACV was used as a vaccine against a disease that was eradicated nearly 40 years ago, there are compelling reasons to continue to study it.

ACKNOWLEDGMENTS

Work in the senior author's laboratory has been supported by the Wellcome Trust, MRC, BBSRC, and Lister Institute. G.L.S. is a Wellcome Trust Principal Research Fellow.

REFERENCES

Aaronson, D.S., Horvath, C.M., 2002. A road map for those who don't know JAK-STAT. Science 296, 1653.

Alcami, A., Smith, G.L., 1995. Vaccinia, cowpox, and camelpox viruses encode soluble gamma interferon receptors with novel broad species specificity. J. Virol. 69, 4633.

Alcami, A., Smith, G.L., 2002. The vaccinia virus soluble interferon-gamma receptor is a homodimer. J. Gen. Virol. 83, 545.

Alcami, A., Symons, J.A., Smith, G.L., 2000. The vaccinia virus soluble alpha/beta interferon (IFN) receptor binds to the cell surface and protects cells from the antiviral effects of IFN. J. Virol. 74, 11230.

Andrade, A.A., Silva, P.N., Pereira, A.C., De Sousa, L.P., Ferreira, P.C., Gazzinelli, R.T., Kroon, E.G., Ropert, C., Bonjardim, C.A., 2004. The vaccinia virus-stimulated mitogen-activated protein kinase (MAPK) pathway is required for virus multiplication. Biochem. J. 381, 437.

Appleyard, G., Hapel, A.J., Boulter, E.A., 1971. An antigenic difference between intracellular and extracellular rabbitpox virus. J. Gen. Virol. 13, 9.

Backes, S., Sperling, K.M., Zwilling, J., Gasteiger, G., Ludwig, H., Kremmer, E., Schwantes, A., Staib, C., Sutter, G., 2010. Viral host-range factor C7 or K1 is essential for modified vaccinia virus Ankara late gene expression in human and murine cells, irrespective of their capacity to inhibit protein kinase R-mediated phosphorylation of eukaryotic translation initiation factor 2alpha. J. Gen. Virol. 91, 470.

Bartlett, N., Symons, J.A., Tscharke, D.C., Smith, G.L., 2002. The vaccinia virus N1L protein is an intracellular homodimer that promotes virulence. J. Gen. Virol. 83, 1965.

Baxby, D., 1981. Jenner's Smallpox Vaccine. The Riddle of the Origin of Vaccinia Virus. Heinemann, London.

Beattie, E., Tartaglia, J., Paoletti, E., 1991. Vaccinia virus-encoded eIF-2 alpha homolog abrogates the antiviral effect of interferon. Virology 183, 419.

Beattie, E., Denzler, K.L., Tartaglia, J., Perkus, M.E., Paoletti, E., Jacobs, B.L., 1995. Reversal of the interferon-sensitive phenotype of a vaccinia virus lacking E3L by expression of the reovirus S4 gene. J. Virol. 69, 499.

Benfield, C.T., Ren, H., Lucas, S.J., Bahsoun, B., Smith, G.L., 2013. Vaccinia virus protein K7 is a virulence factor that alters the acute immune response to infection. J. Gen. Virol. 94, 1647.

Bengali, Z., Townsley, A.C., Moss, B., 2009. Vaccinia virus strain differences in cell attachment and entry. Virology 389, 132.

Blomstrom, D.C., Fahey, D., Kutny, R., Korant, B.D., Knight Jr., E., 1986. Molecular characterization of the interferon-induced 15-kDa protein. Molecular cloning and nucleotide and amino acid sequence. J. Biol. Chem. 261, 8811.

Bowie, A., Kiss-Toth, E., Symons, J.A., Smith, G.L., Dower, S.K., O'Neill, L.A., 2000. A46R and A52R from vaccinia virus are antagonists of host IL-1 and toll-like receptor signaling. Proc. Natl. Acad. Sci. U. S. A. 97, 10162.

Brandt, T.A., Jacobs, B.L., 2001. Both carboxy- and amino-terminal domains of the vaccinia virus interferon resistance gene, E3L, are required for pathogenesis in a mouse model. J. Virol. 75, 850.

Bravo Cruz, A.G., Shisler, J.L., 2016. Vaccinia virus K1 ankyrin repeat protein inhibits NF-kappaB activation by preventing RelA acetylation. J. Gen. Virol. 97, 2691.

Broyles, S.S., 2003. Vaccinia virus transcription. J. Gen. Virol. 84, 2293.

Carter, G.C., Rodger, G., Murphy, B.J., Law, M., Krauss, O., Hollinshead, M., Smith, G.L., 2003. Vaccinia virus cores are transported on microtubules. J. Gen. Virol. 84, 2443.

Carter, G.C., Law, M., Hollinshead, M., Smith, G.L., 2005. Entry of the vaccinia virus intracellular mature virion and its interactions with glycosaminoglycans. J. Gen. Virol. 86, 1279.

Chang, H.W., Watson, J.C., Jacobs, B.L., 1992. The E3L gene of vaccinia virus encodes an inhibitor of the interferon-induced, double-stranded RNA-dependent protein kinase. Proc. Natl. Acad. Sci. U. S. A. 89, 4825.

Chen, R.A., Jacobs, N., Smith, G.L., 2006. Vaccinia virus strain Western Reserve protein B14 is an intracellular virulence factor. J. Gen. Virol. 87, 1451.

Chen, R.A., Ryzhakov, G., Cooray, S., Randow, F., Smith, G.L., 2008. Inhibition of IkappaB kinase by vaccinia virus virulence factor B14. PLoS Pathog. 4, e22.

Colamonici, O.R., Domanski, P., Sweitzer, S.M., Larner, A., Buller, R.M., 1995. Vaccinia virus B18R gene encodes a type I interferon-binding protein that blocks interferon alpha transmembrane signaling. J. Biol. Chem. 270, 15974.

Crotta, S., Davidson, S., Mahlakoiv, T., Desmet, C.J., Buckwalter, M.R., Albert, M.L., Staeheli, P., Wack, A., 2013. Type I and type III interferons drive redundant amplification loops to induce a transcriptional signature in influenza-infected airway epithelia. PLoS Pathog. 9, e1003773.

Cudmore, S., Cossart, P., Griffiths, G., Way, M., 1995. Actin-based motility of vaccinia virus. Nature 378, 636.

de Magalhaes, J.C., Andrade, A.A., Silva, P.N., Sousa, L.P., Ropert, C., Ferreira, P.C., Kroon, E.G., Gazzinelli, R.T., Bonjardim, C.A., 2001. A mitogenic signal triggered at an early stage of vaccinia virus infection: implication of MEK/ERK and protein kinase A in virus multiplication. J. Biol. Chem. 276, 38353.

Der, S.D., Zhou, A., Williams, B.R., Silverman, R.H., 1998. Identification of genes differentially regulated by interferon alpha, beta, or gamma using oligonucleotide arrays. Proc. Natl. Acad. Sci. U. S. A. 95, 15623.

de Weerd, N.A., Nguyen, T., 2012. The interferons and their receptors—distribution and regulation. Immunol. Cell Biol. 90, 483.

Doceul, V., Hollinshead, M., van der Linden, L., Smith, G.L., 2010. Repulsion of superinfecting virions: a mechanism for rapid virus spread. Science 327, 873.

Doceul, V., Hollinshead, M., Breiman, A., Laval, K., Smith, G.L., 2012. Protein B5 is required on extracellular enveloped vaccinia virus for repulsion of superinfecting virions. J. Gen. Virol. 93, 1876.

Downie, A.W., 1939. Immunological relationship of the virus of spontaneous cowpox to vaccinia virus. Br. J. Exp. Pathol. 20, 158.

Doyle, S.E., Schreckhise, H., Khuu-Duong, K., Henderson, K., Rosler, R., Storey, H., Yao, L., Liu, H., Barahmand-pour, F., Sivakumar, P., Chan, C., Birks, C., Foster, D., Clegg, C.H., Wietzke-Braun, P., Mihm, S., Klucher, K.M., 2006. Interleukin-29 uses a type 1 interferon-like program to promote antiviral responses in human hepatocytes. Hepatology 44, 896.

Ember, S.W., Ren, H., Ferguson, B.J., Smith, G.L., 2012. Vaccinia virus protein C4 inhibits NF-kappaB activation and promotes virus virulence. J. Gen. Virol. 93, 2098.

Fahy, A.S., Clark, R.H., Glyde, E.F., Smith, G.L., 2008. Vaccinia virus protein C16 acts intracellularly to modulate the host response and promote virulence. J. Gen. Virol. 89, 2377.

Farrar, M.A., Schreiber, R.D., 1993. The molecular cell biology of interferon-γ and its receptor. Annu. Rev. Immunol. 11, 571.

Ferguson, B.J., Mansur, D.S., Peters, N.E., Ren, H., Smith, G.L., 2012. DNA-PK is a DNA sensor for IRF-3-dependent innate immunity. eLife 1, e00047.

Ferguson, B.J., Benfield, C.T., Ren, H., Lee, V.H., Frazer, G.L., Strnadova, P., Sumner, R.P., Smith, G.L., 2013. Vaccinia virus protein N2 is a nuclear IRF3 inhibitor that promotes virulence. J. Gen. Virol. 94, 2070.

Fitzgerald, K.A., McWhirter, S.M., Faia, K.L., Rowe, D.C., Latz, E., Golenbock, D.T., Coyle, A.J., Liao, S.M., Maniatis, T., 2003. IKKepsilon and TBK1 are essential components of the IRF3 signaling pathway. Nat. Immunol. 4, 491.

Fox, B.A., Sheppard, P.O., O'Hara, P.J., 2009. The role of genomic data in the discovery, annotation and evolutionary interpretation of the interferon-lambda family. PLoS One 4, e4933.

Fujita, F., Taniguchi, Y., Kato, T., Narita, Y., Furuya, A., Ogawa, T., Sakurai, H., Joh, T., Itoh, M., Delhase, M., Karin, M., Nakanishi, M., 2003. Identification of NAP1, a regulatory subunit of IkappaB kinase-related kinases that potentiates NF-kappaB signaling. Mol. Cell. Biol. 23, 7780.

Gao, D., Wu, J., Wu, Y.T., Du, F., Aroh, C., Yan, N., Sun, L., Chen, Z.J., 2013. Cyclic GMP-AMP synthase is an innate immune sensor of HIV and other retroviruses. Science 341, 903.

Geada, M.M., Galindo, I., Lorenzo, M.M., Perdiguero, B., Blasco, R., 2001. Movements of vaccinia virus intracellular enveloped virions with GFP tagged to the F13L envelope protein. J. Gen. Virol. 82, 2747.

Goebel, S.J., Johnson, G.P., Perkus, M.E., Davis, S.W., Winslow, J.P., Paoletti, E., 1990. The complete DNA sequence of vaccinia virus. Virology 179. 247, 517.

Gubser, C., Hue, S., Kellam, P., Smith, G.L., 2004. Poxvirus genomes: a phylogenetic analysis. J. Gen. Virol. 85, 105.

Haas, A.L., Ahrens, P., Bright, P.M., Ankel, H., 1987. Interferon induces a 15-kilodalton protein exhibiting marked homology to ubiquitin. J. Biol. Chem. 262, 11315.

Harte, M.T., Haga, I.R., Maloney, G., Gray, P., Reading, P.C., Bartlett, N.W., Smith, G.L., Bowie, A., O'Neill, L.A., 2003. The poxvirus protein A52R targets Toll-like receptor signaling complexes to suppress host defense. J. Exp. Med. 197, 343.

Hollinshead, M., Vanderplasschen, A., Smith, G.L., Vaux, D.J., 1999. Vaccinia virus intracellular mature virions contain only one lipid membrane. J. Virol. 73, 1503.

Hollinshead, M., Rodger, G., Van Eijl, H., Law, M., Hollinshead, R., Vaux, D.J., Smith, G.L., 2001. Vaccinia virus utilizes microtubules for movement to the cell surface. J. Cell Biol. 154, 389.

Honda, K., Yanai, H., Negishi, H., Asagiri, M., Sato, M., Mizutani, T., Shimada, N., Ohba, Y., Takaoka, A., Yoshida, N., Taniguchi, T., 2005. IRF-7 is the master regulator of type-I interferon-dependent immune responses. Nature 434, 772.

Huang, J., Smirnov, S.V., Lewis-Antes, A., Balan, M., Li, W., Tang, S., Silke, G.V., Putz, M.M., Smith, G.L., Kotenko, S.V., 2007. Inhibition of type I and type III interferons by a secreted glycoprotein from Yaba-like disease virus. Proc. Natl. Acad. Sci. U. S. A. 104, 9822.

Isaacs, A., Lindenmann, J., 1957. Virus interference. I. The interferon. Proc. R. Soc. Lond. B Biol. Sci. 147, 258.

Isaacs, A., Lindenmann, J., Valentine, R.C., 1957. Virus interference. II. Some properties of interferon. Proc. R. Soc. Lond. B Biol. Sci. 147, 268.

Kotenko, S.V., Gallagher, G., Baurin, V.V., Lewis-Antes, A., Shen, M., Shah, N.K., Langer, J.A., Sheikh, F., Dickensheets, H., Donnelly, R.P., 2003. IFN-lambdas mediate antiviral protection through a distinct class II cytokine receptor complex. Nat. Immunol. 4, 69.

Law, M., Carter, G.C., Roberts, K.L., Hollinshead, M., Smith, G.L., 2006. Ligand-induced and nonfusogenic dissolution of a viral membrane. Proc. Natl. Acad. Sci. U. S. A. 103, 5989.

Lee, H.J., Essani, K., Smith, G.L., 2001. The genome sequence of Yaba-like disease virus, a yatapoxvirus. Virology 281, 170.

Leonard, W.J., 2001. Role of Jak kinases and STATs in cytokine signal transduction. Int. J. Hematol. 73, 271.

Li, W.X., 2008. Canonical and non-canonical JAK-STAT signaling. Trends Cell Biol. 18, 545.

Li, X.D., Wu, J., Gao, D., Wang, H., Sun, L., Chen, Z.J., 2013. Pivotal roles of cGAS-cGAMP signaling in antiviral defense and immune adjuvant effects. Science 341, 1390.

Liu, Z., Wang, S., Zhang, Q., Tian, M., Hou, J., Wang, R., Liu, C., Ji, X., Liu, Y., Shao, Y., 2013. Deletion of C7L and K1L genes leads to significantly decreased virulence of recombinant vaccinia virus TianTan. PLoS One 8, e68115.

Malakhova, O.A., Yan, M., Malakhov, M.P., Yuan, Y., Ritchie, K.J., Kim, K.I., Peterson, L.F., Shuai, K., Zhang, D.E., 2003. Protein ISGylation modulates the JAK-STAT signaling pathway. Genes Dev. 17, 455.

Maluquer de Motes, C., Smith, G.L., 2017. Vaccinia virus protein A49 activates Wnt signalling by targetting the E3 ligase beta-TrCP. J. Gen. Virol. 98 (12), 3086–3092.

Maniatis, T., Falvo, J.V., Kim, T.H., Kim, T.K., Lin, C.H., Parekh, B.S., Wathelet, M.G., 1998. Structure and function of the interferon-beta enhanceosome. Cold Spring Harb. Symp. Quant. Biol. 63, 609.

Mann, B.A., Huang, J.H., Li, P., Chang, H.C., Slee, R.B., O'Sullivan, A., Anita, M., Yeh, N., Kiemsz, M.J., Brutkiewicz, R.R., Blum, J.S., Kaplan, M.H., 2008. Vaccinia virus blocks Stat1-dependent and Stat1-independent gene expression induced by type I and type II interferons. J. Interferon Cytokine Res. 28, 367.

Mansur, D.S., Maluquer de Motes, C., Unterholzner, L., Sumner, R.P., Ferguson, B.J., Ren, H., Strnadova, P., Bowie, A.G., Smith, G.L., 2013. Poxvirus targeting of E3 ligase beta-TrCP by molecular mimicry: a mechanism to inhibit NF-kappaB activation and promote immune evasion and virulence. PLoS Pathog. 9, e1003183.

Marq, J.B., Hausmann, S., Luban, J., Kolakofsky, D., Garcin, D., 2009. The double-stranded RNA binding domain of the vaccinia virus E3L protein inhibits both RNA- and DNA-induced activation of interferon beta. J. Biol. Chem. 284, 25471.

Meng, X., Jiang, C., Arsenio, J., Dick, K., Cao, J., Xiang, Y., 2009. Vaccinia virus K1L and C7L inhibit antiviral activities induced by type I interferons. J. Virol. 83, 10627.

Meng, X., Schoggins, J., Rose, L., Cao, J., Ploss, A., Rice, C.M., Xiang, Y., 2012. C7L family of poxvirus host range genes inhibits antiviral activities induced by type I interferons and interferon regulatory factor 1. J. Virol. 86, 4538.

Mercer, J., Helenius, A., 2008. Vaccinia virus uses macropinocytosis and apoptotic mimicry to enter host cells. Science 320, 531.

Meurs, E., Chong, K., Galabru, J., Thomas, N.S., Kerr, I.M., Williams, B.R., Hovanessian, A.G., 1990. Molecular cloning and characterization of the human double-stranded RNA-activated protein kinase induced by interferon. Cell 62, 379.

Montanuy, I., Alejo, A., Alcami, A., 2011. Glycosaminoglycans mediate retention of the poxvirus type I interferon binding protein at the cell surface to locally block interferon antiviral responses. FASEB J. 25, 1960.

Morchikh, M., Cribier, A., Raffel, R., Amraoui, S., Cau, J., Severac, D., Dubois, E., Schwartz, O., Bennasser, Y., Benkirane, M., 2017. HEXIM1 and NEAT1 long non-coding RNA form a multi-subunit complex that regulates DNA-mediated innate immune response. Mol. Cell 67, 387. e5.

Morgan, C., Ellison, S.A., Rose, H.M., Moore, D.H., 1954. Structure and development of viruses observed in the electron microscope. II. Vaccinia and fowl pox viruses. J. Exp. Med. 100, 301.

Moss, B., 1968. Inhibition of HeLa cell protein synthesis by the vaccinia virion. J. Virol. 2, 1028.

Moss, B., 2007. Poxviridae: the viruses and their replicaton. In: Knipe, D.M. (Ed.), Fields Virology, fifth ed. In: vol. 2. Lippincott Williams & Wilkins, Philadelphia, p. 2905.

Moss, B., 2016. Membrane fusion during poxvirus entry. Semin. Cell Dev. Biol. 60, 89.

Mossman, K., Upton, C., Buller, R.M., McFadden, G., 1995. Species specificity of ectromelia virus and vaccinia virus interferon-gamma binding proteins. Virology 208, 762.

Muir, A.J., Shiffman, M.L., Zaman, A., Yoffe, B., de la Torre, A., Flamm, S., Gordon, S.C., Marotta, P., Vierling, J.M., Lopez-Talavera, J.C., Byrnes-Blake, K., Fontana, D., Freeman, J., Gray, T., Hausman, D., Hunder, N.N., Lawitz, E., 2010. Phase 1b study of pegylated interferon lambda 1 with or without ribavirin in patients with chronic genotype 1 hepatitis C virus infection. Hepatology 52, 822.

Nagano, Y., Kojima, Y., 1954. Immunizing property of vaccinia virus inactivated by ultra-violets rays. C. R. Seances Soc. Biol. Fil. 148, 1700.

Nagano, Y., Kojima, Y., Sawai, Y., 1954. Immunity and interference in vaccinia; inhibition of skin infection by inactivated virus. C. R. Seances Soc. Biol. Fil. 148, 750.

Najarro, P., Traktman, P., Lewis, J.A., 2001. Vaccinia virus blocks gamma interferon signal transduction: viral VH1 phosphatase reverses Stat1 activation. J. Virol. 75, 3185.

Paez, E., Esteban, M., 1985. Interferon prevents the generation of spontaneous deletions at the left terminus of vaccinia virus DNA. J. Virol. 56, 75.

Paludan, S.R., 2015. Activation and regulation of DNA-driven immune responses. Microbiol. Mol. Biol. Rev. 79, 225.

Parrish, S., Moss, B., 2007. Characterization of a second vaccinia virus mRNA-decapping enzyme conserved in poxviruses. J. Virol. 81, 12973.

Parrish, S., Resch, W., Moss, B., 2007. Vaccinia virus D10 protein has mRNA decapping activity, providing a mechanism for control of host and viral gene expression. Proc. Natl. Acad. Sci. U. S. A. 104, 2139.

Pereira, A.C., Leite, F.G., Brasil, B.S., Soares-Martins, J.A., Torres, A.A., Pimenta, P.F., Souto-Padron, T., Traktman, P., Ferreira, P.C., Kroon, E.G., Bonjardim, C.A., 2012. A vaccinia virus-driven interplay between the MKK4/7-JNK1/2 pathway and cytoskeleton reorganization. J. Virol. 86, 172.

Perkus, M.E., Goebel, S.J., Davis, S.W., Johnson, G.P., Limbach, K., Norton, E.K., Paoletti, E., 1990. Vaccinia virus host range genes. Virology 179, 276.

Pestka, S., Langer, J.A., Zoon, K.C., Samuel, C.E., 1987. Interferons and their actions. Annu. Rev. Biochem. 56, 727.

Pestka, S., Krause, C.D., Walter, M.R., 2004. Interferons, interferon-like cytokines, and their receptors. Immunol. Rev. 202, 8.

Peters, N.E., Ferguson, B.J., Mazzon, M., Fahy, A.S., Krysztofinska, E., Arribas-Bosacoma, R., Pearl, L.H., Ren, H., Smith, G.L., 2013. A mechanism for the inhibition of DNA-PK-mediated DNA sensing by a virus. PLoS Pathog. 9, e1003649.

Platanias, L.C., 2005. Mechanisms of type-I- and type-II-interferon-mediated signalling. Nat. Rev. Immunol. 5, 375.

Pomerantz, J.L., Baltimore, D., 1999. NF-kappaB activation by a signaling complex containing TRAF2, TANK and TBK1, a novel IKK-related kinase. EMBO J. 18, 6694.

Prokunina-Olsson, L., Muchmore, B., Tang, W., Pfeiffer, R.M., Park, H., Dickensheets, H., Hergott, D., Porter-Gill, P., Mumy, A., Kohaar, I., Chen, S., Brand, N., Tarway, M., Liu, L., Sheikh, F., Astemborski, J., Bonkovsky, H.L., Edlin, B.R., Howell, C.D., Morgan, T.R., Thomas, D.L., Rehermann, B., Donnelly, R.P., O'Brien, T.R., 2013. A variant upstream of IFNL3 (IL28B) creating a new interferon gene IFNL4 is associated with impaired clearance of hepatitis C virus. Nat. Genet. 45, 164.

Rietdorf, J., Ploubidou, A., Reckmann, I., Holmstrom, A., Frischknecht, F., Zettl, M., Zimmermann, T., Way, M., 2001. Kinesin-dependent movement on microtubules precedes actin-based motility of vaccinia virus. Nat. Cell Biol. 3, 992.

Roberts, K.L., Breiman, A., Carter, G.C., Ewles, H.A., Hollinshead, M., Law, M., Smith, G.L., 2009. Acidic residues in the membrane-proximal stalk region of vaccinia virus protein B5 are required for glycosaminoglycan-mediated disruption of the extracellular enveloped virus outer membrane. J. Gen. Virol. 90, 1582.

Ryzhakov, G., Randow, F., 2007. SINTBAD, a novel component of innate antiviral immunity, shares a TBK1-binding domain with NAP1 and TANK. EMBO J. 26, 3180.

Sanderson, C.M., Hollinshead, M., Smith, G.L., 2000. The vaccinia virus A27L protein is needed for the microtubule-dependent transport of intracellular mature virus particles. J. Gen. Virol. 81, 47.

Sato, M., Suemori, H., Hata, N., Asagiri, M., Ogasawara, K., Nakao, K., Nakaya, T., Katsuki, M., Noguchi, S., Tanaka, N., Taniguchi, T., 2000. Distinct and essential roles of transcription factors IRF-3 and IRF-7 in response to viruses for IFN-alpha/beta gene induction. Immunity 13, 539.

Schindler, C., Shuai, K., Prezioso, V.R., Darnell Jr., J.E., 1992. Interferon-dependent tyrosine phosphorylation of a latent cytoplasmic transcription factor. Science 257, 809.

Schmelz, M., Sodeik, B., Ericsson, M., Wolffe, E.J., Shida, H., Hiller, G., Griffiths, G., 1994. Assembly of vaccinia virus: the second wrapping cisterna is derived from the trans Golgi network. J. Virol. 68, 130.

Schrick, L., Tausch, S.H., Dabrowski, P.W., Damaso, C.R., Esparza, J., Nitsche, A., 2017. An early American smallpox vaccine based on horsepox. N. Engl. J. Med. 377, 1491.

Schroder, M., Baran, M., Bowie, A.G., 2008. Viral targeting of DEAD box protein 3 reveals its role in TBK1/IKKepsilon-mediated IRF activation. EMBO J. 27, 2147.

Senkevich, T.G., Ojeda, S., Townsley, A., Nelson, G.E., Moss, B., 2005. Poxvirus multiprotein entry-fusion complex. Proc. Natl. Acad. Sci. U. S. A. 102, 18572.

Sheppard, P., Kindsvogel, W., Xu, W., Henderson, K., Schlutsmeyer, S., Whitmore, T.E., Kuestner, R., Garrigues, U., Birks, C., Roraback, J., Ostrander, C., Dong, D., Shin, J., Presnell, S., Fox, B., Haldeman, B., Cooper, E., Taft, D., Gilbert, T., Grant, F.J., Tackett, M., Krivan, W., McKnight, G., Clegg, C., Foster, D., Klucher, K.M., 2003. IL-28 and IL-29 and their class II cytokine receptor IL-28R. Nat. Immunol. 4, 63.

Shuai, K., Schindler, C., Prezioso, V.R., Darnell Jr., J.E., 1992. Activation of transcription by IFN-gamma: tyrosine phosphorylation of a 91-kD DNA binding protein. Science 258, 1808.

Silva, P.N., Soares, J.A., Brasil, B.S., Nogueira, S.V., Andrade, A.A., de Magalhaes, J.C., Bonjardim, M.B., Ferreira, P.C., Kroon, E.G., Bruna-Romero, O., Bonjardim, C.A., 2006. Differential role played by the MEK/ERK/EGR-1 pathway in orthopoxviruses vaccinia and cowpox biology. Biochem. J. 398, 83.

Silverman, R.H., 2007. Viral encounters with $2',5'$-oligoadenylate synthetase and RNase L during the interferon antiviral response. J. Virol. 81, 12720.

Smith, G.L., Chan, Y.S., 1991. Two vaccinia virus proteins structurally related to the interleukin-1 receptor and the immunoglobulin superfamily. J. Gen. Virol. 72, 511.

Smith, G.L., Symons, J.A., Alcamí, A., 1998. Poxviruses: interfering with interferon. Semin. Virol. 8, 409.

Smith, G.L., Benfield, C.T., Maluquer de Motes, C., Mazzon, M., Ember, S.W., Ferguson, B.J., Sumner, R.P., 2013. Vaccinia virus immune evasion: mechanisms, virulence and immunogenicity. J. Gen. Virol. 94, 2367.

Soulat, D., Burckstummer, T., Westermayer, S., Goncalves, A., Bauch, A., Stefanovic, A., Hantschel, O., Bennett, K.L., Decker, T., Superti-Furga, G., 2008. The DEAD-box helicase DDX3X is a critical component of the TANK-binding kinase 1-dependent innate immune response. EMBO J. 27, 2135.

Stack, J., Haga, I.R., Schroder, M., Bartlett, N.W., Maloney, G., Reading, P.C., Fitzgerald, K.A., Smith, G.L., Bowie, A.G., 2005. Vaccinia virus protein A46R targets multiple Toll-like-interleukin-1 receptor adaptors and contributes to virulence. J. Exp. Med. 201, 1007.

Strnadova, P., Ren, H., Valentine, R., Mazzon, M., Sweeney, T.R., Brierley, I., Smith, G.L., 2015. Inhibition of translation initiation by protein 169: a vaccinia virus strategy to suppress innate and adaptive immunity and alter virus virulence. PLoS Pathog. 11, e1005151.

Stuart, J.H., Sumner, R.P., Lu, Y., Snowden, J.S., Smith, G.L., 2016. Vaccinia virus protein C6 inhibits type I IFN signalling in the nucleus and binds to the transactivation domain of STAT2. PLoS Pathog. 12, e1005955.

Sumner, R.P., Maluquer de Motes, C., Veyer, D.L., Smith, G.L., 2014. Vaccinia virus inhibits NF-kappaB-dependent gene expression downstream of p65 translocation. J. Virol. 88, 3092.

Symons, J.A., Alcami, A., Smith, G.L., 1995. Vaccinia virus encodes a soluble type I interferon receptor of novel structure and broad species specificity. Cell 81, 551.

Symons, J.A., Tscharke, D.C., Price, N., Smith, G.L., 2002. A study of the vaccinia virus interferon-gamma receptor and its contribution to virus virulence. J. Gen. Virol. 83, 1953.

Thacore, H.R., Youngner, J.S., 1973. Rescue of vesicular stomatitis virus from interferon-induced resistance by superinfection with vaccinia virus. I. Rescue in cell cultures from different species. Virology 56, 505.

Thanos, D., Maniatis, T., 1995. Virus induction of human IFN beta gene expression requires the assembly of an enhanceosome. Cell 83, 1091.

Tooze, J., Hollinshead, M., Reis, B., Radsak, K., Kern, H., 1993. Progeny vaccinia and human cytomegalovirus particles utilize early endosomal cisternae for their envelopes. Eur. J. Cell Biol. 60, 163.

Torres, A.A., Albarnaz, J.D., Bonjardim, C.A., Smith, G.L., 2016. Multiple Bcl-2 family immunomodulators from vaccinia virus regulate MAPK/AP-1 activation. J. Gen. Virol. 97, 2346.

Townsley, A.C., Weisberg, A.S., Wagenaar, T.R., Moss, B., 2006. Vaccinia virus entry into cells via a low-pH-dependent endosomal pathway. J. Virol. 80, 8899.

Tulman, E.R., Delhon, G., Afonso, C.L., Lu, Z., Zsak, L., Sandybaev, N.T., Kerembekova, U.Z., Zaitsev, V.L., Kutish, G.F., Rock, D.L., 2006. Genome of horsepox virus. J. Virol. 80 (18), 9244.

Unterholzner, L., Sumner, R.P., Baran, M., Ren, H., Mansur, D.S., Bourke, N.M., Randow, F., Smith, G.L., Bowie, A.G., 2011. Vaccinia virus protein C6 is a virulence factor that binds TBK-1 adaptor proteins and inhibits activation of IRF3 and IRF7. PLoS Pathog. 7, e1002247.

Upton, C., Mossman, K., McFadden, G., 1992. Encoding of a homolog of the IFN-gamma receptor by myxoma virus. Science 258, 1369.

Upton, C., Slack, S., Hunter, A.L., Ehlers, A., Roper, R.L., 2003. Poxvirus orthologous clusters: toward defining the minimum essential poxvirus genome. J. Virol. 77, 7590.

Valentine, R., Smith, G.L., 2010. Inhibition of the RNA polymerase III-mediated dsDNA-sensing pathway of innate immunity by vaccinia virus protein E3. J. Gen. Virol. 91, 2221.

Vanderplasschen, A., Hollinshead, M., Smith, G.L., 1998. Intracellular and extracellular vaccinia virions enter cells by different mechanisms. J. Gen. Virol. 79, 877.

Villarroya-Beltri, C., Guerra, S., Sanchez-Madrid, F., 2017. ISGylation—a key to lock the cell gates for preventing the spread of threats. J. Cell Sci. 130, 2961.

Wack, A., Terczynska-Dyla, E., Hartmann, R., 2015. Guarding the frontiers: the biology of type III interferons. Nat. Immunol. 16, 802.

Ward, B.M., 2005. Visualization and characterization of the intracellular movement of vaccinia virus intracellular mature virions. J. Virol. 79, 4755.

Ward, B.M., Moss, B., 2001. Vaccinia virus intracellular movement is associated with microtubules and independent of actin tails. J. Virol. 75, 11651.

Whitaker-Dowling, P., Youngner, J.S., 1983. Vaccinia rescue of VSV from interferon-induced resistance: reversal of translation block and inhibition of protein kinase activity. Virology 131, 128.

Zhou, Z., Hamming, O.J., Ank, N., Paludan, S.R., Nielsen, A.L., Hartmann, R., 2007. Type III interferon (IFN) induces a type I IFN-like response in a restricted subset of cells through signaling pathways involving both the Jak-STAT pathway and the mitogen-activated protein kinases. J. Virol. 81, 7749.